Aging in the Church

D0580522

Aging in the Church

How Social Relationships
Affect Health

Neal M. Krause

Templeton Foundation Press
West Conshohocken, Pennsylvania

Templeton Foundation Press
300 Conshohocken State Road, Suite 670
West Conshohocken, PA 19428
www.templetonpress.org

© 2008 by Neal M. Krause

All rights reserved. No part of this book may be used or reproduced,
stored in a retrieval system, or transmitted in any form or by any means,
electronic, mechanical, photocopying, recording, or otherwise, without
the written permission of Templeton Foundation Press.

*Templeton Foundation Press helps intellectual leaders and others learn about
science research on aspects of realities, invisible and intangible. Spiritual realities include unlimited love, accelerating creativity, worship, and the benefits of
purpose in persons and in the cosmos.*

Typeset and designed by Glen Burris Book Design

Library of Congress Cataloging-in-Publication Data

Krause, Neal M. (Neal Miller)
  Aging in the church : how social relationships affect health / Neal M.
Krause.
    p. ;   cm.
  Includes bibliographical references and index.
  ISBN-13: 978-1-59947-144-0 (pbk. : alk. paper)
  ISBN-10: 1-59947-144-2 (pbk. : alk. paper) 1. Older people—Religious
life. 2. Aging—Religious aspects—Christianity. 3. Aging—Social aspects.
4. Interpersonal relations—Religious aspects—Christianity. 5. Health—
Religious aspects—Christianity. I. Title.
  [DNLM: 1. Aging—psychology. 2. Aged. 3. Empirical Research. 4.
Interpersonal Relations. 5. Religion and Psychology. 6. Social Environ-
ment. WT 145 K91a 2008]
  BV4580.K73 2008
  261.8'32—dc22   2008008875

Printed in the United States of America

08 09 10 11 12 13 10 9 8 7 6 5 4 3 2 1

Contents

Acknowledgments vii

Chapter 1. Social Relationships in the Church and Health: Problems
and Prospects 3
Religion and Health: What We Know and What We Need to Do Next 4
Setting Boundaries on the Study of Church-Based Social Ties and Health 9
Why Research on Church-Based Social Ties and Health in Late Life Is
Important 11
Overview of the Chapters That Follow 28
Conclusions 31

Chapter 2. Church-Based Social Support: Getting Help during Difficult
Times 33
Conceptualizing and Measuring Informal Church-Based Social Support 35
Stress-Induced Psychosocial Deficits 39
Mobilizing Support from Fellow Church Members 44
Exploring the Benefits of Church-Based Social Support 46
Sharpening the Theoretical Underpinnings of Church-Based Social
Support 53
Less Familiar Dimensions of Church-Based Social Support 65
Bringing Different Kinds of Stressors to the Foreground 70
Conceptual and Methodological Challenges 75
Conclusions 78

Chapter 3. Church-Based Companion Friends 79
Identifying the Basic Nature of Close Companion Friends 80
Measuring Close Companion Friendships at Church 85
Linking Close Companion Friendships with Health and Well-Being 91
Close Companion Friends in Late Life 102
Close Companion Friends and Health: A Preliminary Empirical
Examination 103
Conceptual and Methodological Challenges 106
Conclusions 112

Chapter 4. Social Relationships That Arise from Formal Roles in the
Church 113
Formal Relationships with the Clergy 113
Bible Study Groups and Prayer Groups 127

Formal Relationships in Church Volunteer Programs 134
Formal Assistance for the Homebound 145
Conclusions 151

Chapter 5. Negative Interaction in the Church: Exploring the Dark Side of Religion 155
Measuring Negative Interaction in the Church 157
Prior Research on Negative Interaction in the Church, Health, and Well-Being 160
Negative Interaction in the Church and Health: Examining Conceptual Linkages 162
Negative Interaction with the Clergy 169
Negative Interaction in the Church during Late Life 171
Conceptual and Methodological Challenges 173
Conclusions 185

Chapter 6. Exploring the Pervasive Influence of Social Structural Factors 187
A Strategy for Studying Social Structural Variations in Church-Based Social Ties and Health 189
Variations by Race: Studying Older African Americans 192
Gender, Church-Based Social Ties, and Health in Late Life 203
Church-Based Social Ties and Health: Variations by Socioeconomic Status 216
Conclusions 229

Chapter 7. Conclusions: Taking a Broader Perspective and Identifying Next Steps 232
Core Religious Beliefs and Church-Based Social Relationships 235
General Conceptual and Methodological Challenges 239
Casting a Broader Net: Delving into the Dark Morass of Subjectivity 261

Appendix. Technical Details of the Religion, Aging, and Health (RAH) Survey 267
References 271
Index 303

Acknowledgments

This work is truly a social product, and as a result, there are so many people to thank. It would be impossible to acknowledge them all here, but I wish to make five brief acknowledgments to recognize the individuals who were especially influential. First, I would like to thank all the older men and women who participated in the studies that form the backbone of this volume. What I have learned from them is beyond measure. Second, I would like to thank the National Institute on Aging for funding my research program on religion, aging, and health (RO1 AG014749; RO1 AG026259). I could never have brought my ideas to fruition without their generous support. Third, I am especially grateful to a number of colleagues whose work has had a substantial impact on my own thinking. Among them are Christopher G. Ellison, Harold Koenig, Kenneth Pargament, and Jeffrey S. Levin. Fourth, I would like to express my appreciation to the people at Templeton Foundation Press. I am indebted to them for giving me a free hand in writing this book. Their commitment to fostering creativity and their support of free inquiry made it possible for me to color outside the lines a bit. Finally, but by no means lastly, I wish to thank my wife, Maria, for the love and support she has consistently provided throughout my career. This book would never have been written without her support and encouragement.

Aging in the Church

Chapter 1

Social Relationships in the Church and Health

Problems and Prospects

The purpose of this book is to examine how social relationships that arise in church affect the physical and mental health of older men and women. A number of books have been written about other dimensions of religion and health, such as religious coping (Pargament 1997) and forgiveness (McCullough, Pargament, & Thoresen 2000), but this appears to be the first book that focuses specifically on the health-related consequences of different types of social relationships that are formed by older people in the church. But rather than merely reviewing and critiquing existing studies, the intent of this book is to strike out in a different direction by making a concerted effort to provide researchers with a concrete blueprint for moving forward work on church-based social ties and health. This is accomplished by developing a range of specific and testable hypotheses that link various types of church-based social ties with health and by providing well-developed survey measures that can be used to evaluate them. In the process, a number of methodological and conceptual problems are identified that must be overcome if further progress is to be made. The insights provided in this book arise from the author's extensive experience conducting the first nationwide survey that was devoted exclusively to the study of religion and health in late life. The seven years that it has taken to conduct this research and report the findings that have emerged from it have provided the opportunity for invaluable hands-on experience. When viewed at the broadest level, the intent of this book is to share the insights that were gleaned from this experience with other investigators.

The discussion that follows is divided into four main sections. First, a brief overview of the state of research on religion and health is provided. Problems in this literature are traced to three fundamental short-comings that involve both conceptual and methodological issues. The field of religion and health is vast, and as a result, it would be impossible to cover adequately in a single volume all the work that has been done. Consequently, the second section is devoted to placing boundaries on the scope of this book, which is accomplished by arguing why it is best to focus on religion instead of spirituality and why it makes sense initially to study older Christians only. Section three contains a detailed rationale for why it is important to study religion, why older people are an especially important group to investigate in this context, and why researchers should focus specifically on social relationships that arise in religious settings. Finally, an overview of the chapters that follow is provided in section four.

Religion and Health: What We Know and What We Need to Do Next

An impressive body of research suggests that people who are involved in religion tend to enjoy better physical and mental health than individuals who are not involved in religion (see Koenig, McCullough, & Larson 2001; Lee & Newberg 2005; and Oman & Thoresen 2005 for reviews of this research). Especially convincing evidence is found in studies on the relationship between religion and mortality. This research reveals that people who go to worship services on a regular basis tend to live longer than individuals who do not attend church as often (e.g., Hummer, Rogers, Nam, & Ellison 1999).

Unfortunately, research on religion and health suffers from a number of problems, and as a result, work in this area is not without its critics (e.g., Sloan & Bagiella 2002). Although a number of shortcomings have been identified in the literature, three are especially troubling: the first has to do with the measurement of religion, the second involves the theoretical and conceptual models that have been developed to explain the relationship between religion and health, and the third arises from overlooking the critically important interface between measurement and theory.

Issues in the Measurement of Religion

With respect to measurement, many investigators often rely on single indicators of involvement in religion, especially the frequency of church attendance. However, religion is a vast conceptual domain that cannot be measured adequately with a single item. Evidence of what is missed by relying on limited strategies to measure religion may be found in three sources. First, a panel of experts who were convened by the National Institute on Aging and the Fetzer Institute identified twelve key dimensions of religion that they maintain are important for research on religion and health (Fetzer Institute/National Institute on Aging Working Group 1999). Included among the potentially important dimensions of religion that were identified by the members of this group are religious meaning, forgiveness, and religious beliefs. Second, based on a detailed series of qualitative studies, Krause (2002a) expanded the field of inquiry by identifying fourteen major dimensions of religion. Among the potentially important facets of religion identified by Krause (2002a) are God-mediated feelings of control, religious doubt, and having a close personal relationship with God. Third, Hill and Hood (1999) compiled a comprehensive catalogue of religion measures. This volume comprises seventeen chapters that contain measures of many different facets of religion that may be associated with health and well-being, including scales of religious development (i.e., developing a mature religious faith) and measures of beliefs about death and the afterlife.

Although researchers have made significant progress in measuring religion during the past few years, there are at least two reasons why many investigators have failed to take advantage of these advances. First, a good deal of the work on the conceptualization and measurement of religion is tucked away in specialty journals and books that are outside the mainstream social and behavioral science literature. For example, the Journal of Psychology and Theology contains a number of papers on how to measure various facets of religion, but this journal is not carried by many libraries. As a result, many health-oriented researchers are unaware of the progress that has been made simply because they do not have ready access to the measures that have been developed. The second reason why there are problems with the measures of religion has to do with the wider context in which research on religion and health is often conducted. A good deal of the work in this field is done by investigators who are primary interested in health and who have not received formal training in religion. As a result, these researchers often design questionnaires that devote considerable space to assessing health-related outcomes while leaving much less room for measures of religion. In the process of developing their interview schedules, they often turn to experts on religion and ask them to provide "three or four good questions to measure religion." It is time to stop this practice. If researchers hope to better understand the relationship between religion and health, then more attention must be given to the complex ways in which religion should be measured.

Developing Conceptual Models of Religion and Health

Delving more deeply into the complex multidimensional aspects of religion presents researchers with a significant challenge. Many of the multidimensional batteries of religion were not developed specifically for research on religion and health, and even those that are used in studies of religion and health are often based on underdeveloped theoretical perspectives. This situation led McFadden (2005) to conclude, "Considerable gerontological research has been designed and conducted with little explicit reference to metatheoretical perspectives and frameworks that guided the development of hypotheses, selection of participants, measures and research design, and interpretation of findings" (166).

However, the call for greater conceptual and theoretical development creates yet another challenge. More specifically, researchers must decide whether they want to devise comprehensive models of religion that encompass all the ways religion may influence health in a single conceptual framework (Koenig et al. 2001), or whether they want to develop more focused models that examine the complex ways in which a single dimension of religion may affect health-related outcomes. For example, Pargament (1997) has done outstanding work with conceptual models that show how religious coping responses affect health. Simply put, the dilemma facing researchers is whether to devise grand theories or mid-range theories to study the relationship between religion and health (Merton 1949).

A central premise in the current volume is that it is not advisable at the present time to devise one grand theoretical model of religion and health. Instead, it makes more sense to begin modestly by developing a series of mid-range theories that aim to capture a number of different ways in which specific components of religion may affect health. There are three reasons for recommending that researchers begin by developing more circumscribed theoretical models. The first may be found in the classic work of William James (1902/1997), who argued, "The divine can mean no single quality, it must mean a group of qualities, by being champions of which in alternation, different men may all find a worthy mission.... So a 'god of battles' must be allowed to be the god for one kind of person, a god of peace and home, the god of another. We must frankly recognize the fact that we live in partial systems, and that parts are not interchangeable in spiritual life" (509).

Second, a similar conclusion has been reached in the contemporary literature on causal modeling. More specifically, Bradley and Schaefer (1998) argue, "It is therefore unlikely that there is a single model of any particular situation.... Reality is too complex and models are too limited. It is more likely that several models each shed light on different facets of the real situation" (29).

Third, there are pragmatic reasons for taking a focused approach to building conceptual models of religion and health. In practice, it is difficult to estimate causal models (especially latent variable models) containing more than about six or seven constructs. Put another way, it is hard to imagine what a conceptual model would look like, or how it could be estimated, if it contained all twelve dimensions of religion identified by the Fetzer Institute/National Institute on Aging Working Group (1999).

The goal of the mid-range theories that are explored in the current volume is to identify a manageable set of theoretically circumscribed intervening variables that link various types of social relationships in the church with health and well-being in late life. Two types of intervening variables are examined in this respect. First, some intervening constructs consist of other dimensions of religion that are typically not associated with social relationships in the church. So, for example, an argument is developed in chapter 2 which suggests that social support from fellow church members shapes the selection and implementation of religiously based stress-coping responses, and these coping responses, in turn, influence health and well-being. This approach to model development is important because it provides a point of departure for ultimately developing larger, grand theories of religion and health in late life. The second type of mediating variables presented in the mid-range theories in this volume are secular in nature. Included among them are self-esteem and optimism (see chap. 2) as well as anger (see chap. 5). This approach to theory construction is important because vast bodies of research link these secular constructs with health and well-being across the life course. Embedding them in mid-range models of religion and health will more tightly integrate research on religion into the mainstream literature on physical and mental health.

Although focusing on mid-range conceptual models of religion and health provides a good point of departure, it is important to keep long-range goals in mind. Instead of getting embroiled in a debate about whether grand or mid-range models are best, it makes more sense to rely on an incremental model-building strategy that uses both approaches.

More specifically, a reasonable plan involves the initial development of a series of well-articulated mid-range models that show how specific dimensions of religion are related to health. Then, once the complex relationships involving various aspects of religion are better understood, researchers will be better able to see how they can be fit together to form a larger, more comprehensive conceptual model of religion and health.

Exploring the Interplay between Measurement and Theory

As this discussion of problems in the field reveals, research on religion and health cannot move forward unless adequate attention is paid to measurement and theory. The synthesis of the two is justified because, in the end, they form a seamless whole. This idea is hardly new. The notion was best expressed by Blalock (1982) in his discussion of auxiliary measurement theories. In his view, theory and measurement are inextricably bound. He argued that the selection and development of survey indicators to measure constructs like prayer or social support in church is an inherently theoretical process because embedded in each item are theoretical statements about the nature, meaning, and function of the constructs they are thought to represent. For example, prayer is typically assessed by asking people how often they pray. Therefore, this measurement strategy is based on the assumption that the frequency of prayer is the key factor driving the relationship between prayer and health and that other aspects of prayer, such as the specific content or focus of prayer, are relatively unimportant. But in contrast to measuring how often people pray, other investigators provide evidence that the content of prayer is the critical factor and that meditative prayer (i.e., sitting quietly and contemplating the Divine) may be an especially important correlate of well-being (Poloma & Gallup 1991). Embedded in this alternative measurement strategy is the assumption that the frequency of prayer plays only a secondary role in shaping feelings of psychological well-being.

As this simple example reveals, when insufficient attention is paid to the theoretical underpinnings of study measures, substantive findings from research on religion and health may become ambiguous and difficult to interpret. These problems are especially likely to arise when statistically significant findings fail to emerge from a study. Assume that an investigator relies on a standard measure of the frequency of private prayer and subsequently finds it is not significantly associated with health. Under these circumstances he or she "will not know whether it is the substantive theory, the auxiliary measurement theory, or both that is at fault" (Blalock 1982, 25).

Measurement problems in the social and behavioral sciences are "formidable" (Blalock 1982, 18). This is certainly true of research on religion and health. The only way to overcome these problems is to face them squarely, and for this reason a major emphasis is placed throughout this volume on the interplay between theory and measurement.

Setting Boundaries on the Study of Church-Based Social Ties and Health

Although focusing solely on social relationships in the church clearly narrows the scope of inquiry into the relationship between religion and health, it is, nevertheless, a daunting undertaking. Consequently, two steps were taken to make the task of exploring this facet of religion more manageable.

Religion vs. Spirituality

First, the chapters that follow deal primarily with social relationships that arise in religious settings and not those that are associated with spirituality. Although research suggests that both religion and spirituality may affect health, there are three reasons why it makes sense to concentrate on religion. The first has to do with conceptual issues. Both spirituality and religion involve beliefs about things that are sacred or divine, and both examine the impact of practices that are intended to enhance the experience of the sacred. However, as George, Larson, Koenig, and McCullough (2000) argue, the major difference is that religion is linked to formal institutions whereas spirituality does not necessarily arise in nor is it necessarily associated with a collective or institutional setting. Simply put, "The distinctive character of religion is its collective reinforcement and identity" (George et al. 2000, 104). Because religion is practiced within specialized institutions, the policies and formal teachings that are found in these institutions place boundaries on the beliefs and behaviors of the people who worship there. In contrast, it is much more difficult to determine the boundaries of spirituality because spiritual experiences can arise in an almost limitless number of settings. For example, various ways in which people interact with nature may be construed as a spiritual experience. Evidence of this may be found in the following item from the spirituality index that was developed by the Fetzer Institute/National Institute on Aging Working Group (1999): "I am spiritually touched by the beauty of creation." It is difficult to develop good measures of a phenomena when the boundaries of the phenomena cannot be identified clearly. Stated in more formal terms, it is unlikely that measures of spirituality have good content validity. Content validity has to do with making sure that all the elements that comprise the domain of a construct are adequately represented in scales that are used to assess them (Nunnally & Bernstein 1994). Unfortunately, efforts to differentiate between religion and spirituality may not be as successful as they seem initially. As Fuller (2001) eloquently points out, the two are becoming so tightly bound that elements of spirituality are beginning to reshape the way faith is practiced in many mainstream religious organizations. Perhaps this is one reason why a significant number of individuals indicate that they are both spiritual and religious (see Zinnbauer & Pargament 2005).

The second reason for focusing on religion instead of spirituality arises from the fact that measures of spirituality may be confounded with the measures of psychological well-being they are designed to predict or explain. More specifically, a review of existing measures of spirituality reveals that a number of scales contain items that assess feelings and emotions that arise in the process of searching for the sacred. However, the emphasis on emotions creates methodological problems when studies are designed to assess the relationship between spirituality and mental health or psychological well-being. For example, the following item is included in the spirituality index of the Fetzer Institute/National Institute on Aging Working Group (1999): "I feel deep inner peace and harmony" (16). It is hardly surprising to find that a scale containing this indicator is significantly associated with measures of psychological well-being, including depression and anxiety (Underwood & Teresi 2002). However, this correlation may be explained by the fact that the two scales are essentially measuring the same thing.

The third reason for focusing on religion instead of spirituality is straightforward. So far, most of the studies that have been done with older adults have been concerned solely with religion and not spirituality. As a result, greater insights into the factors that improve health in late life are likely to be found in studies that involve only religion.

Focusing on Christians

In addition to excluding research on spirituality, the scope of the current volume is further restricted by focusing primarily on research that has been conducted with Christian respondents. There are two reasons for concentrating on this particular religion. First, most people in the United States are Christian. According to a recent report by Newport (2004), 82 percent of adult Americans classify themselves as Christians. Given the fact that an additional 10 percent of Americans have no religious preference at all, it is easy to see that the wide majority of people in America who are religious practice the Christian faith. The second reason for restricting the discussion to Christians has to do with the fact that most of the empirical studies on religion and health focus on members of this particular faith.

Why Research on Church-Based Social Ties and Health in Late Life Is Important

A significant investment of resources and effort will be needed to confront the conceptual and methodological problems that face researchers who study the relationship between church-based social relationships and health. Before making these expenditures, it is important to demonstrate they are justified. Justification may be found by addressing three questions that deal with the interface between religion, aging, and church-based social relationships in studies with health-related outcomes: (1) Why study religion? (2) Why study religion and aging? (3) Why study church-based social relationships specifically?

Why Study Religion?

The study of religion is hardly new in the social and behavioral sciences. In fact, research on religion has been an integral part of these disciplines ever since their inception. For example, Durkheim (1915/1965) and Weber (1922/1963) are widely considered to be among the founders of sociology. Both scholars devoted entire volumes to the study of religion. Charles Horton Cooley was an eminent sociologist who played a major role in developing the symbolic interactionist school of social theory. He wrote an entire chapter on religion in his classic work, *Social Organization* (1909/2003). As the following quotation from this chapter reveals, he left little doubt about the important role that religion plays in social life: "Without some regular and common service of the ideal, something in the way of prayer and worship, pessimism and selfishness are almost sure to encroach upon us" (376). Although his research is difficult to classify, the work of Tocqueville is typically included in discussions of classical sociological theory. Many are familiar with the two-volume treatise he wrote while touring the United States shortly after the American Revolution, *Democracy in America* (1835/1960). In this work, he clearly spelled out the core role played by religion in American culture: "There is hardly any human action, however particular it may be, that does not originate in some very general idea men have conceived of the Deity, of his relation to mankind, of the nature of their own souls, and of their duties to their fellow creatures" (21).

However, not all classic sociological theorists took a positive attitude toward religion. Among those with a dim view of religion was Lester Ward, the first president of the American Sociological Association. Writing in one of his most widely cited books, *Dynamic Sociology* (1883), Ward observed, "Each religion regards all others as being wholly false.... This fact... standing alone, could lead the disinterested observer to no other conclusion than that all religions are based upon a fundamental error.... If, then, the very root of the tree consist wholly of error, is it not reasonable to suppose that the branches and the fruit partake of the same nature?" (vol. 2, 266). But even though Ward did not appear to think highly of religion, the fact that he felt compelled to discuss it at length points to the central role that religion plays in social life.

A strong emphasis on religion may also be found in psychology. Many consider William James to be the greatest American psychologist. Like Durkheim and Weber, James (1902/1997) wrote an entire volume on religion. It is interesting to note that James wrote extensively on religion even though his private correspondence indicated he was not deeply involved in formal religion and that he felt awkward praying (Perry 1954). G. Stanley Hall was the first president of the American Psychological Association. Moreover, he trained a number of the first generation of psychologists of religion, including James Leuba and E. D. Starbuck. In 1923, Hall wrote an extensive volume titled *Jesus the Christ in the Light of Psychology*. In addition, it may be surprising for some to learn that Wilhelm Wundt, the founder of experimental psychology, devoted three full volumes to religion in his epic treatise *Volkerpsychologie* (1915).

But the strong emphasis on religion goes beyond sociology and psychology. Two of the founders of psychiatry paid considerable attention to the subject as well. Sigmund Freud (1913) wrote an entire, albeit unflattering, volume on religion, and Carl Jung gave considerable thought to it, too. In fact, Dyer (2000) reports that there are over six thousand references to God in the voluminous writings of Jung. In the process of discussing religious issues, Jung provided one of the most succinct statements about the role it plays in human life, "Everything to do with religion, everything it is and asserts, touches the human soul so closely that psychology least of all can afford to overlook it" (as quoted in Jacobi & Hull 1953, 337).

The broad message from this brief historical overview is straightforward: if so many of the great minds in so many disciplines devoted so much time to the study of religion, then it is imperative that contemporary social and behavioral gerontologists pay attention to religion as well.

Why Study Religion and Aging?

Studying the relationship between religion and health with data provided by older adults is important for two reasons. First, if research ultimately confirms that religion improves health, then the findings from this work may be used to devise interventions that lower healthcare costs among those who use health care services the most: older adults. This is an important goal to strive for because research reveals that in 2000, the mean annual medical expenses for persons age sixty-five and older was ($6,140), nearly three times greater than the corresponding estimate for individuals under the age of sixty-five ($2,127) (U.S. Department of Health and Human Services 2004).

The second reason that research is needed on the relationship between religion and health among older people may be found by reviewing studies on differences in religious involvement across the life course. A number of investigators have argued that religion becomes increasingly important as people grow older. For example, William James (1902/1997) maintained that "the religious age par excellence would seem to be old age" (34, emphasis in original). Writing at about the same time, Starbuck (1899) came to a similar conclusion: "The belief in God in some form is by far the most central conception, and it grows in importance with advancing years" (320). If religion becomes increasingly important with advancing age, and if involvement in religion promotes better health, then it follows that the health-related benefits of religion should be most evident in studies of older adults.

But neither James (1902/1997) nor Starbuck (1899) developed a compelling theoretical rationale for why religion increases with age, nor did they provide empirical evidence to support their claims. Consequently, in order to make a stronger case for studying religion and health in late life it is necessary to address two key issues: (1) Why might religion become increasingly important as people grow older? (2) Is there empirical evidence to support the notion that religious involvement increases with age?

Theoretical Perspectives on Religion and Aging. As Reich (1992) observed some time ago, "There exists no encompassing, generally accepted theory of religious development" (151). This still appears to be true today. Instead, theoretical formulations about age-related change in religion are largely restricted to the work of a few investigators, including Fowler (1981), Kohlberg (1973), and Bahr (1970).

Fowler (1981) identified six stages of progressively deeper and more mature faith development. Although he did not consistently associate each stage with a specific age or age range, the stages nevertheless roughly map onto the life course. For example, he notes that the first stage of intuitive-projective faith is typically observed in children between the ages of three and seven. This type of faith is fantasy-based, imitative, and strongly influenced by the examples, actions, and stories provided by adults. There is little evidence at this time of logical thought as it relates to religious issues. In contrast, the highest stage of faith development (Stage 6—universal faith) is "exceedingly rare" and attained only by individuals of historic importance, such as Gandhi, Martin Luther King Jr., and Mother Teresa (Fowler 1981, 200). As a result, the highest stage of faith development that is reached by the typical adult is Stage 5—conjunctive faith. Fowler (1981) indicates attainment of this stage is "unusual before midlife" (198). Compared to previous stages of faith development, a person who develops conjunctive faith is more reflective and more aware of the paradoxes and contradictions that are inherent in religion. But despite these intellectual challenges, the individual at this stage of development is capable of, and even enjoys, working through these contradictions to attain a deeper and richer understanding. Unfortunately, as McFadden (1999) points out, Fowler's (1981) developmental view of faith has rarely been evaluated empirically, especially with older adults.

Lawrence Kohlberg (1973) is widely known for his theory of moral development. A good deal of attention in his work was paid to tracing the moral development of children, adolescents, and younger adults. But some investigators may not be aware that he also specified a final stage (Stage 7) that he felt was unique to advanced adulthood. According to Kohlberg (1973), people who attain the seventh stage of moral development take on an increasingly religious or cosmic perspective that is concerned with issues involving the infinite and place an emphasis on seeing oneself as part of the larger unified whole of existence.

In contrast to Fowler (1981) and Kohlberg (1973), the Family Life Cycle hypothesis proposed by Bahr (1970) does not specify that the greatest level of involvement in religion occurs in late life. Instead, Bahr (1970) argues that the greatest involvement in religion is found earlier in life when people marry and when they have preadolescent school-age children at home.

Beyond the work of Fowler (1981), Kohlberg (1973), and Bahr (1970), there have been only a few attempts to discuss the development of religiousness across the life course. For example, Levenson and colleagues introduce the notion of self-transcendence that is thought to capture the pinnacle of successful aging (Levenson, Jennings, Aldwin, & Shiraishi 2005). However, the items in the scale they developed to assess self-transcendence appear to deal more with spirituality than religion because they do not mention God or religion explicitly. Other investigators have gone to great lengths to identify the characteristics and components of a mature religious faith, but they typically do not believe that a mature faith is attained only in late life (e.g., Allport 1950; Bidwell 2001; Strunk 1965).

Before researchers invest additional time and effort in developing theories about the development of religiousness over the life course, it is important to address two fundamental issues. First, does the notion that religiousness increases over the life course refer to a universal phenomenon, or does it best describe the experiences of some, but not all older people? Second, even among individuals who become more religious with age, is there a simple linear increase in their faith, or does the history of a person's involvement with religion unfold in other, more complex ways? Simply put, is there more than one trajectory of religious involvement over the life course? Those who assert that all people follow the same pattern of religious development as they grow older subscribe to what developmental psychologists refer to as the assumption of essentialism (Goldhaber 2000). But as Goldhaber (2000) points out, a more plausible approach may have been developed by proponents of the life course cohort perspective. According to their view, development is multidirectional, and the unique influence of historical time and social space creates great variability in the way individual lives unfold over the life course. As the findings reported in the next section reveal, there is some empirical support for adapting the life course cohort perspective to the study of age-related change in religion.

Empirical Research on Age Differences in Religion. Researchers have taken one of three approaches to assess empirically whether people become more religious as they grow older. The first has to do with probing for age differences in current religious involvement with cross-sectional survey data, the second involves longitudinal studies in which the same people are followed over extended periods of time to see if they become more religious as they grow older, whereas the third approach is concerned with reconstructing from retrospective reports lifelong patterns of religious involvement.

By far, the most common way to evaluate age differences in religion empirically is to compare and contrast levels of religious involvement among people who are currently young and individuals who are presently old. The wide majority of these cross-sectional surveys reveal that older people are more religious than younger adults. For example, Barna (2002) reports that older adults attend church more often than younger people, pray more frequently than younger adults, and read the Bible more often than their younger counterparts (see also Gallup & Lindsay 1999). In fact, some investigators argue that this pattern of age differences in religion has consistently emerged in cross-sectional studies for approximately fifty years (Levin 2004).

Although research using cross-sectional data may initially appear to be convincing, there are three reasons that the findings from these studies should be viewed with caution. First, not all cross-sectional studies show greater involvement in religion among older adults. For example, based on data from the 1999 General Social Survey, Spilka, Hood, Hunsberger, and Gorsuch (2003) present evidence that the relationship between age and religious involvement is nonlinear, with the highest levels of religiousness occurring around age thirty or so. Similarly, Maves (1960) reports results from several large-scale cross-sectional surveys that fail to find significant age differences in religiousness. Finally, Hall (1922) reports a study done by Leuba in 1906 which shows that the percentage of people who believed in God and immortality decreased both with age and education.

The fact that cross-sectional studies on age differences in religion have been conducted over a number of decades gives rise to a second problem with the conclusion that people become more religious as they grow older. More specifically, looking at data that have been gathered at a single point in time makes it difficult to distinguish between age, period, and cohort effects. The nature of these problems can be illustrated by focusing on potential cohort effects. Unfortunately, researchers know very little about cohort differences in religion. In fact, it is somewhat surprising to find that some of the more comprehensive studies of differences across multiple cohorts have been conducted by marketing researchers (e.g., Meredith & Schewe 2002), and as a result, only scant attention has been paid to religion. Even so, some intriguing possibilities emerge from this work. More specifically, Meredith and Schewe (2002) present extensive research on seven successive cohorts. Three are important for the current discussion because they deal with people in middle and late life. The first is the Depression Era Cohort (age eighty to eighty-nine in 2001), the second is the World War II cohort (age seventy-four to seventy-nine in 2001), and the third is the Postwar Cohort (age fifty-six to seventy-three in 2001). Meredith and Schewe's research suggests that levels of religious involvement appear to be greater among the Depression Era Cohort and the World War II cohort than among the Postwar Cohort. Meredith and Schewe (2002) attribute these findings to the fact that members of the older cohorts garnered great sustenance from their faith when they encountered the daunting challenges posed by the Great Depression and World War II. In contrast, members of the Postwar Cohort did not have to grapple with such cataclysmic events, and as a result, their involvement in and commitment to religion are not as great. Clearly, much more research is needed on cohort differences in religiousness across the life course.

The third problem with cross-sectional studies on age differences in religion has to do with the limited range of measures that were used in most studies. More specifically, the majority of investigators rely on fairly crude measures of religion, such as the frequency of church attendance and prayer as well as the overall importance of religion. It is especially important to point out that none of these studies examine age differences in church-based social relationships.

Studying change in religiousness with longitudinal data represents a better way to approach research on age differences in religious involvement. A number of noteworthy studies have been done that are based on this type of research design. But once again, the findings from this work are not consistent.

Shand (2000) analyzed data provided by eighty-four male graduates of Amherst College over a period of fifty years. Unfortunately, he focused solely on how certain study participants are that God exists.

Shand (2000) found little change over the course of his study in the certainty that God exists.

Argue, Johnson, and White (1999) performed a sophisticated set of analyses on data provided by the same respondents over a twelve-year period. These investigators report that the importance of religion increases in a nonlinear fashion with age, and that the steepest increase occurs in the middle adult years. This study is noteworthy because the authors controlled statistically for period and cohort effects. Unfortunately, the subjects in this study were between the ages of eighteen and fifty-five at the first interview, making the oldest person at the end of the twelve-year follow-up only sixty-seven years old. This clouds the issue of change in religion over the life course because people are now living well into advanced old age. In fact, there were 4.2 million people age eighty-five and over in 2000 (Federal Interagency Forum on Aging Related Statistics 2004). Truncating the age range in this manner therefore literally excludes twenty or thirty years of the life course, making it impossible to detect a potential resurgence in religious involvement in advanced old age.

Two other longitudinal studies of aging and religiousness were based on well-known data collected in California. The first was conducted by Wink and Dillon (2001) using the famous Berkeley Growth Studies. Data on religion were analyzed for people in their thirties through their seventies. The importance of religion was the only indicator used in this study. Contrary to the results reported by Argue et al. (1999), Wink and Dillon (2001) report that the importance of religion decreased during the early thirties and forties, but then increased in the fifties and early sixties. Although the reason for this pattern of nonlinear change is not clear, the dip in religiousness during the thirties may reflect the waning influence of childhood socialization.

The other longitudinal study that was based on data from California was conducted by McCullough, Enders, Brion, and Jain (2005). These investigators analyzed data from the Terman Study, which involved interviews with very bright individuals (i.e., an IQ above 135) from 1940 through 1991. A complex composite measure of religion was created that consisted primarily of interest in religion and satisfaction with religion. Using sophisticated growth mixture models, these investigators found that instead of one universal pattern of change in religiousness, three distinct trajectories of religious development emerged from their analyses. Study participants in the first trajectory (40 percent of the sample) were characterized by increases in religiousness in early adult life followed by a decline with advancing age. In contrast, members of the second trajectory (41 percent of study participants) exhibited low levels of religiousness in early adulthood and subsequent age-related decline. Only members of the third trajectory (19 percent of the subjects) showed evidence of increasing religiousness with advancing age.

The findings from longitudinal studies of age differences in religion are thought-provoking, but there are two shortcomings in this research. First, the samples used in these studies were not selected at random (e.g., male Amherst College graduates and people with an IQ above 135), and as a result, it is difficult to generalize the findings to the typical or average individual. Second, as with studies using cross-sectional designs, only limited measures of religion were used in this longitudinal research (e.g., the belief that God exists, the importance of religion).

The final way of assessing age differences in religion involves asking older study participants to provide retrospective reports about their level of involvement in religion at specific times in their lives. This means, for example, that researchers might ask older people how important religion was to them when they were twenty years old, forty years old, and sixty years old.

There are at least three studies in the literature that use the retrospective recall design. The first, by Starbuck (1897), was probably the first of its kind. He gathered data on religious involvement from a nonrandom sample of 195 individuals using autobiographies that were written in response to a set of questions he devised. His sample included individuals through age eighty-five. Starbuck (1897) inquired primarily about "religious awakening" and the practice of religious customs at different points in the life course. Like McCullough et al. (2005), Starbuck (1897) found that there was not a single pattern of religious involvement over the life course. Although he did not use sophisticated data analytic procedures, he found that most people experienced a "religious awakening" around age sixteen followed by a period of doubt that was primarily due to the "storm and stress" of adolescence. Following this period of doubt, Starbuck (1897) reported four trajectories of change: (1) people whose faith was "reconstructed," (2) individuals who were struggling to regain their faith but who were making little progress, (3) those who never emerged from doubt, and (4) individuals who were struggling to regain their faith and were making some progress but who had not regained their earlier level of religiousness. Unfortunately, Starbuck (1897) did not fully exploit his data because he truncated the age range in his analyses by collapsing all individuals age forty and older into one category.

Turning to more contemporary research, George, Hays, Flint, and Meador (2004) presented study participants with a series of questions that were designed to assess change over the life course in four dimensions of religion (the frequency of church attendance, private religious practices such as prayer, religious media use, and the importance of religion). Like Starbuck (1897) and McCullough et al. (2005), a complex pattern of multiple trajectories of involvement in religion emerged from their data. For example, some individuals remained highly involved in religion across the life course, other people experienced an increased sense of religiousness, others reported a precipitous decline in religion followed by a rebound, while yet other individuals were never deeply involved in religion at any point in their lifetime.

The notion that there are multiple trajectories of religious involvement over the life course is further reinforced in a qualitative study by Ingersoll-Dayton, Krause, and Morgan (2002). These investigators report four trajectories of change across a range of religious measures, including feelings of closeness to God. These trajectories largely mirror those reported by George et al. (2004).

Unfortunately, the validity of the findings derived from studies using retrospective recall depends, in part, upon the ability of study participants to recall and report accurately their involvement in religion at particular points in the life course. There do not appear to be any studies in the literature that have examined the extent of recall bias in retrospective studies of religiousness across the life course.

Do people become more religious as they grow older? The simple answer is that researchers do not have adequate data to answer this question. The bulk of cross-sectional studies appear to suggest that older people are more religious than younger individuals, but findings from studies using both longitudinal designs as well as studies that rely on retrospective recall do not come to the same conclusion. Instead of revealing that everyone becomes more religious with age, some of these latter studies suggest that people may follow any one of several different trajectories of involvement in religion as they grow older. This complex view of change in religion over the life course is consistent with the basic tenets of Nelson and Dannefer's (1992) aged heterogeneity hypothesis. According to this perspective, there is a general tendency toward greater differentiation among people with advancing age. Their work suggests that this general tendency appears to hold with respect to a wide range of outcomes, including feelings of personal control, self-esteem, and social networks (Nelson & Dannefer 1992). Although it is far too early to draw definitive conclusions, the notion that age-related change in religion is best reflected by multiple trajectories appears to make the most sense and is reinforced by simple observation. Moreover, the fact that some people do not become more religious with age is supported by survey research which shows that 8 percent of people age seventy-five and older feel that religion is not very important in their own lives (Ehmann 1999).

If multiple trajectories best capture the relationship between age and religion, then social and behavioral gerontologists must devise theories that accommodate this complex pattern of findings, and they must gather data and employ statistical procedures (i.e., individual growth curve models) that evaluate them properly. This kind of work is important for the following reason. Although researchers often think about the relationship between religion and health in static terms, and typically analyze this relationship with cross-sectional data, they are really studying an inherently dynamic process in which change is taking place over time both in religious involvement and health. Viewing the issue in this way sharpens the hypothesis that is under investigation by bringing a more dynamic perspective to the foreground. When data on religious involvement are obtained at a single point in time, it is not possible to tell whether an individual is in the process of experiencing an upward, stable, or downward trend in religious involvement.

Although it is not possible at the present time to develop a theory that explains multiple trajectories of change in religion, posing some basic questions about the nature of change in religion over the life course and health highlights the need for more research on this issue. For example, are people who were religious earlier in life but who subsequently drifted away from their faith especially likely to be at risk of developing physical or mental health problems? What about individuals who were never deeply involved in religion at any time in their lives? Is their risk of encountering health-related problems even greater? Or perhaps these people are not more likely to be at risk because they have found a deep sense of meaning in some secular domain, such as work, secular personal relationships, or the arts.

So if there is no consistent pattern of change in religious involvement with age, it may not be clear why it is important to study the relationship between religion and health specifically in late life. As research by Barna (2002) reveals, approximately 80 percent of older adults report that their religious faith is very important in their lives today. This is higher than in any other age group. Similar results are reported by Gallup and Lindsay (1999). Their data suggest that 79 percent of the people age sixty-five to seventy-four indicate that religion is very important in their lives. Once again, the proportion of people who feel that religion is very important in their lives is higher than in any other age group. It is not possible to tell if older people who say their faith is a very important part of their life always felt this way or if religion gradually became more important to them as they grew older. But the fact remains that religion appears to be an extraordinarily important factor in the lives of currently older people, and that it appears to be more important to currently older than currently younger individuals. If greater involvement in religion is associated with better health, then the health-related benefits of religion should therefore be especially evident among people who are presently older. For this reason the current volume focuses on the interface between social relationships and health specifically among older adults.

Why Study Social Relationships in the Church?

There are at least three reasons why it is important to focus specifically on social relationships in the church and health in late life: (1) The first may be found by turning to the work of the grand theoretical masters in sociology, psychology, psychiatry, and philosophy; (2) the second reason has to do with the theoretical insights of contemporary scholars; and (3) the third reason involves findings from research on social relationships and health that have been conducted in secular settings.

Insights from the Grand Theoretical Masters. As discussed earlier in this chapter, many of the grand social and behavioral theorists believed that religion was a core factor in social life. However, in the process of discussing this issue, many argued that religion arises from, and is sustained by, the social relationships that people form in the places where they worship.

The primacy of social relationships in religion is perhaps nowhere more evident than in the classic work of sociologist Georg Simmel (1898/1997). He argued, "The faith that has come to be regarded as the essence and substance of religion is first of all a relationship *between human beings*" (108, emphasis in original).

It is difficult to discuss classic sociological research on religion without touching on the insights of Emile Durkheim. He maintained that the personal strength afforded by religion arises solely from its underlying social foundation. In particular, Durkheim (1915/1965) argued, "The only source of life at which we can morally reanimate ourselves is that formed by the society of fellow beings; the only moral forces with which we can sustain and increase our own are those which we get from others" (473).

Edward Alsworth Ross (1896) was one of the early presidents of the American Sociological Association. He went as far as to define religion solely in terms of its social roots. More specifically, he proposed that religion is *"the conviction of an ideal bond between members of society and the feelings that arise in consequence of that conviction"* (Ross 1896 434, emphasis in original).

The key role played by social relationships in religion was also clearly spelled out in the last volume written by sociologist Charles Horton Cooley (1927). Sounding much like Simmel (1898/1997), Cooley (1927) observed, "Faith in our associates is part of our faith in God" (231).

George Herbert Mead, a sociologist and close associate of Cooley, also recognized the importance of the social dimension of religion. Mead (1934/1962) derived the notion of "universal attitudes" as a way of explaining how social forces give rise to and promote social structure. In the process, he spent a good deal of time focusing on two specific universal attitudes. One was the economic attitude, whereas the other was "neighborliness, which passes over into the principle of religious relationship, the attitude which made religion as such possible" (Mead 1934/1962, 292–293). Of the two universal attitudes, Mead saw religion as being more forceful and more important: "The religious attitude, on the contrary takes you into the immediate inner attitude of the other individual; you are identifying yourself with him in so far as you are assisting him, helping him, saving his soul, aiding him in this world and the world to come—your attitude is that of salvation of the individual. This attitude is far more profound in the identification of the individual with others" (1934/1962, 296–297).

But sociologists were by no means the only scholars to recognize the strong social underpinnings of religion. James Mark Baldwin was an early president of the American Psychological Association. In 1902, Baldwin wrote, "The fact is constantly recognized that religion is a social phenomena. No man is religious by himself, nor does he choose his god, nor devise his offering, nor enjoy his blessings alone" (325).

Referring to Christianity as the "new life," G. Stanley Hall (1923) maintained that "man is gregarious, a socius, and no man lives to himself. The new life is not only intensely inward and solitary, but must have vent and companionship, and the outer kingdom begins in collectivity, sharing things" (363).

Similar views were expressed by psychiatrist Alfred Adler, a student of Freud. The constructs of social feeling and social interest occupied a pivotal position in his theoretical perspective. In Adler's (1933/1956) view, the social feeling involved a sense of community, empathy, solidarity, and interest in others. As the following quotation from his work reveals, he believed these social feelings formed the basis of religion: "The primal energy which was so effective in establishing religious goals was none other than that of social feeling. This was meant to bind human beings closely to one another" (Adler 1933/1956, 462).

It is somewhat ironic to find that some of the strongest statements about the social underpinnings of religion were not made by sociologists or psychologists. Instead, they are found in the work of philosophers. Josiah Royce was a leading philosopher of his time and a close personal friend of William James. Royce wrote a book in 1912, *The Sources of Religious Insight,* that many contemporary social and behavioral scientists who study religion and health have overlooked. In writing this volume, Royce hoped to overcome what he felt were serious oversights in the work of James (1902/1997), especially the role of unconscious processes in the generation of religious insight. Royce (1912/2001) maintained that instead of arising from within the individual, the impetus for religious experiences and sentiments was decidedly social in nature. More specifically, he argued that "our social experience is our primary source of religious insight. And the salvation that this insight brings to our knowledge is salvation through the fostering of human brotherhood. Such salvation accrues to the individual so far as he gives himself over to the service of man" (Royce 1912/2001, 58).

Although many of the grand masters believed that the foundations of religion are found in social relationships, not all agreed with this view. For example, Alfred North Whitehead, an eminent philosopher wrote, "Religion is solitariness; and if you are never solitary, you are never religious. Collective enthusiasm, revivals, institutions, churches, rituals, bibles, codes of behavior are trappings of religion, its passive forms" (1926/1996, 17). Nevertheless, the widespread and broad-based interdisciplinary endorsement of the social basis of religion suggests that opinions such as Whitehead's are not shared widely.

The extensive work of the grand masters is important for several reasons. First, it helps trace the intellectual roots of contemporary research on social relationships in the church, thereby imbuing it with a rich sense of history and continuity. Doing so underscores the notion that investigators who are presently working in the field are laboring with issues that leading scholars have wrestled with for centuries. This helps more firmly establish their intellectual identity and imparts a sense that contemporary investigators may be on the right track when they look to church-based social relationships for insights into the fundamental nature of religion. Second, turning to the classic works in the field reminds contemporary researchers that some of the discoveries they think are new may in fact be centuries old. As Alfred North Whitehead so aptly put it, "Everything of importance has been said before by somebody who did not discover it" (1917, 127) This realization opens up the scope of the scholarship that must be covered and illustrates why it is important to consider not only contemporary, but classic research in studies of church-based social relationships. Third, the fact that the views of the grand masters are so consistent, yet come from a range of disciplines that are so dissimilar in the approach they take to the study of human life, instills conviction in the belief that research on social relationships in the church is of fundamental, if not universal importance.

Although the theoretical insights of the grand masters are invaluable, there are at least two problems with the work they have done. First, their views on the social foundations of religion lack specificity. As the literature on social relationships has evolved, it has become increasingly clear that this is also a vast conceptual domain in its own right, and there are a number of different ways in which social relationships may develop (Krause 2006a). As a result, it is difficult to translate a good deal of the work of the grand theoretical masters into specific research hypotheses that can be evaluated empirically. Second, the grand masters never set out to study the relationship between religion and health, nor were they interested in studying older adults specifically. As a result, their perspectives provide an important point of departure, but a significant amount of work must be done to infuse their insights into research on church-based social relationships and health in late life.

Even though there may be limitations in the work of the grand theorists, these shortcomings should not overshadow the debt that is owed to these early pioneers. This sense of indebtedness was captured succinctly in the twelfth century by Bernard of Chartres, who wrote, "We are like dwarfs seated on the shoulders of giants: We see more things than the ancients and things more distant, but this is due neither to the sharpness of our own sight, nor to the greatness of our own stature, but because we are raised and borne aloft on that giant mass" (as quoted in Fremantle 1954, ix).

Views of Contemporary Scholars. A number of contemporary scholars have expressed views about the social underpinnings of religion that are remarkably similar to those found in the works of the grand theoretical masters. For example, C. S. Lewis (1942/2001) was regarded as one of the most influential Christian writers of his day. He argued, "God can show Himself as He really is only to real men. And this means not simply men who are individually good, but to men who are united together in a body, loving one another, helping one another, showing Him to one another.... Consequently, the one really adequate instrument for learning about God is the whole Christian community" (Lewis 1942/2001, 165).

Similar notions of community figure prominently in the work of Paul Tillich, a noted liberal theologian. More specifically, he argued that "the act of faith, like every act in man's spiritual life, is dependent upon language, and therefore the community. For only in the community of spiritual beings is the language alive" (Tillich 1987, 27).

In his comprehensive view of research on religion, spirituality, and health, Levin (2001) set out to explain why more frequent church attendance is associated with better health. He concludes, "I believe that the supportive relationships provided through active religious fellowship best explain the findings we have examined" (58). However, Levin (2001) goes on to argue that even though church-based social relationships may explain the potentially important health-related effects of church attendance, they provide less insight into how other dimensions of religion may influence health. Given the current state of the literature, this conclusion is not unwarranted. Even so, as subsequent chapters in the current volume reveal, there are sound reasons for arguing that social relationships in the church influence health through a number of other religious factors that were not considered by Levin (2001).

Over the course of the past several decades, Christopher G. Ellison has made an enormous contribution to our understanding of the relationship between religion and health. In this research, he argues that social relationships in the church may play an especially important role in explaining the health-related benefits of religion. Ellison attributes these benefits to the fact that "participants in religious communities may enjoy larger, denser, more satisfying social networks, and greater access to support than do their unchurched counterparts" (Ellison & George 1994, 47).

Taylor, Chatters, and Levin (2004) recently published an influential book on religion among African Americans. These investigators report that rich interpersonal networks arise within church settings and that "assistance from church members is not trivial and appears to be especially important for particular groups, such as the elderly" (Taylor et al. 2004, 165). They go on to point out that church-based social support systems may improve the health of older blacks by helping them cope more effectively with the noxious effects of stress.

The insights provided by contemporary scholars on social relationships in the church have moved the field to new heights. Even so, there are at least two ways in which their work can be improved. First, as noted in the previous section, different kinds of social relationships may be found in the church, yet there have been relatively few attempts to delineate the content domain of church-based social relationships, and there has been little effort to compare and contrast how different types of church-based social ties may influence health and well-being in late life. Second, in order to take research in the field to the next level, researchers must begin to specify and empirically evaluate the intervening constructs that link social relationships in the church with health. For example, we need to know precisely how social support from fellow church members helps older adults cope more effectively with the deleterious effects of stress. This, as well as a range of other issues, is explored in the chapters that follow.

Research on Social Relationships and Health in Secular Settings. A vast number of studies that have been conducted in secular settings suggest that people with strong interpersonal relationships have better physical and mental health, and they tend to live longer than individuals who do not maintain strong ties with others (Berkman, Glass, Brissette, & Seeman 2000; Cohen 2004; Krause 2006a). The enthusiasm with which social and behavioral scientists view these findings and the depth of their conviction in these results are reflected in the astounding conclusion reached some time ago by House, Landis, and Umberson (1988). More specifically, these investigators report that the age-adjusted relative risk ratios from research on social relationships and mortality "are stronger than the relative risk for all cause mortality reported for cigarette smoking" (House et al. 1988, 543). Further evidence of the enthusiasm for research on social relationships and health may be found in the work of Rowe and Kahn (1998). Based on findings from the widely cited MacArthur Foundation Study, these investigators conclude that being embedded in a strong social support system is a vitally important component of successful aging.

The sheer volume and uniformity of secular research findings provides compelling justification for examining the relationship between church-based social relationships and health. If social relationships play a pivotal role in the maintenance and improvement of health in secular settings, and if social relationships are even more well developed in the church, then it follows that the health-related benefits of maintaining strong ties with others should be especially evident in religious settings.

Overview of the Chapters That Follow

As defined by Krause (2006a), social relationships are recurrent patterns of interaction with other individuals. Church-based social relationships may therefore be viewed as recurrent patterns of interaction that take place within formal places of worship. However, even a moment's reflection reveals that church-based social relationships are a complex multidimensional phenomena, and it is therefore necessary to identify the major components or dimensions that are subsumed under the rubric of this vast conceptual domain. Doing so provides the organizing theme for the chapters that follow.

Unfortunately, the task of staking out the content domain of church-based social relationships is formidable, which is perhaps one reason that such taxonomy has yet to appear in the literature. It is unlikely that this goal will be accomplished successfully in a single volume. Instead, as Kaplan (1964) recommends, it may be best to follow an iterative approach in which initial efforts to specify the content domain of a given construct are subsequently refined by other investigators. Because so little effort has been made to take a comprehensive look at social relationships in the church, the framework that forms the backbone of this volume does not represent the final word on the matter. Instead, it is an initial step that is taken in full awareness of the fact that what is proposed is likely to be in need of further refinement.

In the discussion that follows, a chapter is devoted to each of four types of social relationships in the church. These dimensions of church-based social ties are introduced only briefly here. However, their fundamental nature and functions are examined in detail in the following chapters. As in the current chapter, the ones that follow draw from a wide range of disciplines and sources, including sociology, psychology, psychiatry, public health, philosophy, nursing, theology, history, and literature. Throughout, the intent was to leave no stone unturned so that social relationships in the church could be viewed from the most comprehensive vantage point possible. A question may be raised about why literature is cited and discussed in a text that aims to take a scientific look at the relationship between social relationships in the church and health. The answer is straightforward. Issues involving social relationships and religion have occupied scholars long before the social and behavioral sciences emerged. As a result, many valuable insights were garnered by these fine literary minds. It would therefore be unfortunate to overlook their labors, and, as shown in subsequent chapters, it would be disingenuous to lay claim to insights that are in fact centuries old.

Informal church-based social support is examined in detail in chapter 2. This refers to assistance provided by fellow church members for the explicit purpose of helping an older congregant cope more effectively with the deleterious effects of stress.

Close companion friendships in the church are explored in chapter 3. These informal social ties are pursued primarily for the purpose of enjoyment. Yet as Rook (1987) and others show, close companion friends may play an important role in the maintenance and improvement of health and well-being across the life course.

Because the church is an institution, formal social roles have developed within it that link the individual with the wider congregation. The norms and values associated with these roles shape the nature of the social relationships that arise from them. Although formal relationships that arise around any number of church roles could be examined, four are discussed in chapter 4 because there is reason to believe they may influence health and well-being in late life. First, members of the clergy occupy a pivotal position in the church. Although they perform many important functions, one—pastoral counseling—is especially relevant for the health and well-being of older adults. The second type of formal relationship that may be found in the church arises in groups that are designed to provide specialized religious functions. More specifically, careful attention will be given to Bible study groups and prayer groups. Third, many churches provide the opportunity to become involved in volunteer activities that are designed to help people in need. Many times, these programs are developed to help church members as well as people who are not affiliated with a given congregation. Fourth, there is another type of formal relationship in the church that is especially important for some older people: help for the homebound. This refers to formal outreach programs that attend to the religious and secular needs of older church members who are unable to leave their homes due primarily to their own illness or the illness of a significant other (e.g., a spouse). Although the formal relationships that arise around this type of service have rarely been discussed in the literature, a small cluster of studies has emerged recently which suggests that they warrant further investigation.

Researchers have known for some time that social relationships in the church do not always follow a smooth course. Instead, congregations may become rife with interpersonal conflict and dissension (Becker 1999). This is important because a number of studies that have been conducted in secular settings suggest that negative interaction may have an especially pernicious effect on health and well-being in late life (Rook 1984). Consequently, chapter 5 is devoted to taking an in-depth look at interpersonal conflict in the church.

Each chapter on the four types of social relationships in the church follows the same format. Formal definitions are presented first, and key characteristics of each type of social relationships are examined in detail. Then, whenever possible, survey measures of each type of social relationship are provided. Following this, extensive efforts are made to show how each type of social relationship may influence health and well-being in late life. Finally, each chapter closes with a discussion of methodological and conceptual challenges that must be met in order to move research forward on each construct.

Once the four main types of church-based social relationships have been examined in detail, an effort is made in chapter 6 to cast research in this field in a wider context by bringing to the foreground the pervasive influence of social structural factors. Age, race, gender, and socioeconomic status (SES) form the pillars of social structure. However, since age-related issues are woven throughout the entire volume, chapter 6 is devoted to exploring the impact of race, gender, and SES on church-based social relationships and health in late life. A chapter on social structural factors is imperative because a considerable amount of research suggests that these social structural factors influence religion and health across the life course. As a result, religion (and especially social relationships in the church) may help explain how at least part of the potentially important effect of social structural factors on health is conveyed.

The final chapter, chapter 7, is devoted to summarizing what has emerged from this extensive undertaking and identifying gaps in the perspectives and methods that have been discussed. In the process, an effort is made to trace broader themes that envelop the study of church-based social relationships and health in late life.

As noted earlier, empirical and theoretical support for the mid-range theories that are examined in this volume come from a wide array of sources. However, a good deal of this work has been done by the author. A number of his studies have been published, but some of the work that is discussed in the following chapters has not. Instead, this latter body of research is ongoing and represents work in progress. Since this research has not been peer-reviewed, it should obviously be viewed cautiously. Nevertheless, this work is included in the current volume because there do not appear to be any studies in the literature that examine the questions and issues that are investigated with this data. All this unpublished research comes from an ongoing longitudinal nationwide survey of older whites and older African Americans that the author has been conducting since 2002 (Krause 2002a). Although this study has not been given a formal name or acronym, it will be referred to throughout this volume as the Religion, Aging, and Health Survey (i.e., the RAH Survey). A detailed overview of the mechanics of this study (e.g., the sampling frame and sampling strategy) is provided in the Appendix.

Conclusions

Social relationships stand at the pivotal juncture between the individual and society: It is through social relationships that society influences the individual, and it is primarily through social relationships that the individual influences society (Berger & Luckman 1966). This dialectic between the individual and society is played out in a number of different social settings, including the family, the neighborhood, and formal institutions. But among these, social relationships that arise within institutions are among the most important, and among the most important and enduring institutions is the church. The church stands at this critical juncture because many of the formal doctrines that religion is built upon are intended to promote better social relationships. Included among these core precepts are the benefits of forgiveness (Rye, Pargament, Ali, Beck, Dorff, Hallisey, Narayanan, & Williams 2000) and the importance of helping people who are in need (Wuthnow 1991). In the process of adhering to these fundamental tenets, some investigators have observed that at least some individuals may derive health-related benefits (Ellison & Levin 1998). There do not appear to be any volumes in the literature that examine the impact of social relationships in the church on health and well-being in late life, even though it is an area with immense potential.

Over the centuries, religion has had no shortage of critics. For example, John Dewey (1922/1950) wrote, "Religion has lost itself in cults, dogmas, and myths. Consequently the office of religion as a sense of community and one's place in it have been lost" (330). Even more scathing views on religion may be found in the work of Upton Sinclair, who was a well-known muckraker. Writing in his book, *The Profits of Religion* (1918/2000), Sinclair claimed, "The supreme crime of the church to-day is that everywhere and in all its operations and influences it is on the side of sloth of mind; that it banishes brains, it sanctifies stupidity, it canonizes incompetence" (55). But perhaps the most boldly outspoken critic of religion is the widely cited philosopher Friedrich Nietzsche. The last book he wrote, *The Anti-Christ,* dealt solely with the dangers of the Christian religion. In this work, Nietzsche (1895/1999) bitterly argued, "The Christian church has left nothing untouched by its depravity; it has turned every value into worthlessness, and every truth into a lie, and every integrity into baseness of soul" (90). Yet despite these acerbic criticisms, religion continues to endure. And because it has, religion must be performing some essential functions and meeting some fundamental needs. The overall intent of the discussion in the chapters that follow is to suggest that at least some of these functions and needs may be found by taking a closer look at social relationships that arise in the church.

Chapter 2

Church-Based Social Support

Getting Help during Difficult Times

Stress is ubiquitous. Virtually everyone experiences the death of a loved one, and many people encounter a range of other major problems, such as significant financial difficulty. In fact, as research by Krause (1994) reveals, the typical older person is exposed to approximately two stressful events in an eighteen-month period alone. Given the widespread nature of stress, it is not surprising to find that many older adults rely on a range of coping resources to help them either avoid or alter the course of unwanted events in their lives. Researchers have argued for decades that religion is one such coping resource. For example, writing eighty years ago, Charles Horton Cooley (1927) maintained that religion "often exists without our being aware of it, until some crisis brings it out" (254). In fact, a good deal of the Old and New Testaments in the Christian Bible involves stories and lessons that are intended to help people deal more effectively with stressful life events (e.g., the story of Job). Although there are a number of ways in which religion may help people confront the stressors in their lives, a core premise in this chapter is that assistance provided by fellow church members plays an especially important role in this respect.

The notion that older adults turn to others for help during difficult times is hardly new (Eckenrode & Wethington 1990). In fact, a vast amount of research that has been done in secular settings indicates that stress exerts a deleterious effect on the physical and mental health of older people, but that the pernicious effects of stress are offset, or buffered, by assistance that is provided by social network members (Krause 2001). Among these potential support providers are family members, friends, and neighbors. But some investigators maintain that

support provided by fellow church members may be especially efficacious because social relationships that develop in the church are particularly close and highly supportive (Ellison & Levin 1998).

It is surprising to find that there are relatively few studies in the literature that empirically evaluate the potential stress-buffering function
of church-based social support. Instead, some investigators provide evidence that stress and social support explain the relationship between religious involvement and depression, but they rely on measures that simultaneously assess support received from church members and assistance
from family members and friends who may or may not be involved in
religion (e.g., Eliassen, Taylor, & Lloyd 2005). This measurement strategy
makes it difficult to isolate the effects of church-based social support per
se. In contrast, other investigators, like Maton (1989), study the stress-
buffering role of perceived support from God, but it is not clear if getting
support from God is the same thing as receiving assistance from fellow
church members. One of the few studies to examine explicitly whether
church-based social support offsets the effects of stress was conducted
by Ellison, Boardman, Williams, and Jackson (2001). These investigators were unable to find evidence that support from fellow church members helps buffer the pernicious impact of stress on either psychological
well-being or psychological distress. However, church-based social support was measured in this study with a single item that asked about assistance in a rather general way (i.e., "How often do people in your church
or place of worship help you out?"). As the discussion provided below
reveals, there is far more to church-based social support than this.

The purpose of this chapter is to explore the potential stress-buffering properties of church-based social support in detail. However, this is a
formidable task because people at church can help each other in a number of different ways when difficult times arise. Put another way, church-
based social support is a complex multidimensional phenomenon in
its own right. Consequently, a necessary first step is to stake out the
vast content domain of this construct by examining the different ways
in which church-based social support may be conceptualized and measured. Once the content domain of church-based support is fleshed out,
a detailed discussion will be provided about how the potentially beneficial effects of more well-known types of church-based support arise.
Thinking in terms of the natural history of a stressful experience helps
frame this discussion. This perspective traces the course of a stressor
from its inception to its potential resolution. More specifically, the natural history approach identifies the deficits or needs that are initially cre-

ated by a stressor, describes how people subsequently react to these deficits by mobilizing or seeking support from fellow church members, and specifies the precise ways in which assistance from people at church offsets or counterbalances the deficits created by the stressor. Throughout, an effort is made to show that a number of the stress-buffering mechanisms that are fostered by fellow church members have a uniquely religious character.

Once a general outline of the natural history of the stress process has been developed, the scope of inquiry will be expanded by bringing to the foreground lesser-known facets of church-based social support. Then issues involving the nature of stress will be examined. Like social support, stress is also a complex multidimensional phenomenon. Simply put, there are several different kinds of stressful experiences. Consequently, a discussion of different types of stressors will be provided, and an effort will be made to show how various aspects of church-based social support may help older people cope with them. Following this, the chapter closes with an examination of methodological and conceptual issues that face investigators who study church-based social support.

Conceptualizing and Measuring Informal Church-Based Social Support

Although it is not hard to find good theoretical discussions of the health protective effects of church-based social support (e.g., Ellison & Levin 1998), relatively few investigators have empirically examined the relationship among these constructs. The reason for this is relatively straightforward. Until recently, good measures of church-based social support have not been available. Evidence of this may be found by turning to the work of Hill and Hood (1999). These investigators provide one of the most comprehensive efforts to date to catalog various measures of religion. This massive undertaking resulted in a volume consisting of seventeen chapters that are devoted to issues like religious attitudes and values, as well as forgiveness and beliefs about the afterlife. But a chapter on church-based social support does not appear in this volume, nor do the authors identify a scale that has been designed specifically for this purpose.

The Fetzer Institute/National Institute on Aging Working Group (1999) was among the first to develop a set of indicators to assess multiple dimensions of church-based social support. This group of scholars devised nine closed-ended survey questions to assess three dimensions of church-based social support. One dealt with emotional support received from fellow church members, whereas another focused on emotional support that is provided by a respondent to the people with whom he or she worships. Emotional support is defined as the provision of empathy, caring, love, and trust during difficult times (Barrera 1986). The third dimension of church-based social support that was devised by this working group is anticipated support, which is defined as the belief that people at church would be willing to help out in the future should the need arise (Wethington & Kessler 1986).

More recently, Krause (2002a), in the RAH Survey, made what is perhaps the most comprehensive effort to assess religion in late life. Deriving measures of church-based social support was a major focal point of this extensive item development program. Seven dimensions of church-based social support emerged from this work. These dimensions, and the twenty-four indicators used to assess them, are provided in Table 2-1. Research by Krause (2002b) reveals that the internal consistency reliability of these scales is good. Some dimensions of church-based social support will be familiar to most investigators because they appear frequently in research on social support that has been conducted in secular settings. One is emotional support that is exchanged with (i.e., provided to and received from) fellow church members. Another is tangible help. Tangible support is instrumental behavior that is designed to help a person directly. Here, the support provider intervenes personally in a problem situation by taking practical action, such as helping with household chores or yard work, or by providing transportation (Barrera 1986).

In contrast to emotional support and tangible help, Krause (2002b) devised measures of other aspects of the church-based social support that may not be recognized immediately by some investigators. Included among these lesser-known dimensions are spiritual support, anticipated support, and satisfaction with support. Spiritual support, which is relatively unique to religious institutions, is assistance that is specifically intended to increase the religious commitment, beliefs, and behavior of a fellow church member. There are a number of ways in which church members may exchange spiritual support. For example, they may share their own religious experiences with a coreligionist, they may show them how to apply their religious beliefs in daily life, or they may help them find solutions to problems they encounter by turning to the Bible (Krause 2002b).

The other two lesser-known types of church-based social support are more perceptual in nature; they reflect an individual's subjective

Table 2-1. Measures of Church-Based Social Support from the RAH Survey

1. Emotional Support Received from Fellow Church Members[a]
    A. Other than your minister, pastor, or priest, how often does someone in your congregation let you know he or she loves and cares for you?
    B. How often does someone in your congregation talk with you about your private problems and concerns?
    C. How often does someone in your congregation express interest and concern in your well-being?

2. Satisfaction with Emotional Support Received from Fellow Church Members[b]
    A. During the past few moments, we've been talking about emotional support you may have received from members of your congregation. How satisfied are you with the emotional support you've received from the people in your church?

3. Tangible Support Received from Fellow Church Members[a]
    A. How often does someone in your congregation give you a ride to church services?
    B. How often does someone in your congregation provide you with transportation to other places, like the grocery store or the doctor's office?
    C. How often does someone in your congregation help you with things that need to be done around your home, such as household chores or yard work?
    D. How often does someone in your congregation help out when either you or a family member is ill?

4. Satisfaction with Tangible Support from Fellow Church Members[b]
    A. During the past few moments we've been talking about practical things that people in your congregation might have done for you, such as providing you with transportation or helping out when you were ill. How satisfied are you with this type of help?

5. Emotional Support Provided to Fellow Church Members[a]
    A. How often do you show someone in your congregation that you love and care for them?
    B. How often have you talked with someone in your congregation about his or her private feelings and concerns?
    C. How often have you expressed interest and concern in the well-being of someone in your congregation?

6. Tangible Support Provided to Fellow Church Members[a]
    A. How often do you provide transportation to church for someone in your congregation?
    B. How often do you provide transportation for someone in your congregation to other places, like the grocery store or the doctor's office?

Table 2-1. *continued*

    C. How often have you helped someone in your congregation with things that need to be done around his or her home, such as household chores or yard work?

    D. How often have you helped take care of someone in your congregation when he or she was ill?

7. Anticipated Support from Fellow Church Members[c]

    A. If you were ill, how much would someone in your congregation be willing to help out?

    B. If you needed to talk to someone about your problems and private feelings, how much would someone in your congregation be willing to listen?

    C. If you needed to know where to go to get help with a problem, how much would someone in your congregation be willing to help you find it?

8. Spiritual Support Received from Fellow Church Members[a]

    A. Not counting Bible study groups, prayer groups, or church services, how often does someone in your congregation share his or her own religious experiences with you?

    B. Not counting Bible study groups, prayer groups, or church services, how often does someone in your congregation help you find solutions to your problems in the Bible?

    C. Not counting Bible study groups, prayer groups, or church services, how often do the examples set by others in your congregation help you lead a better religious life?

    D. Not counting Bible study groups, prayer groups, or church services, how often does someone in your congregation help you to know God better?

---

[a] These items are scored in the following manner (coding in parentheses): never (1); once in a while (2); fairly often (3); very often (4).

[b] These items are scored in the following manner: completely dissatisfied (1); not very satisfied (2); fairly satisfied (3); very satisfied (4).

[c] These items are scored in the following manner: not at all (1); a little (2); some (3); a great deal (4).

evaluation of the supportiveness of fellow church members. The first, anticipated support, was defined above. The second is satisfaction with support. The indicators of emotional and tangible support in Table 2-1 assess how often fellow church members have provided assistance. But these measures fail to capture all there is to the social support process because researchers have known for some time that there are substantial individual variations in the need for support; some individuals require a good deal of help to confront a stressor, whereas other people can resolve problems with relatively little assistance from others (Krause,

Liang, & Yatomi 1989). Therefore, in addition to knowing how often support has been provided, it is also important to assess whether an individual's need for assistance has been met. Measures of satisfaction with support from fellow church members were designed to address this issue. These measures are based on the assumption that a person will be satisfied with the emotional or tangible support he or she receives if his or her need for assistance has been met.

As this brief overview of church-based social support reveals, people at church can help each other in a number of different ways when stressors arise in life. Although the various types of church-based support may convey similar benefits, they may also help in ways that are relatively unique. But before these benefits can be discussed in detail, it is necessary to identify the problems or needs that stressors create in the first place. For this reason the psychosocial deficits created by stressful experiences are examined in the following section.

Stress-Induced Psychosocial Deficits

Although stress may affect health and well-being in a number of ways, a substantial number of studies that have been conducted primarily in secular settings suggest that three psychosocial pathways may be especially important. More specifically, stress may exert an adverse effect on health and well-being because it erodes a person's sense of self-esteem and because it diminishes their feelings of personal control (Pearlin, Menaghan, Lieberman, & Mullan 1981). In addition, a small cluster of studies suggest that stress may also create physical and mental health problems because it tends to diminish a person's sense of meaning in life (Krause 2004a). This is an especially important issue to study in church settings because a number of investigators have argued that one of the primary functions of religion is to provide a sense of meaning in life (Pargament 1997; Spilka et al. 2003). Each of these intervening mechanisms is discussed below in greater detail.

Self-Esteem

Some time ago, Coopersmith (1967) defined self-esteem as "a personal judgment of worthiness that is expressed in the attitudes the individual holds toward himself" (5). The critical role that feelings of self-worth play in social life is highlighted by Kaplan's (1975) formulation of the self-esteem motive. He maintains that the need to develop and maintain positive self-feelings is one of the primary motivating forces in social life and one of the factors that shapes a good deal of human behavior. These self-assessments are important because a number of studies indicate that a positive sense of self-worth is associated with better mental health, better physical health, and the use of a number of positive health behaviors (see Trzesniewski, Donnellan, & Robins 2003 for a review of this research).

There is now considerable evidence that stressful life events tend to erode or diminish feelings of self-worth (e.g., Krause & Borawski-Clark 1994). This problem arises because stressors can often be stigmatizing or embarrassing (e.g., divorce or losing a job). In addition, people sometimes play a role in bringing about the undesirable events that confront them, and the awareness that they are the architects of their own misfortune reflects poorly on the self. The essence of these issues is captured succinctly by Pearlin and his colleagues, who observe that stress "can confront people with dogged evidence of their own failures—or lack of success—and with inescapable proof of their inability to alter the unwanted circumstances of their lives" (Pearlin et al. 1981, 340).

The loss of self-esteem in the face of stress is important because a number of investigators maintain that self-esteem is a key resource for dealing with the noxious effects of stress. For example, research reviewed by Hoyle, Kernis, Leary, and Baldwin (1999) reveals that people with high self-esteem tend to disregard or emotionally offset negative feedback associated with undesirable life events. In contrast, this research further indicates that individuals with low self-esteem are more likely to readily accept negative feedback, and the internalization of these negative self-images interferes with their ability to handle adverse events efficaciously. Similarly, as Baumeister, Tice, and Hutton (1989) point out, people with low self-evaluations are characterized by uncertainty and confusion, which may lead to ineffective coping efforts. Finally, researchers who study stressful life events have known for some time that it is possible to ward off or avoid some stressors before they arise, which is sometimes referred to as anticipatory coping. This understanding is important because a study by Newby-Clark (2004) indicates that people with low self-esteem are less likely than individuals with high self-esteem to engage in anticipatory coping efforts. The failure of persons with low self-esteem to take this kind of action is attributed to a lack of confidence in their own abilities.

Viewed from a broader vantage point, research on self-esteem provides one way of showing why the effects of stress are so pernicious: stressful life events tend to erode the very resources (i.e., self-esteem) that are needed to cope more effectively with them. Research on the

interface between stress and self-esteem in late life is especially important because a number of studies suggest that feelings of self-worth tend
to decline across the life course (Robins, Trzesniewski, Tracy, Gosling, &
Potter 2002). As a result, health practitioners need to find ways to shore
up the self-esteem of older people when stressful events arise. But self-
esteem is not the only resource that is adversely affected by stressful
experiences. As discussed in the next section, undesirable life events also
tend to diminish another critical coping resource: feelings of personal
control.

Feelings of Personal Control

The construct of control has played a central role in social and
behavioral science research for nearly fifty years (Zarit, Pearlin, & Schaie
2003). In fact, some investigators claim that feelings of personal control may be a more important determinant of psychological well-being
than any other psychosocial construct (Ross & Sastry 1999). Therefore,
finding that a strong sense of personal control is considered to be a
key marker of successful aging (Rowe & Kahn 1998) is not surprising.
Although researchers have devised numerous ways to conceptualize the
construct of control (e.g., locus of control, mastery, self-efficacy), these
different perspectives nevertheless share a common conceptual core.
Embedded in each view is the notion that individuals with a strong sense
of personal control believe the things that happen to them are responsive to and contingent upon their own choices, efforts, and actions (Ross
& Sastry 1999). In contrast, people with a weak sense of personal control believe the events in their lives are shaped by forces outside their
influence, and they feel they have little ability to regulate the things
that happen to them. A vast literature indicates that, much like self-
esteem, strong feelings of personal control are associated with better
physical health, better mental health, and the adoption of beneficial
health behaviors (see Krause 2003a, for a review of this research).

A number of studies suggest that stressful life events may erode a
person's sense of control (Pearlin et al. 1981; Krause & Borawski-Clark
1994). There are at least two ways this may happen. First, by definition,
stressful events are unwanted and undesirable. Therefore, the very fact
that an unwanted event has arisen may be construed as evidence of a
person's inability to maintain control over the things that happen in
his or her life. The second way in which stress may erode feelings of
personal control is found in Caplan's (1981) classic paper on the stress
process. He maintains that the distress and disorientation created by

a stressor erodes an individual's usual cognitive and problem-solving abilities, thereby making it more difficult for him or her to take control of the situation by initiating effective coping responses. These insights reveal that, as with self-esteem, the effects of stress are especially noxious because life events tend to erode the very psychosocial resources (i.e., feelings of personal control) that are needed to confront them. It is especially important to focus on the factors that influence personal control in late life because a number of studies suggest that feelings of control decline at an accelerating rate as people grow older (Mirowsky 1995).

Meaning in Life

Reker (1997) defines meaning in life as "having a sense of direction, a sense of order, and a reason for existence, a clear sense of personal identity, and a greater social consciousness" (710). Researchers have argued for decades that deriving a sense of meaning lies at the very heart of life itself. For example, Frankl (1959/1985) maintained that the desire to find a sense of meaning is one of the primary motivating forces in life, and Maslow (1971) placed constructs that are closely akin to meaning (i.e., self-actualization) at the top of his widely cited hierarchy of needs. Research on meaning is important because a small cluster of studies that have been done in secular settings suggest that deriving a well-developed sense of meaning is associated with better mental health (Reker 1997) and better physical health (Krause 2004a) in late life. Perhaps more important, research by Krause (2004a) that has been conducted in secular settings suggests that stressful life events may erode an older person's sense of meaning in life.

The widely cited theoretical framework devised by Erikson (1959) helps show why it is especially important to focus on meaning in late life. He maintained that as people approach late life, they enter into the final stage of development that is characterized by the crisis of integrity versus despair. This is a time of deep introspection when older people survey their lives, attempt to reconcile the things they have done, and make sense of the experiences they have had. Ultimately, the goal of this process is to weave the story of one's life into a more coherent whole. Doing so imbues life with a deep sense of meaning and purpose. However, if people are unable to resolve this developmental challenge successfully, Erikson (1959) argues that they will slip into despair.

As Reker (1997) points out, a sense of meaning in life can arise from a number of sources, including personal relationships, work, hobbies, and religion. However, given the focus of the current volume, it is important to examine meaning that arises specifically from involvement in religion. Krause (2003b) defines religious meaning as the process of turning to religion in order to find a sense of purpose in life, a sense of direction in life, and a sense that there is a reason for one's existence. However, there are two problems with the way that the interface between religion and meaning has been handled in empirical research. First, most researchers who study the relationships among religion, meaning, and health rely on indicators of a general sense of meaning in life. For example, Peterson and Roy (1985) found that religious salience (i.e., the importance of religion) is associated with a greater sense of general meaning in life. However, the survey measures in these studies do not assess meaning that arises specifically from religion. The nature of this problem may be seen more clearly by turning to the following item, which comes from the widely cited scale developed by Battista and Almond (1973): "I feel like I have found a really significant meaning for leading my life" (427). In contrast, Krause (2003b) devised measures of meaning in life that are anchored specifically within the context of religion: "My faith gives me a sense of direction in my life" (S164). Second, researchers have yet to fully explore the content domain of religious meaning. Although Krause (2003b) made an initial effort to devise a measure of religious meaning, his work did not go far enough because the items he developed focus solely on whether religion helps older people find a sense of purpose and direction in life, as well as a reason for their existence. Although this represents a reasonable point of departure, other facets of meaning that are unique to religion are not captured in his scale. For example, researchers need to know whether beliefs in salvation and divine grace are important components of meaning for older Christians.

Even though there are limitations in the measurement of religious meaning, researchers can ill afford to overlook this core construct in their empirical research. As noted above, a number of investigators argue that one of the primary functions of religion is to provide a sense of meaning in life. Evidence of this may be found in the classic work of Clark (1958), who maintained that "religion, more than any other human function satisfies the need for meaning in life" (419). Similarly, in the process of developing his thought-provoking discussion of significance, Pargament (1997) observed, "In essence, religion offers meaning in life" (49; see also Berger 1967). If religion plays a role in the wider stress process, then it makes sense to focus on meaning that arises specifically from involvement in religion. If items that assess a general sense of meaning are used instead, it would be more difficult to know if the stress-buffering effects of meaning can be attributed to religion, or whether they might arise from other sources, such as work or interpersonal relationships outside the church.

Unfortunately, very little empirical research focuses specifically on religious meaning. In fact, there appears to be only one study in the literature that examines the relationship between religious meaning and well-being (Krause 2003b). Krause (2003b) found that older people who derive a sense of meaning in life from religion tend to have higher levels of life satisfaction, self-esteem, and optimism than older individuals who do not have a strong sense of religious meaning.

But the study by Krause (2003b) did not focus explicitly on religious meaning and stress. Moreover, there do not appear to be any other studies that explicitly examine the interface between these constructs. Even so, there are several ways in which stress may threaten or diminish an older person's sense of religious meaning. When stressful events arise, it may become more difficult for an older person to believe that God has a purpose for his or her life, and it may be harder to find a reason for what has happened, which is why Pargament and his colleagues found that some people react to stressful events by wondering if God was trying to punish them, by questioning the power of God, and by believing that God had abandoned them (Pargament, Koenig, & Perez 2000).

Having a low sense of self-worth, diminished feelings of personal control, and an inability to find meaning in life is a painful state that motivates older people to take action. Because stress tends to erode the very resources that people need to deal with it (i.e., self-esteem, feelings of personal control, and religious meaning), they are often unable to resolve problems on their own. When this happens, they may turn to significant others for assistance; and for those involved in religion, fellow church members are an important source of support. For this reason the process of mobilizing support from fellow church members is examined in detail in the next section.

Mobilizing Support from Fellow Church Members

According to the prevailing view in the secular literature, people actively seek out, and gratefully receive, assistance from significant others during difficult times. But as research reviewed by Eckenrode and Wethington (1990) reveals, this may not always be true. Instead, as these investigators argue, people sometimes feel reluctant to take their problems to others, which may happen for several reasons. First, as noted earlier, some stressful events are stigmatizing and embarrassing. For example, admitting that a spouse, child, or grandchild has a problem with drugs or alcohol is difficult. Second, as discussed above, people sometimes play a role in bringing about their own misfortune. More specifically, an individual's action (or inaction) may cause a stressor to arise. For example, inappropriate or unsupportive behavior may help bring about a divorce. Older people may therefore be reluctant to seek support when they have played a role in causing the stressors that confront them, because doing so brings their own shortcomings to the foreground and lays their faults and limitations in the open for others to see. Simply put, ego-related costs are associated with seeking assistance from others. Third, social support is not an unlimited resource; potential support providers may begin to feel they are being taken advantage of if subject to repeated requests for assistance (see La Gaipa 1990, for a review of this research). Taken as a whole, this brief overview of the support mobilization process indicates that people may need assistance from others, but they may not always be willing or feel comfortable in asking for it. Unfortunately, the factors that influence the decision to seek help from others are not clearly understood. However, turning to relatively unique aspects of social relationships in the church may provide valuable insight into this issue.

The basic tenets of religion create an environment that may help older people overcome the reluctance to ask for support in time of need. As Coward (1986) points out, helping those who are confronted by adversity is a central tenet in virtually every religion in the world. Moreover, the Christian faith eschews negative judgments of those in distress, extols the virtues of altruistic or selfless helping behaviors, and places a strong emphasis on the importance of forgiving people for things they have done wrong. The essence of this orientation was discussed over one hundred years ago by sociologist Edward Alsworth Ross (1896). Recall from chapter 1 that he defined religion in terms of an ideal bond among members of society. Ross (1896) went on to argue that the basis of this ideal bond among people arises from "the idea of an All-Father having those social qualities—love, goodness, mercy, truthfulness, faithfulness—which characterize the soul in its perfect state. He is at once source and goal of man's life. Men are brothers because they are his sons" (438). Ross (1896) believed that this sense of ideal brotherhood inspired sympathy among people and instilled a sense of the "underlying oneness" among them (441). To the extent that the views of Ross (1896) are correct, it is not difficult to see why the social relationships fostered in the church create a welcoming and trusting interpersonal environment that makes it easier for fellow church members to reach out to each other during difficult times.

The ease with which the helping process may be initiated in the church is further enhanced by a practice found in a number of Christian denominations. In order for people to help someone in need, they must first be aware that their assistance is required. Time is often set aside during worship services for the identification of people in the congregation who are faced with difficult circumstances. Then, once these individuals are identified, the congregation offers a prayer on their behalf. Church members who are in need are also often identified in church bulletins and newsletters. As these examples reveal, a number of mechanisms are in place in the church that help older persons receive assistance without having to ask explicitly for it. This consideration is especially important for older people because a number of investigators maintain that members of the current cohort of older adults view their independence highly, and they do not like to think of themselves as the type of individual who must rely on others for help (Lee 1985). The simple face-saving devices that the church provides may go a long way toward ensuring the ultimate success of assistance.

Exploring the Benefits of Church-Based Social Support

Having identified the psychosocial deficits that are created by stress and the factors that influence subsequent help-seeking behavior, it is time to turn to the issues that lie at the heart of this chapter. More specifically, the goal of this section is to delve into the precise ways in which support provided by fellow church members offsets the deleterious effects of stress. A two-step strategy is used to address this issue, moving from more general to more specific points. Focusing on more general principles in the first step will show that support from fellow church members helps bolster and replenish feelings of self-worth, personal control, and meaning in life that undesirable life events have eroded. Turning to the second step helps flesh out the finer points of this process by identifying the intervening constructs that link church-based social support with self-esteem, control, and meaning. As this discussion reveals, religious coping responses play an especially important role in this respect. In the process, an effort is made to show how other seemingly unrelated facets of religion—such as prayer, forgiveness, and gratitude toward God—can be folded into the emerging perspective by highlighting their common social underpinnings and their relevance to the coping process. Following an examination of these issues, this section closes with a discussion of how anticipated support as well as giving (rather than receiving) assistance to people at church helps older people cope more effectively with their own stressful experiences.

Church-Based Support and Feelings of Self-Worth

If stress erodes self-esteem, then a key issue involves identifying the ways in which this important coping resource is replenished. A basic premise in this chapter is that fellow church members play an especially important role in this respect. In order to see how this happens, it is necessary to take a closer look at how feelings of self-worth arise. One of the most fundamental principles in social psychology specifies that a sense of self-worth comes from feedback offered by significant others. Many attribute this classic insight to Charles Horton Cooley's (1902/2003) classic notion of the looking-glass self, but the roots of this principle go back much further. For example, many believe that Johann Wolfgang von Goethe possessed one of the greatest minds of his time. Writing in 1823, Goethe began with the simple notion that one of the most important tasks in life is for people to understand themselves better. He went on to argue that, in pursuing this goal, "the greatest help comes from other people; they have the advantage of being able to compare us with the world from their own standpoint, and thus they know us better than we ourselves can" (as quoted in Naydler 2000, 102). Then, presaging Cooley (1902/2003), Goethe maintained that other people therefore serve as "so many mirrors" (as quoted in Naydler 2000, 102). But the earliest discussion of the looking-glass self may actually have been written by Adam Smith. Many are familiar with his classic work in economics—*An Inquiry into the Nature and Causes of the Wealth of Nations* (1776). However, few may be aware that Smith first wrote a treatise on fundamental aspects of human nature: *The Theory of Moral Sentiments* (1759/2002). In it, Smith (1759/2002) explicitly notes that "we either approve or disapprove of our own conduct...when we place ourselves in the situation of another man, and view it, as it were, with his eyes and from his station....This is the only looking glass by which we can, in some measure, with the eyes of other people, scrutinize the propriety of our own conduct" (128, 131).

There have been many elaborations and extensions of the looking-glass self since Cooley (1902/2003), Goethe (1823/2000), and Smith (1759/2002) discussed this construct. One of the most significant developments has been the realization that instead of having one sense of self, people have many, and some of these selves are valued more highly than others. The origins of this perspective go back at least to the classic work of William James (1892/1961). He argued that a person has "as many different social selves as there are distinct *groups* of persons about whose opinion he cares" (James 1892/1961, 40, emphasis in original). But James (1892/1961) went on to point out that people tend to value oneself more highly than others: "So the seeker of his truest, strongest, deepest self must review the list carefully and pick out the one on which to stake his salvation. All other selves thereupon become unreal, but the fortunes of this self are real" (53). If individuals have multiple selves that are grounded in the groups to which they belong, then people who go to church are likely to have a sense of self associated with their faith (i.e., a religious self). Depending upon the level of commitment to one's faith, this religious self may be valued more highly than any other self.

Focusing on the beliefs that define and guide the religious self helps more clearly specify how fellow church members may help an older person who is grappling with a stressful event. Although it is not possible to stake out here the full content of these beliefs, some beliefs about the religious self are especially relevant for studying the stress process. The basic tenets of Christianity teach that God has unconditional love for all people and that even though they may do things that fall short of God's law, they are nevertheless forgiven and valued highly (Rye et al. 2000). Perhaps more important, the precepts of the faith further maintain that people should emulate the example set by God and show unconditional love and forgiveness toward each other (Koenig 1994). Knowing there is a source of forgiveness and unconditional love may go a long way toward replenishing feelings of self-worth that have been depleted by a stressful event, but it is not clear how individuals who are in the throes of a stressor avail themselves of these insights. Although these religious teachings may be derived from a number of sources (e.g., sermons or reading the Bible privately), the theoretical rationale provided above suggests they may also come from the reflected appraisals of fellow church members who reinforce the importance and salience of the religious self and show an older individual who is confronted by a stressor how the basic teachings of the faith underscore his or her value as a person.

Earlier, several different types of church-based social support were identified. Two may help replenish and bolster an older person's sense of self-worth that has been eroded by a stressful experience. First, as the discussion of the work by Ross (1896) reveals, people who are religious strive to integrate the ideal qualities of their faith into the relationships they have with others. Loving and caring for others are among these God-like qualities. This point is reflected in the items contained in Table 2-1 that capture emotional support provided by fellow church members (e.g., "How often does someone in your congregation let you know they love and care for you?"). If older people are confronted by stressful events that erode their feelings of self-worth, then knowing that people at church love and care for them may help shore up their depleted sense of self-esteem.

Evidence that there may be something special about church-based emotional support can be found in a recent study by Krause (2006c). The findings from this study reveal that emotional support from fellow church members offsets the pernicious effects of ongoing financial problems on self-rated health. In contrast, this study further indicates that emotional support received from people outside the church fails to provide a similar stress-buffering function.

The second type of church-based support that may help replenish feelings of self-worth is spiritual support. For an older person facing a stressor, significant others may remind that person of Bible passages which underscore the love that God has for each of us, or they may discuss personal experiences in which they came to this realization themselves. The messages reinforced through spiritual support may go a long way toward soothing a bruised sense of self-esteem.

Church-Based Support and Feelings of Personal Control

A number of studies conducted in secular settings suggest that support from family members and close friends tends to replenish and bolster feelings of personal control that have been depleted by stressful life events (see Krause 2003a, for a review of this research). Caplan (1981) provides a succinct overview of how this takes place. He argues that when stressors arise, social network members help define the problem situation, help develop a plan of action, assist in implementing the plan, and provide feedback and guidance as the plan is being executed. Because of this assistance, the stressed person comes to believe that the problem situation can be controlled and overcome. This brief theoretical overview underscores the pervasive influence of social factors in the stress process; social factors (i.e., stressful life events) erode feelings of personal control, and other social factors build feelings of control back up again (i.e., social support).

Turning to the theoretical perspective developed by Schulz and Heckhausen (1996) provides a way to delve more deeply into the relationship between church-based social support and control that takes a uniquely religious character. The distinction between primary and secondary control figures prominently in their work. Viewed in general terms, primary control refers to efforts aimed at changing the external world, whereas secondary control is concerned with changing internal cognitions (e.g., one's attitudes, attributions, and perceptions) rather than the external social environment. Following the theory of selection, optimization, and compensation (Baltes 1991), Schulz and Heckhausen (1996) argue that as people age, and as their resources dwindle, people gradually relinquish primary control in some areas of life so available resources can be devoted to maintaining primary control in other domains.

Although the theoretical perspective developed by Schulz and Heckhausen (1996) is thought provoking, there are problems with the way in which they conceptualize secondary control. As Skinner (1997) argues persuasively, the internal cognitions that form the bedrock of secondary control in their framework may not capture efforts to exercise control at all. Instead, efforts geared solely toward changing cognitions and emotions reflect feelings of passivity and helplessness, and culminate in the relinquishing of control. But there is another way to approach the study of secondary control that is intrinsically social in nature and that explicitly addresses two specific ways in which the role played by fellow church members comes into play. The first is best illustrated with an example. Assume an older woman in church is having trouble with the upkeep of her home, so her fellow church members pitch in and help out by doing things like mowing her lawn. As a result, the older woman is likely to feel that her affairs at home are under control. But because she has little to do with this directly, it is difficult to see why she would feel that she is personally in control of her household. Instead, her fellow church members are in control of it. As this example reveals, secondary control is a sense of confidence that the challenges arising in a specific domain of life are turning out in a desired way because significant others (e.g., fellow church members) are working to ensure this outcome. This perspective on church-based support and secondary control shows how tangible support from fellow church members may help an older person feel as though their life is under control. This notion of secondary control is not without precedence in the literature. Similar principles were espoused some time ago in the secular literature by Bandura (1982), when he introduced the notion of proxy control.

But there is another way in which secondary control may be manifest specifically in religious settings. More specifically, older people may attempt to cope with diminishing age-related resources by relying on a concept known in the literature as God-mediated control (Berrenberg 1987). A good definition of God-mediated control is difficult to provide, because this construct has been conceptualized in different ways. One approach is found in the discussion of divine control by Schieman, Pudrovska, and Milkie (2005). According to this view, people turn over control of their lives completely to God. The essence of this perspective is captured in the following item that was taken from their scale: "God has decided what your life shall be." However, Krause (2005a) takes a different approach. He maintains that people do not completely surrender control of their lives to God. Instead, they work collaboratively with God to master the social environment. The following item taken from the work of Krause (2005a) reflects the essence of this view: "All things are possible when I work together with God." This notion of collaboration with God is also embedded in Pargament's religious coping scale (Pargament, Koenig, & Perez 2000).

The extensive qualitative research reported by Krause (2002a) helps reconcile the two different perspectives of God-mediated control. When the subjects in his study discussed God-mediated control, they initially indicated their belief that God controls everything that happens in their lives, which is consistent with the notion of divine control (Schieman et al. 2005). However, study participants were subsequently asked if this meant that no action or involvement was required on their part. A number of older respondents indicated this was not the case. Instead, they said that they did all they could to resolve a problem and then turned to God for help after that. Others said it meant that they kept on trying to solve the problem, while God also became involved and lightened the burden created by the stressor. For this reason, Krause (2005a) focused on collaborative God-mediated control. However, given the initial response of subjects in the qualitative studies, measures of divine control are likely to be correlated highly with indicators of collaborative God-mediated control.

Findings from the study by Krause (2005a) indicate that older people with a strong sense of God-mediated control have higher levels of life satisfaction, are more optimistic, and have greater feelings of self-worth and lower levels of death anxiety than older people with a weaker sense of God-mediated control. However, there do not appear to be any studies in the literature that explicitly assess whether feelings of God-mediated control help offset the noxious effects of stress on health and psychological well-being.

Although the discussion provided up to this point helps stake out the essential nature of God-mediated control, the role that fellow church members play in bolstering this potentially important coping resource is still not entirely clear. Fortunately, a recent longitudinal study by Krause (2007b) helps clarify this issue. He examined a number of factors in the church that influence change in God-mediated control. One emerged as being especially important. The findings from this study reveal that spiritual support from fellow church members helps sustain feelings of God-mediated control over time. These findings are consistent with the widely cited theory of religion devised by Stark and Finke (2000), who maintain that interaction with fellow believers exerts a vitally important influence on a wide range of religious beliefs. Referring to religious belief systems or religious models of reality as "religious explanations," these researchers propose, "An individual's confidence in religious explanations is strengthened to the extent that others express their confidence in them" (Stark & Finke 2000, 107).

Church-Based Support and Meaning in Life

In addition to restoring feelings of self-worth and personal control that have been depleted by stressful life events, support from fellow church members may also help shore up an older person's sense of meaning in life. Evidence of this may be found in a recent longitudinal study by Krause (2007c). Research conducted in secular settings by Debats (1999) reveals that significant others are an important source of meaning in life (see also Krause 2004a). These findings are consistent with arguments developed by Berger in his classic work, *The Sacred Canopy* (1967). In it, Berger asserts that a sense of meaning in life, or *nomos*, is "built up in the consciousness of the individual by conversation with significant others" (Berger 1967, 16). Berger goes on to maintain that a good deal of this conversation takes place within religious settings, but how conversations that take place in the church perform this vitally important function is not entirely clear. At least part of the problem arises from the fact that social relationships in the church are a complex multidimensional phenomena (see Table 2-1), and as a result, the ties that older people develop with fellow church members may influence religious meaning in a number of ways.

Two types of church-based social support—spiritual support and emotional support from fellow church members—figured prominently in Krause's study (2007c), because there is reason to believe they play an especially important role in restoring and maintaining a sense of religious meaning in life. As defined earlier, spiritual support is assistance that is intended to increase the religious commitment, belief, and behavior of a fellow church member. If a core function of religion is to promote a sense of meaning in life, and church members encourage an older person to adopt religious principles and beliefs, then spiritual assistance from fellow church members should be an important source of religious meaning.

In contrast to spiritual support, it may be less evident why emotional support provided by coreligionists may also bolster an older person's sense of meaning in life. However, as a study that Krause (2004a) conducted in a secular setting reveals, emotional support operates in a more general way by helping people appreciate that the ties they have developed with others integrates them more tightly into a larger social whole, thereby fostering a sense of purpose and meaning in life. The findings from the survey by Krause (2007c) suggest that both emotional and spiritual support from fellow church members tend to bolster a sense of religious meaning in life. But of the two, spiritual support appears to have the greatest effect.

Sharpening the Theoretical Underpinnings of Church-Based Social Support

The argument that has been developed up to this point suggests that church-based social support may help older people deal more effectively with stressful life events because it replenishes and maintains feelings of self-worth, personal control, and meaning in life that have been eroded by difficult circumstances. But deeper reflection reveals that something is still missing from this theoretical framework because it is not clear what significant others do specifically that bolsters an older person's sense of personal control, self-worth, and meaning in life. Self-esteem, feelings of control, and a sense of meaning reflect more general orientations to life: these psychosocial resources arise from and are encouraged by more specific cognitions and behaviors that directly confront problems created by difficult circumstances in life. As the discussion in this section reveals, religious coping responses play an especially important role in this respect. In the process, a different way of studying religious coping responses is introduced that highlights challenges that are inherent in this important conceptual domain.

Religious Coping Responses

Lazarus and Folkman (1984) define coping responses as the specific thoughts and behaviors that people rely on to manage internal and external demands that they appraise as stressful. It follows from this definition that religious coping responses arise explicitly from, and are motivated by, religious principles and beliefs.

No one has done more research on religious coping responses than Pargament (1997). His distinguished research program reveals two broad ways to classify religious coping responses: positive and negative. Perhaps the best way to illustrate the meaning of these constructs is to turn to the indicators that are used to assess them in his widely cited scale: the RCOPE (Pargament et al. 2000). The following items capture the essence and basic nature of positive religious coping responses: "I asked God to help me find a purpose in life," "I sought help from God in letting go of my anger," "I looked to God for strength, support, and guidance." In contrast, the following indicators capture the underlying nature of negative religious coping responses: "I wondered whether God had abandoned me," "I questioned the power of God," "I disagreed with what the church wanted me to do or believe" (Pargament et al. 2000).

Pargament's (1997) extensive research program reveals that people who turn to positive religious coping responses when adversity arises tend to enjoy better physical and mental health than individuals who do not rely on positive religious coping responses. In contrast, his work further indicates that individuals who use negative religious coping responses are especially at risk for developing physical and mental health problems. In fact, the size of the impact of negative religious coping responses is greater than that of positive religious coping responses. The greater impact of negative aspects of religion will come to light again in chapter 5, when negative interaction in the church is examined.

A number of problems have been identified with the way researchers handle coping responses in studies that have been conducted in secular settings (see, for example, Coyne & Racioppo 2000; Folkman & Moskowitz 2004). Although reviewing all these shortcomings here is not possible, one is especially important. Comprehensive checklists of religious coping responses subsume a broad array of religious cognitions and behaviors, but aggregating a wide range of coping responses in the same inventory makes it easy to overlook potentially important causal relationships among them; as a result, it is possible to miss important ways in which these coping responses may operate. Although much is to be gained from the broad vista afforded by the global approach to assessing religious coping, coupling this measurement strategy with a finer-grained approach is also important. The benefits associated with this alternative strategy are addressed below in two ways. First, religious coping checklists typically contain items referring to church-based social support. However, an effort will be made to show that fellow church members can be a source of religious coping responses rather than a coping response per se. Second, religious coping indices also often contain references to prayer and forgiveness. But as the discussion provided below reveals, these are complex conceptual domains in their own right that also have strong social underpinnings. Embedding them in checklists with other coping responses may therefore obfuscate the wider social process in which they operate.

Fellow church members can exert a profound influence on the nature of the religious coping responses that older adults rely on to reduce the deleterious effects of stress. The theoretical underpinnings of this issue may be found by recasting Caplan's (1981) discussion of the stress process in the lexicon of coping responses. As discussed earlier, Caplan shows how significant others help define the problem situation (i.e., they shape primary stress appraisals), suggest a plan of action (i.e., they identify specific coping responses), and provide feedback and guidance as the plan is being implemented. But it is difficult to appreciate the finer nuances of this process when items involving church-based social support are embedded in comprehensive religious coping checklists. For example, Pargament, Koenig, and Perez (2000) include items in their index of religious coping that acknowledge the influence of fellow church members in the stress process (e.g., "I sought support from members of my congregation"). Although clearly recognizing the potentially important influence of coreligionists, this strategy falls short in two respects. First, this item shows that a respondent turned to fellow church members for help, but it does not reveal what happened and what they received once they did. Simply put, it is not possible to tell what people at church may have suggested or what they may actually have done. Knowing what significant others have actually provided is important, because the secular literature is replete with examples of how the social support process may go awry, and how the well-intentioned efforts of others may be a source of further difficulty instead of a source of solace (Coyne, Wortman, & Lehman 1988). By keeping church-based support separate from religious coping responses, it is possible to identify what they have done explicitly, thereby making it possible to explore the circumstances under which assistance from others is helpful and when well-intentioned support from people at church merely adds to the problem.

The second issue also has to do with knowing what transpired in a potentially supportive encounter. As noted earlier in this chapter, people at church may help in several ways. They may, for example, provide emotional support. This direct coping response requires no further action on the part of the recipient because emotional support may, for example, directly enhance an older individual's sense of self-worth. But fellow church members may also provide spiritual support, which is not a coping response per se. Instead, it is a form of informational support designed to encourage and inspire a person who is confronted by a stressor to engage in other, more explicit religious coping responses. This means, for example, that fellow church members may tell an older person who is in the throes of some difficulty to pray or seek solutions to their problems in the Bible. Since praying and finding solutions to problems in the Bible are measured elsewhere in religious coping response inventories, in essence, this means that causal relationships exist between one religious coping response (i.e., seeking religious support) and another religious coping response (i.e., praying).

Evidence that church-based social support may be associated with other religious coping responses can be found in a study by Krause, Ellison, Shaw, Marcum, and Boardman (2001). Based on data provided by a nationwide survey of Presbyterians of all ages, these investigators compared and contrasted the effects of three types of church-based support on positive religious coping responses: emotional support from fellow church members, spiritual support from fellow church members, and emotional support from the pastor. The data suggest that more spiritual support from fellow church members was strongly associated with greater use of positive religious coping responses, whereas the influence of emotional support from a member of the clergy was fairly minimal, and emotional support from fellow church members failed to exert a statistically significant effect.

The discussion provided up to this point suggests that greater insight into the religious coping process may be found by looking for potentially important causal relationships among religious coping items. So far, this argument has been illustrated by showing that even though some investigators consider church-based social support to be a coping response, it may be a source of other, more specific religious coping responses as well. However, relatively little has been said about the specific coping responses that significant others might encourage an older person to adopt. Although there is not sufficient space to explore a full range of coping responses, three are especially important and are considered below: prayer, forgiveness, and feeling grateful toward God. It should be emphasized at the outset that there is an extensive literature on each of these constructs. However, a good deal of this work is not grounded explicitly in the stress process. So, for example, Poloma and Gallup (1991) wrote an entire volume on prayer, but they say relatively little about its potential stress-buffering properties. Consequently, no effort is made here to discuss in detail all the research that has been done on prayer, forgiveness, and gratitude. Instead, the intent is to focus on linking each facet of religion with stress and church-based social support. Those interested in exploring the wider literature on these constructs may wish to read the detailed overview of prayer by Brown (1994); the in-depth examination of forgiveness by McCullough, Pargament, and Thoresen (2000); and the extensive review of research on gratitude by Emmons and McCullough (2004).

Prayer as a Coping Response

A number of prominent theologians and classical theorists have maintained that prayer lies at the very heart of religion. For example, Martin Luther argued that faith is "prayer and nothing but prayer" (as reported by Heiler 1932, xiii). Similarly, William James maintained that prayer is "the very soul and essence of religion" (James 1902/1997, 486). Describing prayer as "religion in action," James believed that prayer is the arena in which the real work of religion is done (James 1902/1997, 486). Recent studies on the frequency of prayer are consistent with these classic views because this work suggests that prayer is the most common form of religious practice. More specifically, Gallup and Lindsay (1999) report that over 90 percent of American adults pray, and 74 percent report they pray daily. Significantly, older people appear to pray more often than younger adults (Barna 2002). Given the central role played by prayer in religious life, it is not surprising to find that a number of investigators have attempted to see if more frequent prayer is associated with better physical and mental health. Extensive reviews of this research suggest that this is the case (Levin 1996a; McCullough & Larson 1999).

A key issue that has yet to be determined conclusively involves how the potential health-restoring and health-enhancing effects of prayer arise. One possibility is that prayer helps people cope more effectively with stress. However, surprisingly few studies have directly evaluated the potential stress-buffering properties of prayer. One of the few studies in this area examined the relationship between stress and prayer from a different perspective. Instead of seeing whether prayer for oneself during times of stress was a factor, Krause (2003c) assessed whether praying for others reduced the effects of stress. The findings from this study suggest that the deleterious effects of financial strain on physical health status are reduced significantly for older people who pray for others.

Despite the paucity of research on the stress-buffering properties of prayer, religious coping inventories typically list prayer as a religious coping response. For example, the RCOPE index (Pargament et al. 2000) contains numerous references to prayer. One item in this inventory asks respondents who have been faced by a stressor if they prayed for a miracle, whereas another asks if they prayed to find a new reason to live. But why some people decide to pray when stressors arise and others do not is not entirely clear, nor is it clear where beliefs about prayer and the content or text of a prayer originate. There are two ways to address these issues: the first comes from a general sociological perspective, whereas the second involves empirical data that speak more directly to the social underpinnings of prayer.

Prayer, like any other form of human behavior, arises in a social context. The underlying social nature of all human behavior is perhaps best expressed by Berger and Pullberg (1965) in their discussion of how the social world is created: "*men together* engage in constructing the world, which then becomes their dwelling. Indeed, since sociality is a necessary element of human being, the process of world production is necessarily a social one" (Berger & Pullberg 1965, 201, emphasis in original). They went on to argue that efforts to develop definitions of social reality are not a one time effort. Instead, "The world must be confirmed and re-confirmed *by others*" (Berger & Pullberg 1965, 201, emphasis in original). Cast within the context of the current chapter, views on the value of prayer and beliefs about where, when, and how to pray are social products that are jointly constructed during social interaction. Moreover, once beliefs and practices involving prayer have been set in place, they are maintained and reinforced by further interaction with significant others. This is consistent with the views of Tillich (1987), who noted that "the act of faith, like every other act in man's spiritual life, is dependent on language and therefore the community" (27). But the social influences on prayer are perhaps nowhere more evident than in formal prayer groups that tend to thrive in religious settings (Wuthnow 1994). The explicit purpose of these groups is to provide a place where people encourage and motivate each other to pray and discuss a range of issues related to prayer. It is not hard to see how the social principles described by Berger and Pullberg (1965) would be at work in this context. More about formal prayer groups in the church is discussed in chapter 4.

Empirical evidence of the informal social underpinnings of prayer was provided in an unpublished set of analyses from the RAH Survey (Krause 2002a). The purpose of these longitudinal analyses was to see whether formal as well as informal social relationships in the church influence change in the frequency of private prayer over time. More specifically, the analyses evaluated the impact of the following indicators of church-based social ties on prayer: attendance at worship services, attendance at Bible study groups, attendance at prayer groups, and informal spiritual support from fellow church members. The impact of a range of demographic control variables was taken into consideration as well. An examination of bivariate correlations coefficients revealed that each of the church-based social relationship measures was significantly associated with prayer. But when they were evaluated with multivariate procedures (i.e., a multiple regression model), the data suggest that only two exerted a statistically significant effect. More specifically, the findings indicate that more frequent attendance at worship services (Beta = .118; $p < .005$) and more frequent informal spiritual support from fellow church members (Beta = .116; $p < .005$) are associated with more frequent private prayer over time.

Forgiveness and the Process of Coping

Virtually all checklists of stressful life events contain a number of stressors that deal with interpersonal difficulties. For example, the widely used scale devised by Holmes and Rahe (1967), the Social Readjustment Rating Scale, lists marital separation and divorce, as well as trouble with in-laws and trouble with the boss, as stressful events. Although older people may grapple with interpersonal difficulties in a number of ways, one strategy lies at the very heart of religion: forgiveness. Forgiveness figures prominently in the Christian tradition. The basic tenets of the faith encourage people to repent and seek forgiveness from God (Brown 1997). Moreover, a central message in the New Testament involves the importance of forgiving other people for the things they have done (Rye et al. 2000). As the literature on forgiveness continues to evolve, researchers have assessed forgiveness from a number of different perspectives, including forgiveness of others, forgiveness of self, and the belief that one has been forgiven by God. However, the greatest amount of attention in the literature has been devoted to forgiving others. Enright, Freedman, and Rique (1998) define forgiveness of others as "a willingness to abandon one's right to resentment, negative judgment, and indifferent behavior toward one who has unjustly injured us, while fostering the undeserved qualities of compassion, generosity, and even love toward him or her" (46–47). Given the close conceptual link between interpersonal stress and forgiveness, it is not surprising to find that religious coping indices often contain forgiveness as a coping response. For example, the RCOPE (Pargament et al. 2000), asks participants who have been faced with a stressor if they sought God's help in trying to forgive others and whether they asked God to help them be more forgiving.

A number of studies have been conducted to see if forgiving others is associated with psychological well-being. For example, Maltby, Macaskill, and Day (2001) report that people who are able to forgive others are less likely to experience symptoms of psychological distress than individuals who are unable or unwilling to forgive. Further support for the potentially beneficial effects of forgiving others is found in studies done by clinical psychologists. They have devised a number of psychotherapeutic programs designed explicitly to enhance a person's ability to forgive others, and it appears that adopting these coping techniques is associated with greater psychological well-being (Worthington, Mazzeo, & Canter 2005).

Many researchers who study forgiveness and well-being merely ask respondents if they forgive others. However, as research by Krause and Ellison (2003) reveals, the benefits of forgiving others may arise only under certain circumstances. Consistent with previous studies, their work reveals that older adults who forgive others tend to report greater life satisfaction, fewer symptoms of depression, and less death anxiety than older people who do not forgive others; but the findings from this study further indicate that how older people go about forgiving others is important. More specifically, the results suggest that older adults who require transgressors to perform acts of contrition (e.g., apologize, promise not to repeat the offense, and make restitution whenever possible) experience more psychological distress than older people who forgive unconditionally and do not require transgressors to perform acts of contrition in order to be forgiven. This study further reveals that forgiveness by God may be involved in this process because older people who feel they are forgiven by God for the things that they have done are less likely to expect transgressors to perform acts of contrition. Important causal linkages may thus exist among the different types of forgiveness as well.

Researchers have yet to explore fully the factors that promote forgiveness, but some evidence is present that significant others play a role in this process. If forgiveness is a core tenet in the Christian faith, and significant others at church informally encourage the adoption of religious principles, then greater spiritual support should be associated with more frequent forgiveness of others. Unpublished data from the RAH Survey is consistent with this view. Controlling for the effects of the frequency of church attendance and private prayer, as well as a number of demographic variables, these analyses suggest that older people who report receiving more spiritual support from their fellow church members also indicate they are more likely to forgive others for the things they have done (Beta = .106; $p < .001$).

The Stress-Buffering Function of Gratitude

Gratitude refers to feelings of thankfulness toward a specific person or entity for the benefits that individual or entity has provided (Peterson & Seligman 2004). Recently, as Emmons and McCullough (2004) point out, researchers are showing increasing interest in studying feelings of gratitude toward God, which are not typically contained in inventories of religious coping responses. However, as the discussion provided below reveals, there are theoretical and empirical grounds for thinking about gratitude toward God as a religious coping response. Moreover, exploring the nature of gratitude toward God provides yet another way to illustrate how church-based social support may help older people deal more effectively with the deleterious effects of stress.

Research on feelings of gratitude toward God is important for two reasons. First, as a study by Emmons and McCullough (2003) reveals, people who are grateful tend to experience fewer symptoms of physical illness than individuals who are not grateful. Second, feelings of gratitude are cultivated by all the major religions in the world (Emmons & Crumpler 2000). If gratitude is associated with better health, and religion promotes feelings of gratitude, then delving more deeply into the study of gratitude may help explain how the potentially health-related benefits of religion arise. Emmons and Crumpler (2000) suggest one way to approach this complex issue: specifically, they argue that gratitude may help people cope more effectively with the deleterious effects of stress. However, very few empirical studies have been conducted to explore this issue. One of the few to do so, conducted by Krause (2006c), is helpful because it explains how feelings of gratitude toward God may reduce the pernicious effects of stress and provides the results of a preliminary test of this emerging theoretical perspective. After examining these issues here, an effort is made to trace the social underpinnings of feelings of gratitude toward God.

Secular research on finding growth in the face of adversity serves as a good point of departure for showing how feelings of gratitude toward God may benefit older people who are confronted by stressful experiences. As Tedeschi and Calhoun (2004) maintain, "The evidence is overwhelming that individuals faced with a wide variety of difficult circumstances experience significant changes in their lives that they view as highly positive" (223). The notion that stress serves a beneficial function in life is hardly new. Epictetus was a Stoic who lived in the first century ce. Although he never committed his philosophical insights to writing, one of his students recorded the following quotation that speaks directly to growing in the face of adversity: "It is the critical moment that shows the man. So when the crisis is upon you, remember that God, like a trainer of wrestlers, has matched you with a rough and stalwart antagonist—'To what end' you ask. That you may prove the victor in the Great Games. Yet without toil and sweat this may not be!" (Plato & Eliot 1909, 173). Writing centuries later, in 1851, the influential German philosopher Schopenhauer expressed essentially the same view when he argued, "One can even say that we *require* at all times a certain quantity of care or sorrow or want, as a ship requires ballast, in order to keep on a straight course" (1851/2004, 43, emphasis in original).

McMillen (1999) discusses a number of the benefits that arise from adversity. He points out, for example, that when people are faced with adversity, they either gain new coping skills or they realize they possess coping skills they did not know they had. In addition, stressors often trigger self-examination, leading people to channel their lives in more positive directions. Life events also help people develop a deeper appreciation for their social network members, especially when they have been a source of support during difficult times. Finally, McMillen (1999) points out that even the most severe types of adversity may help people develop a sense of meaning in life. The last two points made by McMillen are important because they begin to lay the groundwork for showing how significant others replenish a sense of meaning in life that has been challenged by stressful experiences.

The discussions provided by McMillen (1999), as well as Tedeschi and

Calhoun (2004), are helpful, but their viewpoints were developed out-side the context of religion. Instead, these investigators are concerned with the almost limitless ways in which growth may take place in sec-ular settings. But stress may help people grow in more religious or spir-itual ways as well. Therefore, it is important to explore growth in the face of adversity specifically as it arises within a religious context. For-tunately, theologians and religious scholars have been discussing this issue for centuries. The work of two individuals is especially helpful in this respect. The first is Moses Maimonides, whom some regard as one of the greatest Jewish theologians of all time. In 1190 he wrote a fasci-nating volume, *The Guide for the Perplexed,* that speaks directly to the issue of religious or spiritual growth through adversity: "The sole object of all the trials mentioned in Scripture is to teach man what he ought to do or believe; so that the event which forms the trial is not the end desired; it is but an example for our instruction and guidance" (Mai-monides 1190/2004, 514). Josiah Royce (1912/2001) provides a more recent discussion of growth in the face of adversity within the context of religion. Royce firmly believed that instead of trying to eliminate or avoid stressful experiences, people should embrace them because stress is necessary for religious growth. More specifically, he argued that evil and suffering are "true sources of [religious] insight. They reveal to us some of the deepest truths about what loyalty, and spiritual triumph, and good really are. They make for salvation. They drive away the clouds and bring us face to face with the will of the world" (Royce 1912/2001, 237).

The observations made of Maimonides (1190/2004) and Royce (1912/2001) are well founded because the Old and New Testaments of the Christian Bible contain numerous stories of people who were faced with significant adversity but emerged from it better off than they were before the stressor was encountered. In fact, as Koenig (1994) points out, one of the core messages in the Christian faith involves trusting that God has a purpose and plan for one's life, and that even though this plan involves exposure to difficult experiences and adversity, it is nec-essary for greater spiritual and personal development. If people believe that the problems they face are part of God's plan to strengthen them and help them grow, then they are likely to feel grateful to God when adversity arises and they begin to see the benefits that arise from it. Fur-ther, if these feelings of gratitude toward God are deeply and sincerely felt, then the deleterious effects of stress are likely to be offset.

But it is still not entirely clear how feeling grateful to God in the face of adversity may lead to better health. When people are confronted by adverse situations, they often experience a flood of negative emotions. One way that gratitude may buffer stress is by offsetting these negative emotions with positive feelings. In fact, as Emmons and McCullough (2003) point out, feelings of gratitude tend to promote a sense of contentment, happiness, pride, and hope. These emotions are important, because research reviewed by Ryff and Singer (1998) suggests that positive emotions have a direct and beneficial physiological effect on the body by bolstering immune functioning (see also Marques & Sternberg 2007). Moreover, as research by McCarty and Childre (2004) reveals, feelings of appreciation and gratitude may have especially beneficial cardiovascular effects because they tend to lower a person's blood pressure and heart rate.

Krause (2006c) recently conducted the first study to examine whether feelings of gratitude toward God help older people deal more effectively with the pernicious effects of stress. The findings from this study suggest that the noxious effects of one particular type of stressor (i.e., living in a rundown neighborhood) on health are reduced for older people who feel more grateful to God.

If feelings of gratitude toward God are an efficacious coping response, then it is important to reflect on how they arise. Consistent with the overall theme of this chapter, the support provided by fellow church members may have something to do with it. The intellectual roots of this perspective go back at least to the seminal work of Simmel (1898/1997). In the following quotation from his work, Simmel (1898/1997) first underscores the social basis of religion, then grounds emotions that are remarkably close to gratitude in this social foundation:

> The individual feels himself bound to a universal, to something higher, from which he came and into which he will return, from which he differs and to which he is nonetheless identical. All these emotions, which meet as in a focal point in the idea of God, can be traced back to the relationship the individual sustains with the species.... Thus the humility with which the pious person acknowledges that all that he is and has comes from God, recognizes in Him the source of his existence and strength, is properly traced to the relationship of the individual to the whole. (115–116)

Unfortunately, contemporary researchers have yet to follow up on the insights provided by Simmel (1898/1997) and empirically evaluate the social underpinnings of gratitude toward God. Nevertheless, the theoretical insights that have been developed in the current chapter provide a useful point of departure for addressing both issues. Viewed broadly, the following specific linkages can be derived from this framework: (1) Older people who encounter adversity turn to their fellow church members for assistance; (2) significant others at church provide help by encouraging them to look for growth in the midst of adversity; (3) finding growth in difficult times fosters a sense of gratitude toward God; and (4) older adults who feel gratitude toward God are more likely to enjoy better physical and mental health. By linking growth through adversity and gratitude toward God, it is possible to derive testable hypotheses that clearly spell out one way in which the potentially important stress-buffering properties of church-based social support operate.

Less Familiar Dimensions of Church-Based Social Support

The discussion so far has focused primarily on the emotional and spiritual support of fellow church members. An emphasis was placed on these specific types of assistance perhaps because more empirical work has been done with them and because it is easier to identify the theoretical role they play in the stress process. But as the information contained in Table 2-1 reveals, support may be exchanged at church in several other ways. Although reviewing all of the remaining dimensions of church-based social support is not possible here, focusing on two may help deepen our understanding of the role that religion plays in the stress process: anticipated support from fellow church members and the provision of informal support to others at church.

Anticipated Support

As defined earlier, anticipated support is the belief that others will provide assistance in the future if it is needed. Wethington and Kessler (1986) show why this type of support may be especially useful during stressful times. These investigators point out that when a stressor arises, people do not always turn immediately to significant others for assistance. Instead, they often try to resolve their problems on their own. Trying to solve problems without the intervention of others serves three important functions. First, it helps people avoid the ego-related costs associated with having to disclose and discuss one's problems with others. Second, it helps older people avoid becoming overly dependent upon social network members. Third, it helps avoid burnout among significant others that can arise from repeated requests for assistance.

Even though an older person may put off seeking support from significant others at church, fellow church members may nevertheless exert an influence on the coping process. As Wethington and Kessler (1986) point out, the realization that significant others stand ready to help if the need arises constitutes a social safety net that promotes risk taking and encourages older adults to resolve problems on their own. Older people will be willing to try new solutions to problems if they know they can count on social network members to set things straight should these new solutions fall short. Being able to work out problems and meet needs without the direct intervention of others is important because the skills that are gained through these self-initiated actions are likely to enhance an older person's sense of self-worth as well as his or her feelings of personal control.

But other benefits are associated with anticipated support also. More specifically, the belief that others stand ready to assist may foster the perception that even though difficult times are at hand, there is a chance that things will improve in the future. In this way, the social safety net afforded by anticipated support from fellow church members promotes a sense of hope and a more optimistic view of the future, which is important, because some evidence exists that individuals can endure adversity as long as they have hope and they believe things will eventually turn around (Nunn 1996). Perhaps this is one reason why Peterson and his colleagues found that people who are optimistic tend to live longer than individuals who are pessimistic (Peterson, Seligman, & Vaillant 1988).

There is good reason to believe that a sense of anticipated support may be stronger in religious settings than in the secular world. As noted earlier, the Christian church strongly advocates helping people who are in need and providing assistance in a nonjudgmental way. Knowing that significant others at church share these basic beliefs may help older people feel more confident that support will be forthcoming if it is needed.

Providing Support to Others

Older people often give as well as receive support from their fellow church members (Krause 2006d). This is not surprising, because the importance of helping others has been advocated in the Christian faith since its inception and has been discussed by prominent theologians for hundreds of years. For example, writing in 1536, John Calvin argued that "all the endowments which we possess are divine deposits entrusted to us for the very purpose of being distributed for the good of our neighbor" (as quoted in Thornton & Varenne 2006, 86). Since then, scholars from many different disciplines have reiterated, elaborated, and extended the notion that people should help each other. For example, Albert Schweitzer (1933/1990), the well-known philanthropist and Nobel laureate, argued that, "One can save one's life as a human being... if one seizes every opportunity, however unassuming, to act humanly toward those who need another human being" (90–91). In fact, Schweitzer (1933/1990) believed that the success and worth of entire civilizations depends upon this virtue. More specifically, he maintained that great and successful civilizations emerge only when the will toward material progress is matched with an equally strong will toward ethical progress. But the precise nature of ethical progress is difficult to pinpoint and define. Schweitzer (1933/1990) clarified this elusive notion by defining an ethical society in terms that highlight the importance of helping others. He illustrated this through the notion of what he called the "Reverence for Life," which "comprehends within itself everything that can be described as love, devotion, and compassion in suffering, the sharing of joy and common endeavors" (158). He went on to elaborate on the notion of Reverence for Life in his widely read two-volume treatise, *The Philosophy of Civilization* (1949).

Although it is the subject of some debate, Koltko-Rivera (2006) presents evidence that shortly before his death, Abraham Maslow, the highly acclaimed former president of the American Psychological Association, posited that helping others is part of a new motivational state—self-transcendence—that sits atop his hierarchy of needs. Based on a thorough reading of Maslow's private diaries, Koltko-Rivera (2006) concluded that individuals with a strong motivation toward self-transcendence "seek a benefit beyond the purely personal and seek communion with the transcendent, perhaps through mystical or transpersonal experiences; they come to identify with something greater than the purely individual self, often engaging in service to others" (306). The strong quasi-religious underpinnings of this motivation to help others (i.e., mystical experiences) are especially noteworthy in this passage.

Researchers in the contemporary social and behavioral sciences have begun to examine empirically the process of helping people who are faced with difficult times, and have discovered that helping others may provide somewhat surprising and unanticipated benefits. More specifically, a small, but intriguing, cluster of studies done primarily in secular settings indicate that helping others may benefit the support provider as well as the support recipient (Krause, Herzog, & Baker 1992; Midlarsky 1991).

The notion that people may benefit from helping others is hardly new. In fact, the roots of this perspective are thousands of years old. For example, Lao-tzu wrote the seminal work on Taoism sometime during the fourth century BCE. In this brief volume, Lao-tzu (400 BCE/1988) argued that helping others is essential for the help-provider's own happiness and well-being:

> The Master has no possessions.
> The more he does for others,
> the happier he is.
> The more he gives to others,
> the wealthier he is. (81)

The notion that helping others benefits the help-giver was also evident centuries later in a classic poem by Alexander Pope (*An Essay on Man*, 1731/1965). Some consider this poem to be one of the most succinct statements about the essence of human nature that has ever been written (Brady 1965). Four lines in this poem speak directly to the benefits arising from the help-giving process:

> Heav'n forming each on other to depend,
> A master, or a servant, or a friend,
> Bids each on other for assistance call,
> Till one Man's weakness grows the strength of all. (Pope 1731/1965, 26)

Three main points about the process of helping others emerge from these lines. First, people are by their very nature dependent upon others. Second, as a result, people cannot live without both giving and receiving support. Third, in the process of helping others, support providers become stronger themselves.

Thus, the insights of theologians, physicians, philosophers, poets, and social scientists suggest, benefits accrue to those who help others. However, the precise ways in which these benefits are manifest are not entirely clear in their writings. Fortunately, Reissman (1965) addressed this issue some time ago. He identified three ways in which support providers benefit from helping others. The principles discussed by Reissman (1965) are important because they speak directly to the deficits created by stressful experiences that were discussed earlier in this chapter. First, Reissman (1965) argues that helping other people enhances the self-esteem of the support provider. Providing assistance to those who are less fortunate or those who are in need makes a clear and unambiguous statement about the support provider because it highlights basic aspects of his or her character that are admired widely in American culture, especially in religious settings. This is an important consideration because renewed evidence of one's own self-worth may come at a time when a support provider's self-esteem has been diminished by a stressful experience. Second, Reissman (1965) maintains that seeing support recipients overcome problems with assistance they have been given tends to make support providers believe they may be able to resolve their own difficulties with the help of significant others as well. In this way, helping others may increase a support provider's own feelings of personal control. Third, Reissman (1965) points out that assisting people who are in need provides a psychological sense of respite from the support provider's own difficulties: it shifts the focus of attention away from the self and the problems with which a support provider may be wrestling. This benefit is noteworthy because being able temporarily to escape one's own problems may have salubrious effects on health and well-being, especially when a stressor does not dissipate quickly (Gottlieb 1997).

Although the principles identified by Reissman (1965) were meant to apply to people of all ages, there is some evidence that older adults may be especially likely to profit from helping others. Some time ago, Rosow (1976) described aging as a "roleless role." Baltes and Smith (1999) picked up and expanded this theme, writing that "relatively speaking, old age is young; therefore neither biological nor cultural evolution has had sufficient opportunity to evolve a full and optimizing scaffolding (architecture) for the later phases of life" (158). Embedded in these perspectives is the notion that as people enter late life, they encounter a social and psychological vacuum, and as a result, they must find ways to profitably invest their energy and efforts so they may continue to enjoy the benefits and security associated with occupying a meaningful place in the social order. Perhaps this is one reason for Rowe and Kahn (1998) reporting that giving support to others is a more important factor in successful aging than receiving assistance from social network members. If helping others is a major avenue for leading a productive life and for being tightly integrated into society, then the benefits of being involved in the help-giving process should be especially important for older adults.

Although Reissman (1965) conducted his research in a secular setting, there is reason to believe that the benefits of helping others may be particularly evident among people who are more deeply involved in religion. In order to see why this may be so, it is important to delve more deeply into the process of helping others. At the most basic level, one person cannot provide effective assistance to another without first understanding the situation of the individual who is in need. Otherwise, the support they provide may be either inappropriate or, at best, ineffective. Although a number of factors may come into play, there is some evidence that help-giving is more effective when support providers view the circumstances of the support recipient with empathy and compassion. In fact, this approach to helping formed the cornerstone of Carl Rogers's outlook on psychotherapy. Based on years of clinical experience, he concluded that effective help-giving in the therapeutic setting is contingent upon the empathy, caring, and compassion of the therapist (Rogers 1986). These virtues are important because, as Wuthnow (1991) points out, they lie at the heart of biblical teachings. More specifically, Wuthnow (1991) observes, "The biblical tradition teaches compassion as a duty to divine law, as a response to divine love, and as a sign of commitment to the Judeo-Christian ethic" (50). If empathy and compassion are essential for effective help-giving, and these virtues are strongly supported by religious teachings, then the health-related benefits of helping others should be especially evident among those who are more deeply involved in religion.

A study by Krause (2006d) offers recent evidence that helping others benefits support providers. The purpose of this study was to see if support provided to and received from fellow church members offsets the deleterious effects of financial strain on mortality. The findings indicate that ongoing economic problems increase an older person's odds of dying. However, the data further reveal that providing emotional support to fellow church members reduces the effects of the support provider's own financial problems on mortality. In contrast, the results also suggest that receiving support from people at church did not have the same stress-buffering effect.

Bringing Different Kinds of Stressors to the Foreground

Although a considerable effort has been made in this chapter to discuss different kinds of church-based social support and how they offset the noxious effects of stress, stress has been treated in a fairly generic way. However, problems arise when stress is viewed in a general way because doing so overlooks the fact that researchers have known for decades about several different kinds of stressful experiences. Recognizing the different kinds of stressors is important because it raises the possibility that church-based social support may be more helpful in dealing with some kinds of stress than others. After identifying and exploring the interface between different kinds of stress and church-based social support, an effort is made here to examine one type of stress that is unique to the study of religion: religious doubt.

Over the course of the past fifty years or so, researchers who have studied stress in secular settings have identified at least four different types of stressful experiences. Unfortunately, there are no widely agreed-upon definitions for these stressors. Moreover, an examination of how these stressors are measured reveals significant overlap among them. No effort is made here to resolve these long-standing difficulties. Instead, the intent is to identify the stressors and develop loose boundaries between them so a case can be made for the notion that church-based social support may be more likely to buffer the effects of some kinds of stress than others.

The first type of stress identified in the literature is typically called "stressful life events" (Turner & Wheaton 1995). These events are thought to have a clear beginning and endpoint. For example, an older person may move from one neighborhood to another. Although the process of moving may be stressful, it has a relatively clear beginning and end. Based on the way stressful events have been measured in the literature, it appears that most investigators believe that stressors arising roughly in the past year to eighteen months are the most consequential for health and well-being (Turner & Wheaton 1995).

The second type of stressor that emerged in the literature is "daily hassles" (Kanner, Coyne, Schaefer, & Lazarus 1981). Daily hassles are thought to be relatively minor events that often emerge and dissipate in the same day. Getting caught in a traffic jam or receiving a speeding ticket are good examples of daily hassles.

The third kind of stressor goes by different names, but is often referred to as "chronic strains" (Pearlin et al. 1981). As opposed to stressful events and daily hassles, chronic strains are thought to be continuous and ongoing. So, for example, some older people may encounter ongoing financial problems that never dissipate and that remain a source of significant difficulty for the rest of their lives. Some investigators who study chronic strains maintain that the effects of this type of stressor are more pernicious than the effects of either stressful life events or daily hassles (Lepore 1995).

The final type of stressor is sometimes referred to as "lifetime trauma." As Wheaton (1994) points out, traumatic events are "spectacular, horrifying, and just deeply disturbing experiences" (90). Included among traumatic events are sexual and physical abuse, witnessing violence, the premature loss of a parent, and participation in combat. Traumas are distinguished from the other types of stressors by their imputed seriousness; their impact is thought to be far worse than the impact of stressful events, daily hassles, or chronic strain. In fact, traumatic life events are thought to differ from other kinds of stressors because the effects of traumatic events may last for an entire lifetime (Wheaton 1994). Support for this contention came from a study by Krause, Shaw, and Cairney (2004). Their research reveals that traumatic events arising between the ages of eighteen and thirty appear to have a more adverse effect on the current health status of people aged sixty-five and over than traumatic events arising at any other point in the life course.

There do not appear to be any studies in the literature that systematically compare and contrast the stress-buffering properties of church-based social support across all four types of stressors discussed here. Research on this issue should be a high priority in the future. Even though little is known about this differential stress-buffering issue, Gottlieb (1997) provides some useful insights. He speculates that religion may be most useful for helping people cope with the effects of stressors that cannot be resolved and that do not dissipate. Gottlieb maintains that this happens, in part, because involvement in religion helps people accept what cannot be changed. After all, continued efforts to change something that cannot be altered may do little more than lead to further frustration. Instead, finding a religious explanation for the problem and a religious response to handling the fallout from it may help a person accept the situation and avoid additional pain and distress.

If Gottlieb's (1997) explanation is valid, then church-based social support may be more likely to help older people who are confronted by chronic strain and traumatic events because these stressors are less likely to be altered, and they are less likely to dissipate than stressful life events or daily hassles. This is especially true with respect to lifetime trauma, because these events may have taken place decades ago. The notion that religion may help people deal with stressors that are especially difficult to resolve may help explain why Krause (2006d) found that helping others at church offsets the effects of ongoing (i.e., chronic) financial strain on mortality and why his research also shows that gratitude buffers the effects of living in a rundown neighborhood (Krause 2006c). The insight provided by Gottlieb (1997) may also show why Mattlin and his colleagues found that religious coping responses were more effective for buffering the effects of death of a loved one than any other kind of stressful experience (Mattlin, Wethington, & Kessler 1990). After all, death is a final and irreversible event. Moreover, evidence suggests that the effects of bereavement may last longer than many researchers suspect. For example, a study by Wortman, Silver, and Kessler (1993) reveals that depressive symptoms arising from the death of a spouse were evident nearly two decades after the event occurred. This may be one reason why the sudden and unexpected death of a family member is listed by the American Psychiatric Association as a traumatic life event (American Psychiatric Association 1994).

Only one study apparently has explored whether religion helps people deal more effectively with lifetime trauma (Krause 2008). This research, based on data from the RAH study, reveals that prayer tends to reduce the deleterious effects of traumatic events on psychological distress in late life.

So far, the stressors that have been discussed could affect people who are not religious as well as those who are religious. However, other stressors are unique to religious individuals. One that has received some attention in the literature is religious doubt. Hunsberger and his colleagues define religious doubt as "a feeling of uncertainty toward, or questioning of, religious teachings and beliefs" (Hunsberger, McKenzie, Pratt, & Pancer 1993, 28). Hecht (2003) recently published a comprehensive volume on the history of doubt. In this fascinating book, she maintains that doubt is as old as religion itself, and having doubts about one's faith appear to be an inescapable part of leading a religious life. Evidence of the long history of religious doubt may be found, for example, in the play *Hippolytus*, written in 428 BCE by the famous Greek playwright Euripides (1960). In it, a chorus chants the following lines: "Verily, it is a great thing to believe in gods that care; it soothes the griefs of the believer. Though my secret heart hopes in an intelligent Providence, yet when I look at the fortunes of men and their actions, hope fails me" (Euripides 1960, 91).

Although religious doubt is a difficult and complex topic to tackle, viewing it as a stressful experience is justified. Years ago, Holmes and Rahe (1967) defined stress as occurrences that are likely to bring about significant readjustment in a person's usual activities. Religious doubt clearly fits this definition because it is a difficult and challenging experience that often requires a significant readjustment in thoughts, feelings, beliefs, and behaviors. If this challenge is not met successfully, it is capable of generating significant psychological distress (Krause, Ingersoll-Dayton, Ellison, & Wulff 1999; Krause 2003d; Krause 2006e), as well as physical health problems (Krause & Wulff 2004; but see Hunsberger,

Pratt, & Pancer 2002). In fact, Exline and Rose (2005) explicitly refer to such spiritual struggles as a significant strain. The deep sense of despair that is fostered by religious doubt was captured succinctly by Saint John of the Cross, who referred to wrestling with religious doubt as the "dark night of the soul" (Coe 2000).

Research reveals that religious doubt, like many other stressors, may not affect all people in the same way (Krause et al. 1999; Krause & Wulff 2004). Instead, some individuals have resources they can rely upon to help them cope more effectively with the noxious effects of religious doubt. Evidence of this may be found in longitudinal research by Krause (2006e) which suggests that greater religious doubt is associated with a diminished sense of life satisfaction, self-esteem, and optimism. However, the findings further indicate that older people with higher levels of educational attainment are less likely to suffer from the pernicious effects of religious doubt than older people who have fewer years of schooling. These findings may be explained by reflecting more deeply on the fundamental nature of religious doubt. When viewed in the simplest terms, religious doubt is a cognitive problem that arises because the world is filled with contradictory evidence and experiences (Hecht 2003). For example, some people may have a hard time believing in a loving and protecting God while at the same time recognizing that there is a great deal of pain, suffering, and injustice in the world (Krause et al. 1999). The resolution of these contradictions and inconsistencies therefore requires a certain amount of insight, reasoning, and other cognitive abilities. As Mirowsky and Ross (2003) point out, education provides precisely these traits. More specifically, they maintain that a good education develops a host of sound habits and skills, including

> inquiring, discussing, looking things up, and figuring things out. It develops analytic skills of broad use such as mathematics, logic, and, on a more basic level, observing, experimenting, summarizing, synthesizing, interpreting, classifying, and so on. Because education develops the ability to gather and interpret information and to solve problems on many levels, it increases control over events and outcomes in life. (26–27)

But it seems unlikely that older people will rely solely on their own cognitive abilities to resolve doubts they may have about their faith. Consistent with the resource mobilization perspective discussed earlier (Eckenrode & Wethington 1990), an older person who is confronted by religious doubt may reach out to a trusted other at church to help resolve the problem. Then, based on the principles discussed by Berger

and Pullberg (1965), both the older person and his or her trusted coreligionist may use their reasoning and cognitive abilities to arrive at a new,
jointly negotiated resolution of the problem. Put another way, spiritual
support may be an especially important resource for coping with the
effects of religious doubt.

Conceptual and Methodological Challenges

One of the major challenges facing those who work in the field
is to determine whether church-based social support provides unique
health-related benefits, or whether the benefits of support from fellow
church members is roughly comparable to assistance that people might
exchange in the secular world. There are two ways to approach this
problem.

The first involves identifying types of support that are not likely to
be found outside the context of religion. Krause's (2002a) measure of
spiritual support is a good example of a uniquely religious type of assistance. Spiritual support can then be compared with a type of assistance
that may be found inside and outside the church (e.g., emotional support from fellow church members). If spiritual support has a beneficial
effect on health whereas emotional support does not, then there would
be some evidence of something special about the unique type of assistance (i.e., spiritual support) found in religious settings, which is precisely what the study by Krause (2002c) reveals. His work shows that
spiritual support is related to the self-rated physical health status of older
adults, whereas emotional support from fellow church members fails to
exert a significant effect.

The second strategy was developed in a more recent paper by Krause
(2006b). As discussed earlier, the purpose of this study was to see if emotional support provided by fellow church members is more likely to offset the deleterious effect of financial strain on health than emotional
support received from people outside an older person's place of worship.
The data suggest that emotional support from fellow church members
buffers the pernicious effect of financial strain on health, but emotional
support from secular sources fails to have a significant effect.

Although Krause's two studies (2002c, 2006b) appear to suggest that
there may be something unique about church-based social support, a
subtle, but critical issue arises in the way the data for these studies were
obtained. The questions about church-based support ask study participants only about assistance they have received from the people in their
congregation. But even a moment's reflection reveals that religiously

motivated or religiously based support may be exchanged in other social settings as well. However, expanding the scope of inquiry beyond the congregation raises a host of tricky problems about the boundaries between church-based support and secular support. Three challenging conceptual problems involving this issue are as follows.

The first issue has to do with differentiating between support from fellow church members and assistance from family members who worship in the same congregation. Clearly family members help each other inside and outside of church. If a husband and his wife worship in the same congregation, and the wife provides emotional support to her husband, is the support she gives him religiously based or is it merely secular support? Must this assistance be given specifically within the church edifice in order for it to be religious support? What if she helps her husband at home? Is that religious or secular support? Initially, it might appear that simply asking study participants to make the distinction would suffice, but it is not clear if respondents consciously differentiate between the two. Moreover, different study participants may not use the same criteria or the same referents to distinguish between religious and secular support.

What if a deeply religious man provides emotional support to his neighbor who is an atheist? Is this religious or secular support? What if a devout Methodist exchanges emotional support with his neighbor, who is a devout Catholic? These examples point to fundamental challenges in the way religious support is defined. As these examples reveal, focusing on support that is exchanged solely within a single congregation may be inadequate because this measurement strategy may exclude religiously based assistance that is provided in the wider secular world.

The second problem with setting the boundaries of church-based support arises from living in a technologically sophisticated age. More specifically, when it becomes too difficult for older people to leave their homes to attend worship services, they often watch religious services on the television or listen to them on the radio (see Hayes, Landerman, Blazer, Koenig, Carroll, & Musick 1998, for a discussion of the "electronic church"). Sometimes these programs allow people to mail in or phone in their problems and concerns. The pastor, as well as the congregation, may then pray specifically for them. The pastor may also offer specific religious advice during the broadcast that is designed to help them deal with their problems. This approach may lead some older people to claim the congregation on television as their own and view the help they get over the airways as church-based emotional or church-based spiritual support.

The third problem in setting the boundaries of church-based support has to do with beliefs that some people have about God. Some individuals believe that God is right there with them physically each day, and they believe that God hears them and answers them directly. As a result, these older people feel that they have developed a deep personal relationship with God (Krause 2002a). If this is true, then, as Maton (1989) argues, is the assistance they believe they get from God a meaningful type of church-based support?

In addition to problems associated with determining the boundaries of church-based social support, another issue must be addressed in order to determine if social support in the church provides unique health-related benefits. Church-based social support is clearly assistance that arises in and is supported by an organization. Therefore, it is important to determine whether the effects of assistance received in church is more efficacious than help provided by members of organizations that are not associated with religion, such as the Rotary Club or the Elks Club. The subtle issue embedded in this proposition is whether the philosophy, structure, and activities of any formal organization promote better social ties or whether the explicit religious principles and religious activities found in the church foster social relationships that are more efficacious than those found in the wider secular world. This research question differs from the one investigated by Krause (2006b), because he compared the effects of church-based support with informal assistance that did not specifically arise within the context of a secular organization. Some investigators argue that studies should be done to compare and contrast support in the church with support in secular organizations (e.g., Kirkpatrick 2005), but no one to date appears to have examined this issue empirically. Doing so should be a high priority.

As the discussion of problems encountered in determining the potentially unique effects of church-based social support reveal, researchers must come to grips with some significant conceptual challenges. Perhaps the best way to tackle issues involving the boundaries of church-based social support is to conduct a detailed series of qualitative studies to see how respondents differentiate between church-based and secular social support. Finding out whether support received in the church differs from assistance provided in secular organizations must also be addressed, but the choice of secular organizations to use as a point of comparison must be done with great care, because all secular organizations do not place a similar emphasis on support-related issues, such as the importance of helping others.

Conclusions

The discussion of church-based social support provided in this chapter boldly underscored the social underpinnings of religion by showing how different types of assistance from fellow church members offset the psychosocial damage inflicted by stressful experiences. More specifically, a theoretical perspective was developed which suggests various ways in which informal assistance from rank-and-file church members helps replenish and maintain feelings of self-worth, personal control, and a sense of meaning in life that have been depleted by stress. In the process, an effort was made to integrate more tightly previously unrelated aspects of religion into the emerging theoretical framework. More specifically, an argument was developed that links the study of church-based support with research on religious coping responses. The intent was to show that one way significant others at church help older people deal with stress is by encouraging the use of religious coping responses. Empirical support was provided for some, but not all, of these insights. Clearly, a good deal of work remains to be done. Nevertheless, the current chapter provides a way to move the field forward by identifying explicit hypotheses that can be evaluated empirically as well as the measures that are necessary to do so.

Chapter 3

Church-Based Companion Friends

Although people at church often help each other when stressful events arise, the social relationships they develop and maintain involve much more than crisis management. Instead, a good deal (if not most) of the time spent with others is likely to take place outside the context of the stress process. One of the most important types of social ties that are formed in this respect is close companion friends (Cocking & Kennett 1998). Unfortunately, research on companion friends is in a state of disarray (Adams, Blieszner, & De Vries 2000). The terms "friendship" and "companionship" are used interchangeably; there is no agreed-upon definition of either term, and researchers have not reached a consensus on the key characteristics and functions of companion friends. No attempt will be made to resolve these long-standing problems here. Instead, the goal of this chapter is to identify key characteristics of close companion friends that are most likely to be found in the church and that are likely to have the greatest effect on the health and well-being of older church members.

The definition of companion friends provided by Rook (1987) provides a useful point of departure for getting into the field. She defines companionship as social relations that involve "shared leisure activities that are undertaken primarily for the intrinsic goal of enjoyment" (Rook 1987, 1133). Rook points out that companions provide the opportunity for self-disclosure, the discussion of personal aspirations, and the sharing of private jokes and stories. Although Rook's research makes a valuable contribution to the literature, there are three reasons why it does not fully inform our understanding of companion friendships that develop specifically within the church. First, Rook's (1987) work was done solely in secular settings, and as a result, the potentially unique functions of companion friends at church are largely unknown and unexamined. Second, a key element is missing from Rook's (1987) definition: the closeness of the relationship. As it stands, casual acquaintances may share leisure activities solely for the purpose of enjoyment. But, as the discussion provided later in this chapter reveals, it seems unlikely that casual acquaintances affect health and well-being to the same extent as close companion friends. Third, because the nature and content domain of close companion friends has not been explored fully, Rook's (1987) measures of this potentially important construct are underdeveloped.

The discussion provided in this chapter is divided into six main sections. First, an effort is made to delve more deeply into the precise nature and functions of close companion friends at church. This step is accomplished by focusing specifically on what companion friends do for each other and give to each other. Second, in order to illuminate more fully the nature of these potentially important social relationships, a discussion of the measurement of close companion friends is provided. New measures from the RAH Survey (Krause 2002a) are introduced at this point, and the psychometric properties of these indicators are evaluated. Third, the ways in which companions at church may influence the health and well-being of older adults are examined. Fourth, several reasons why close companion friends may be especially important in late life are provided. Fifth, new data from the RAH Survey (Krause 2002a) are presented that provide a preliminary assessment of the relationships between companion friends and a number of health-related outcomes. Finally, this chapter closes with a discussion of conceptual and methodological challenges in the study of close companion friends at church.

Identifying the Basic Nature of Close Companion Friends

Unfortunately, a good discussion of close companion friends at church is not available in the literature. Consequently, the discussion provided here begins by focusing on research that comes from a number of secular sources. However, once the basic elements of secular companion friendships have been identified, an effort is made to specify the relatively unique ways in which these relationships are manifest in the church.

Close Companion Friends in Secular Settings

Although a number of characteristics of companion friends have been identified in the literature (Ueno & Adams 2006), several core factors seem to cut across the discussions that have appeared in print so far. Four interrelated functions of companion friends that may be especially important are examined below.

First, companion friendships are characterized by a relatively high degree of self-disclosure that arises from a deep sense of trust (Patterson, Bettini, & Nussbaum 1993). This means, for example, that close companion friends tell each other things that they would not usually share with other individuals (Rook 1987). This issue was discussed by imminent French philosopher Michel de Montaigne. Some regard him as the quintessential skeptic (Hecht 2003), but Montaigne was hardly skeptical when it came to the subject of close friendships. Writing in the late 1500s, Montaigne discussed some of the core characteristics of close friendships. Trust and self-disclosure figured prominently in his view: "The secret I have sworn to reveal to no other man, I can impart without perjury to the one who is not another man: he is myself" (Montaigne 2003, 172). Clearly, this kind of intimate self-disclosure cannot take place without a high degree of openness, honesty, and truthfulness. The importance of truthfulness as a prerequisite for the development of close companion friendships was discussed by the famous essayist Ralph Waldo Emerson (1841/1983), who was an ordained minister. Emerson wrote, "There are two elements that go to the composition of friendship.... One is truth. A friend is a person with whom I may be sincere. Before him I think aloud" (347).

Second, as Cocking and Kennett (1998) argue, companion friends share things they value highly. For example, as Rook (1987) maintains, they share plans, hopes, dreams, and ambitions. And as the degree of intimacy grows between companion friends, they share private jokes and discuss private stories that arise from their mutual experiences (Rook 1987). But there is disagreement in the literature about the nature of the values and interests that companion friends share. Some investigators, like Rook (1987), argue that companion friends share common interests (see also Adams et al. 2000). However, other researchers, such as Cocking and Kennett (1998), maintain that the interests shared by companion friends do not necessarily have to be the same. Instead, what matters most is that companion friends share with each other what they value the most and that each person expresses interest in whatever his or her friend values highly. The notion that companion friends appreciate and develop what is unique in each other is stated succinctly by Emerson (1841/1983): "Let him not cease an instant to be himself. The only joy I have in his being mine, is that the not mine is mine. I hate, where I looked for a manly furtherance, or at least a manly resistance, to find a mush of concession. Better be a nettle in the side of your friend than his echo" (350).

Third, companion friends inspire each other, and they strive to emulate what they admire in their counterpart. As Sherman (1993) argues, "Each is inspired to develop himself more completely as he sees admirable qualities, not fully realized in himself, manifest in another whom he esteems. . . . Character friends, as extended yet different selves, are eminently suited as models to be emulated" (105–6).

The final core characteristic of companion friends is related to the previous one. It has to do with the self-development and personal growth that arise from emulating a close companion friend. Instead of merely providing the opportunity to emulate admirable qualities, companion friends actively encourage and spur the other on to greater self-awareness and greater personal growth. In essence, companion friends provide each other with a view of how they should be; they motivate each other to pursue an ideal self (Sherman 1993).

Church-Based Close Companion Friends

A key issue involves determining whether close companion friends at church differ in any appreciable way from close companion friends in the secular world. There is reason to believe they may. More specifically, close companion friendships may be more likely to arise in religious settings, and they may function more effectively when they emerge within the social environment of the church. In addition, the nature of the ideal self that is fostered by church-based companion friends may be relatively unique.

Recall that close companion friendships are characterized by a high degree of openness, trust, and honesty. Unfortunately, researchers have known for some time that people are often defensive, they deliberately withhold information, and they may even manipulate situations in an effort to create a more favorable impression of themselves (Goffman 1959). However, fundamental aspects of the social milieu in the church may help overcome this sort of defensive behavior. Thomas Oden (1969), a noted theologian, shows why this may be so. He wrote, "It is only amid a community of genuine acceptance where unconditional forgiveness is mediated that persons find the freedom to put down their self-righteous defenses and freely enter into a responsible covenant with their neighbors" (117).

Writing over a century ago, Ross (1896) further illuminated how religious institutions foster especially close companion friendships. He maintained, "To have the same gods, to be watched, loved, and protected by the same deities, to be destined to join the same unforeseen company at death—these created fellowship" (Ross 1896, 437). His choice of words is important because the *New American Webster Dictionary* (1982) defines "fellowship" as "companionship." Ross (1896) went on to argue that companions at church become so close that they assume the qualities of close family members: "conviction of our fundamental identity in nature and destiny... [is]... the modern counterpart of the old blood bond" (441).

The views of Oden (1969) and Ross (1896) are consistent with more recent research on the homophily principle (McPherson, Smith-Lovin, & Cook 2001). According to this perspective, similarity promotes greater interpersonal connectivity. Consequently, it is not surprising to find that McPherson et al. explicitly discuss religious settings in the process of garnering support for their homophily principle. Similarity between fellow church members arises from at least two sources. The first involves shared beliefs, such as those mentioned by Oden (1969). But in contrast, the other is more general in nature. Researchers have argued for decades that congregations are often quite homogeneous with respect to race (Bartkowski & Matthews 2005) as well as socioeconomic status (SES) (Davidson & Pyle 2005). This point is important because, as McPherson and his colleagues point out, social relationships in groups that are homogeneous with respect to race and SES tend to be more tightly knit (McPherson et al. 2001).

As discussed earlier, Sherman (1993) argued that companion friends encourage each other to pursue and attain an ideal self, but she failed to provide a clear sense of the precise nature of the ideal self that arises from these relationships. Sherman was concerned with companion friends in the secular world, and as a result, the type of ideal self that may be encouraged in this context is virtually limitless; but this may not necessarily be true when it comes to close companion friends in the church. Religious teachings and principles often specify how an ideal person should feel, think, and act. Because these religious precepts and values are shared by fellow congregants, they are likely to encourage each other to pursue and adopt them. Viewed in this way, close companion friendships in the church may be seen as an important vehicle in the search for, and attainment of, a particular type of ideal self—the religious self. Striving to attain an ideal religious self is likely to be quite important for older churchgoers because research indicates that 74 percent of elderly people believe their religious faith is very important in daily life (Barna 2002).

During the past decade, a number of researchers have relied on rational choice theory to make significant inroads in the study of various facets of religious life (e.g., Iannaccone 1995). Rational choice theory is concerned with how individuals make decisions about how to practice their faith, including whether to switch to another congregation, how often to attend religious services or participate in other formal church activities, and how much money they should contribute to their congregation. According to adherents of this theoretical perspective, people approach these issues rationally by carefully weighing the costs and benefits of different options, and ultimately selecting the action that maximizes their net benefit. However, as Ellison (1995) points out, proponents of rational choice theory often overlook the influence other people may exert on the decisions made by an individual. Although Ellison (1995) provides many valuable insights in his discussion of social underpinnings of rational choice theory, the particular individuals in church who are likely to hold the greatest sway over the religious choices that are made by rank-and-file congregants are not identified clearly. One way to remedy this situation is to think in terms of the different kinds of social relationships that are found within the church. Although a case could be made for demonstrating how any number of different church-based social ties may play a role in this respect (e.g., formal relationships with the clergy), it seems that close companion friends at church may be especially influential. More specifically, the sense of trust, openness, and mutual respect that forms the bedrock of close companion friendships is likely to be a necessary prerequisite for sharing the deeply personal issues that often emerge around questions of how to practice one's faith.

With data provided by older adults, McFadden, Knepple, and Armstrong (2003) have conducted what appears to be the only study that compares close friendships that develop in church with close friendships that are forged in the wider secular world. Contrary to the rationale provided above, they find little evidence that friendships arising in these two settings differ appreciably. More specifically, they fail to find that older people receive more emotional support from close friends at church nor are they more likely to feel more comfortable sharing emotions with close friends at church than with close friends who are not fellow church members. However, as these investigators note, their sample contained a disproportionately greater number of older women than is found in the general population. More specifically, 77 percent of the participants in their study were older women. This is problematic because, as research discussed in chapter 6 reveals, older women are more likely than older men to be more deeply involved in social relationships that arise in the church and the secular world (Antonucci 2001). In addition, the sample obtained by McFadden et al. (2003) consisted of ninety-three older people who attend three congregations in two midwestern cities, making it difficult to determine if the results can be generalized to the typical older church member. Nevertheless, a high priority should be placed on determining whether relationships that are formed with church-based social companion friends are more efficacious than ties with secular companion friends.

Measuring Close Companion Friendships at Church

Identifying the key characteristics of close companion friends at church is an important first step, but in order to conduct high-quality empirical research in this field, good measures of the core facets of this construct must also be in place. There have been a number of attempts to derive closed-ended survey measures of friendships in secular settings (Ueno & Adams 2006). Unfortunately, as Ueno and Adams (2006) point out, these indices sometimes merge social support with other functions that are performed by companion friends. As discussed below, this measurement strategy blurs the distinction between social support and companion friends, thereby creating problems for those who wish to study the relatively unique aspects of companion friendships in the church. Because measures of friendships have been developed primarily within secular settings, no attempt is made to review them here. Instead, the measurement strategy employed by Rook (1987) will be used as a point of departure for discussing how to assess close companion friendships in the church.

Rook's (1987) initial research on companions was based on the secondary analysis of several different surveys. As a result, companionship is measured in different ways in her paper. In one set of analysis, companionship is operationalized by counting the number of leisure activities that are shared with others. Included among these activities are going to someone's home for a meal, or going with someone to a restaurant, movie, or park. In a more recent paper, Sorkin, Rook, and Lu (2002) measure companionship with two indicators. The first assesses whether respondents know someone they could visit, chat with over the phone, or laugh and have fun with, whereas the second is a count of the number of people who have actually provided these types of companionship activities.

Rook's (1987) research is noteworthy because she focuses on behavioral indicators of companionship. However, there are two problems with the measurement strategy she employs. First, as discussed earlier, it is difficult to know, for example, whether the person with whom someone shared a meal was a casual acquaintance or whether this individual was a close companion friend. Second, behavioral indicators assess whether social contact was made with a potential companion, but they reveal little about what transpired when this interaction took place. For example, just because an individual went to the home of another for a meal, it does not necessarily follow that he or she necessarily had a pleasant time. If we want to understand how companionship affects health and well-being in late life, then it is important not to rely solely on measures of social contact. Instead, researchers must also measure what companion friends actually do for each other. The problems that arise from ignoring the specific functions of companion friends make it difficult to define the boundaries of this key construct. For example, Rook (1987) argues that companionship does not involve assistance that is intended to help a significant other deal with adversity. She correctly points out that social support performs this important stress-buffering function. Yet Rook (1987) provides empirical data showing that both companions and social support offset the deleterious effects of minor stressful events. This makes it difficult to distinguish between the two types of social relationships, thereby obfuscating their relatively unique characteristics and functions.

New measures of close companion friendships in the church were developed recently by Krause for the third wave of the RAH Survey. The items in this index are provided in Table 3-1. This scale was designed to capture the core elements of companion friendships discussed in the previous sections. As shown in Table 3-1, the indicators in this scale were designed to be administered in a two-step process. First, an item was devised to see if an older person has a close companion at church. Second, older study participants who said they had a close companion friend at church were asked a series of questions that assess the nature and functions of this relationship. Included among these items are questions about how often there is frequent self-disclosure with this trusted other, how often the older study participants share things they value highly with their companion friend, how often they pursue common interests, whether their companion friend has characteristics they try to emulate, and whether the relationship with their close companion friend has led to greater self-awareness and personal growth.

Because the church-based companion friendship items in Table 3-1 have not appeared before in the literature, a number of technical issues involving the factor structure and psychometric properties of this scale are reported below in an effort to encourage further use of these measures by other investigators. An exploratory factor analysis was conducted with the thirteen items in the new companionship scale. Three distinct factors emerged from this work. The initial insights provided by this work were extended by conducting a confirmatory factor analysis of the church-based companionship indicators. The confirmatory factor analysis was performed with Version 8.71 of the LISREL statistical software program (du Toit & du Toit 2001).

The three factors that emerged from the data are consistent with the way church-based companion friendships have been discussed in the current chapter. The three factors and the indicators that assess them are provided in Table 3-2. The first factor reveals whether older study participants feel they can share secrets, hopes, and interests with their companion friend (i.e., intimacy). The second reflects whether the older adults in the RAH Survey feel they can be open and honest with their companion friend, and whether they feel their companion friend understands them (i.e., openness). The third factor assesses whether church-based companion friends change the way older study participants view themselves and their worlds (i.e., self-enhancement).

Based on the initial findings from the exploratory factor analysis, two indicators were excluded from the confirmatory factor model. The first ("How often does [name of companion] express interest in your opinions even if they are different from his/her own?") was eliminated because the factor loadings of this indicator on all three factors were roughly the same. The second ("How often do you look forward to spending time with [name of companion]?") was dropped from the confirmatory factor model because it did not appear to cover the same content domain as the other indicators that loaded on the same underlying factor (i.e., the intimacy factor).

The standardized factor loadings and measurement error terms that were derived from the confirmatory factor analysis are also provided in

Table 3-1. Measures of Church-Based Companion Friendships

1. Not counting your minister, pastor, or priest, is there someone in your congregation you feel especially close to—someone who is a good friend and valued companion?[a]

2. Now I'd like to ask you to think about your very good friend or valued companion when you answer the following questions.[b]
   A. How often do you share your plans, hopes, and dreams with (NAME OF COMPANION)?
   B. How often do you share private jokes or private stories with (NAME OF COMPANION)?
   C. How often do you tell things to (NAME OF COMPANION) that you wouldn't share with other people?
   D. How often do you discuss common interests with (NAME OF COMPANION)?
   E. How often do you feel like you can be yourself around (NAME OF COMPANION) without having to worry about what he/she might think?
   F. How often do you feel you can be completely honest and open with (NAME OF COMPANION)?
   G. How often does (NAME OF COMPANION) express interest in your opinions and views even if they are different from his/her own?
   H. How often do you feel like (NAME OF COMPANION) really understands you?
   I. How often do you think you would like to be more like (NAME OF COMPANION)?
   J. How often do you feel like (NAME OF COMPANION) has changed the way you feel about yourself?
   K. How often do you feel that (NAME OF COMPANION) has helped you learn more about yourself?
   L. How often do you feel like (NAME OF COMPANION) has changed the way you view the world?
   M. How often do you look forward to spending time with (NAME OF COMPANION)?

[a] This variable is scored in the following manner (coding in parentheses): yes (1), no (0).
[b] These variables are scored in the following manner: very often (4), fairly often (3), once in a while (2), never (1).

Table 3-2. Before turning to a discussion of the underlying meaning of the factors, it is important to examine the fit of the model to the data. The findings reveal that the fit of the model to the data is acceptable. More specifically, the Bentler-Bonett Normed Fit Index (NFI, Bentler & Bonett 1980) estimate of .955 is above the recommended minimum cut-point of .900. Similarly, Bollen's (1989) Incremental Fit Index (IFI) value

Table 3-2. Confirmatory Factor Analysis of Close Companions Friendship
Functions (N = 332)

Item	Intimacy	Openness	Self-Enhancement	Measurement Error Term
Share plans[a]	.747[b]			.442
Share jokes	.652			.575
Tell things	.690			.524
Discuss interests	.720			.481
Be yourself		.764		.416
Be honest		.814		.337
Understands you		.674		.546
Be more like			.578	.666
Feel about yourself			.826	.317
Learn more about			.816	.334
Changed worldview			.824	.321

[a] Item paraphrased for purposes of identification. See Table 3-1 for the complete item text.
[b] Factor loading from the completely standardized solution. All factor loadings and
measurement error terms are significant at the .001 level. The first-listed item in each factor was
fixed at 1.0 in order to set the scale of the factor.

of .969 is reasonably close to the ideal target value of 1.0. Finally, as Kelloway (1998) points out, values of the root mean square error of approximation (RMSEA) that fall below 0.10 indicate a good fit of the model to the data, whereas values below 0.05 reveal a very good fit to the data. The RMSEA value of .082 for the confirmatory factor model reported in Table 3-2 lies between the two cutpoints, suggesting that the fit is acceptable.

The factor loadings and measurement error terms reported in Table 3-2 are important because they provide preliminary information about the reliability of the newly devised church-based companionship measures. Although there are no firm guidelines in the literature, Kline (2005) recommends that factor loadings in excess of .600 tend to have reasonable reliability. As shown in Table 3-2, only one standardized factor loading falls just short of this target (.578). However, it should be emphasized that the value of .600 recommended by Kline (2005) is a rule of thumb and is not based on rigorous simulation studies. Moreover, the difference between .587 and .600 is trivial.

Although the factor loadings and measurement error terms associated with the observed indicators provide useful information about the reliability of each item, it would be helpful to know something about the reliability of each factor or sub-scale taken as a whole. Fortunately, it is possible to compute these estimates with a formula provided by DeShon (1998). This procedure is based on the factor loadings and measurement error terms in Table 3-2. Although it is not discussed often in the literature, there is a problem with the way reliability estimates are typically reported. As Vacha-Haagse, Kogan, Tani, and Woodall (2001) point out, the reliability of an instrument cannot be assessed directly. Instead, data from a sample of study participants are used to obtain estimates of reliability. However, because these data come from a sample, and not an entire population, reliability estimates fluctuate from sample to sample. Consequently, it is important to derive confidence intervals for reliability estimates so researchers may get a better sense of where the true population-based reliability coefficients are likely to fall. Fortunately, 95 percent confidence intervals (C.I.) for reliability estimates can be obtained by following the procedures discussed by Raykov (1998).

Applying the procedures described by DeShon (1998) and Raykov (1998) to the church-based companionship data yields the following reliability estimates and confidence intervals for the three factors that are embedded in this scale: intimacy (reliability = .796; lower C.I. = .756; upper C.I. = .829), openness (reliability = .796; lower C.I. = .755; upper C.I. = .832), and self-enhancement (reliability = .850; lower C.I. = .820; upper C.I. = .874). As these estimates reveal, the reliability of the church-based companionship sub-scales is acceptable.

The correlations among the underlying church-based companionship factors are important because they provide evidence of the multidimensional nature of this complex construct and the relative independence of the factors that compose it. More specifically, the correlation between the intimacy and openness factors is .664 (the LISREL software program does not provide tests of statistical significance for these bivariate estimates), the correlation between the intimacy and self-enhancement factors is .617, and the correlation between the underlying openness and self-enhancement concepts is .233.

As shown in Table 3-1, a screening question was used to identify older people who had a close companion friend at church. If he or she indicated they had such a friend, then the items in the remainder of the table were administered to find out more about the nature of this relationship. Analysis of the responses to the screening question revealed that 61.8 percent of the older participants in the RAH Study reported having a close companion friend in the church where they worship. This figure is important because it reveals that many, but by no means all, older people have a close friendship with a fellow church member.

The fact that all older study participants do not have a close companion friend at church raises a host of questions about who has and who has not been able to develop this type of relationship. Even so, as the discussion in the following section reveals, older people who have had the good fortune to develop a close companion friend at church may enjoy better health and have a more enhanced sense of well-being than older adults who do not have a companion friend where they worship.

Linking Close Companion Friendships with Health and Well-Being

As Mendes de Leon (2005) observed recently, the mechanisms that link secular friendships with health remain poorly understood. The same is certainly true with respect to church-based companion friends. Even so, there are a number of ways in which having close companions at church may influence the health and well-being of older people. Undoubtedly, close companion friendships may influence health through a number of the mechanisms that were discussed in the chapter on church-based social support (see chap. 2). For example, companion friends at church are quite likely to bolster the self-esteem of an older person, and a reasonable argument could be developed to show that close companion friends at church help older adults find a deeper sense of religious meaning in life. This may be especially true with respect to two dimensions of meaning that have been identified in secular studies: developing goals and plans (Krause 2004a). But these overlapping intervening mechanisms are not discussed in the current chapter so an emphasis may be placed on the potentially unique benefits that arise from having close companion friends at church.

Consistent with this goal, six unique intervening pathways that may link church-based companion friends with health and well-being are examined in the discussion that follows:

1. Companion friends may help promote a sense of belonging.
2. Companion friends may encourage the adoption of positive health behaviors.
3. Self-disclosure among close companions may provide health-related benefits.
4. Further beneficial effects on health may arise from self-expressiveness among companion friends.
5. The sense of trust that arises between close companion friends may also enhance health and well-being.

6. Having a close companion may discourage excessive self-preoccu-
    pation (i.e., self-absorption), which may be an especially important
    issue in late life.

Reviewing these health-related benefits of church-based companion
friends gives new meaning to Emerson's (1841\1983) observation that
friendship is a masterpiece of nature.

When coupled with the relevant intervening mechanisms discussed
in chapter 2, it is evident that there are a number of potentially important ways in which close companion friends at church may influence
health and well-being in late life. Unfortunately, empirical assessments
of church-based companions and health, as well as the factors that link
the two, have yet to appear in the literature. As a result, some of the
pathways linking companion friends with health may ultimately prove
to be invalid. In the end, this question is empirical. But when a field is as
underdeveloped as the study of church-based close companion friends,
then a necessary first step involves identifying all the possible ways that
make the most sense from a theoretical point of view. Doing so serves as
a blueprint for moving the field forward, which is precisely the intent of
the discussion that follows.

Belonging

One important benefit of having a close companion friend at
church arises from the fact that this relationship may make an older person feel that he or she belongs in his or her place of worship. The construct of belonging has a long history in the social and behavioral sciences, but not enough has been said about it in the context of religion.
Over half a century ago, Maslow (1954) identified belonging as one of
the most basic human needs. Given the central role of belonging in life,
it is not surprising to find that some investigators, such as Baumeister
(1991), argue that one of the most important functions of religion is to
help people find a sense of belonging.

Although it appears logical to argue that having a close companion
friend at church fosters a sense of belonging in a congregation, the essential nature and meaning of belonging presents a challenge for those who
wish to examine it empirically. As Carrier (1965) points out, belonging involves much more than a stated religious preference or religious
affiliation (e.g., "I am a Catholic"). Instead, it is an attitude, a psychological reality, that encompasses a set of positive emotions and cognitions that arise from playing a meaningful role in a group. More specif-

ically, Carrier (1965) argues that when a person believes that he or she belongs in a church, "The member sees himself taking part in his group; he identifies himself with it, he participates in it, he receives his motivation from it; in a word, he is in a state of disposition of interaction with the group which understands, inspires, and welcomes him" (58). Carrier's (1965) choice of words is important; by pointing out that people at church understand, inspire, and welcome each other, Carrier is, in essence, touching on some of the key characteristics of companion friends.

Unfortunately, there is confusion in the literature about how to measure a sense of belonging in a congregation. This problem arises because researchers seem unsure about how to cast belonging in the wider context of social relationships. And until this issue is resolved, investigators may be overlooking an important way to explain the relationship between church-based companion friends and health. More specifically, some researchers, such as Fiala, Bjorck, and Gorsuch (2002), maintain that belonging is a dimension of church-based social support, and is therefore synonymous with it. As a result these investigators embed measures of belonging in their index of church-based social support. Sorkin, Rook, and Lu (2002) also equate companionship with a sense of belonging in the secular literature. But belonging arises from and is produced by church-based companion friendships, and as a result, it is not part of the conceptual domain of companionship per se. Instead, it reflects something that companion friends promote.

In order to see why this may be so, it is helpful to turn to a study by Krause and Wulff (2005). These investigators argue that if a sense of belonging can arise from factors other than informal relationships in the church, then belonging cannot be part of the content domain of church-based social ties. Krause and Wulff (2005) provide empirical support for this point by focusing on attendance at worship services. More specifically, they argue that regular attendance at church services may also bolster a person's sense of belonging in a congregation. When an individual attends worship services, he or she is exposed to a number of basic tenets of the faith. Messages embedded in group prayer, sermons, hymns, and rituals (e.g., communion) continually remind them that they are part of a larger family that is bound together by a shared faith. Data provided by Krause and Wulff (2005) reveal that the frequency of church attendance exerts a positive effect on a sense of belonging above and beyond the impact of informal relationships with fellow church members.

Unfortunately, the measure of social ties in the church that Krause and Wulff (2005) used did not focus specifically on companionship. Instead, these investigators assessed emotional support and negative interaction with fellow church members. As a result, this study does not directly evaluate the notion that church-based companion friends specifically bolster a sense of belonging. Fortunately, support for this link is found in a recent study by Winseman (2005). His research reveals that 84 percent of study participants who report they have a best friend at church are also more likely to feel they belong in their congregation.

Although companions in church may contribute to an older person's sense of belonging in a congregation, it is important to show that belonging is, in turn, associated with health. Krause and Wulff (2005) provide what appears to be the first study in the literature to examine this relationship. Data provided by a nationwide survey of religiously diverse congregations reveals that individuals who feel they belong in their congregation tend to be more satisfied with their health than people who do not feel they belong in the place where they worship. It should be emphasized, however, that this study included adults of all ages. Consequently, the relationship between church-based companionship, belonging, and health specifically in late life remains largely unexamined in the literature.

Health Behaviors

A growing number of studies suggest that people who are more involved in religion tend to have better health because they are more likely to engage in positive health behaviors (e.g., maintaining a good diet) while avoiding negative or undesirable health behaviors (e.g., alcohol abuse) (Hill, Burdette, Ellison, & Musick 2006). This is important because an extensive literature suggests that adopting positive health behaviors lowers the risk of developing a wide range of illnesses and may even reduce the odds of dying as well (U.S. Department of Health and Human Services, 1992).

A good deal of the research on religion and health behavior focuses on the use of alcohol. A fairly large number of these studies suggest that greater involvement in religion is associated with either the moderate use of alcohol or the avoidance of alcoholic beverages altogether (e.g., Herd 1996). But the influence of religious involvement extends to other health behaviors also. For example, research by Idler and Kasl (1997) indicates that older adults who attend worship services more frequently have a lower probability of having ever used tobacco. However, one study on religion and health behavior stands out above the rest. This research was conducted by Hill et al. (2006). These investigators examined the relationship between the frequency of church attendance and twelve health behaviors. Their findings reveal that regular attendance at worship services (especially weekly church attendance) is significantly associated with eleven of the twelve health behaviors they examined. Included among these health behaviors was the avoidance of tobacco, the moderate use of alcohol, engaging in strenuous exercise, seat belt use, vitamin use, the utilization of preventive health-care services (e.g., physical and dental examinations), sleeping well, and walking.

As Hill et al. (2006) point out, many religions adhere to the notion that "the body is the temple of God." As a result, various religious groups advocate the use of certain types of health behavior while discouraging the practice of others (Sabate 2004). For example, the Seventh-Day Adventists strongly encourage the pursuit of sound dietary practices, while Southern Baptists strictly prohibit the use of alcohol. But it is not entirely evident how these religious teachings and beliefs are transmitted to rank-and-file church members. Undoubtedly, a number of mechanisms are involved (see Krause 2006f, for a discussion of several mechanisms), but the purpose of the discussion in this section is to argue that close companion friends at church may have something to do with it. Simply put, religious rules and teachings regarding health behaviors may be transmitted and reinforced through informal social interaction with like-minded companion friends. It is important to reflect on precisely how this takes place.

Some insight into the role that companion friends may play in the adoption of beneficial health behavior may be found in an intriguing paper by Rook (1990). She turned to the notion of social control to explain the relationship between social ties and health behavior. Social control is defined simply as interaction with significant others that involves influence and regulation (Lewis & Rook 1999). As Rook (1990) points out, the roots of this social control perspective go back to the work of Durkheim (1897/1951), who maintained that close social relationships involve enduring responsibilities and obligations, and that these responsibilities and obligations are thought to influence health behaviors. When people feel bound to others, they are more likely to engage in better self-care, and they are more likely to avoid self-destructive behavior because doing so may create health problems that limit their ability to fulfill their obligations. But Rook (1990) takes this a step further by suggesting that other, more overt influences may be at work as well. More specifically, she maintains that significant others may take steps to prompt or persuade an individual to adopt health-enhancing behavior and discourage them from engaging in behaviors that compromise health. This more overt influence may even take the form of threats and negative sanctions.

But it is not entirely clear from Rook's (1990) discussion whether anyone who is acquainted with an individual can exercise health-related social control or whether this function arises only in certain kinds of relationships. It seems likely that casual acquaintances may feel uncomfortable trying to exert this kind of influence, and if they did, it is even more likely that an older person would resist and even resent their efforts to do so. Instead, a person who is closely associated with an elder, one he or she can trust, is in the best position to exert this kind of influence. Simply put, close companion friends may be more likely to regulate health behavior overtly because this type of relationship possesses the intimacy and trust that are necessary for the exercise of effective social control. In fact, the high degree of contact and intimacy among close companion friends helps ensure that they will know which health behaviors an older person is practicing in the first place.

But it is still not entirely evident why efforts to influence the health behavior of older adults would be especially likely to come from close companion friends at church. There are two ways to address this issue. The first reason may best be found by using research on religion and alcohol use as an example. Earlier, based on the work of Herd (1996), it was noted that some denominations have strong prohibitions against the use of alcohol. For members of these congregations, avoiding alcohol is therefore a basic religious precept (i.e., a fundamental religious truth). If friendships are built on truth, as Emerson (1841/1983) maintains, then it follows that close companion friends at church should be especially likely to provide the impetus for reinforcing religious truths that form the cornerstone of their shared faith.

The second reason that close companion friends at church may be more likely to influence the health behavior of an older fellow congregant may be found in studies on controlling health behaviors that have been conducted in secular settings. For example, research done in secular settings by Tucker and Mueller (2000) suggests that a spouse is likely to resent efforts to influence his or her health behaviors if he or she believes that the partner has ulterior motives for doing so, such as the desire to control or manipulate. It seems that questionable motives such as these are less likely to arise in the church when both companion friends share a common faith that underscores the virtues of selfless helping. Nevertheless, the work of Tucker and Mueller (2000) and others helps signal the fact that attempting to control the health behavior of another is a delicate process. Consequently, researchers wishing to study the influence of companion friends in church on health behavior would be well advised to pay careful attention to the conditions under which such efforts are likely to succeed and when they may be likely to fail.

Self-Disclosure

Self-disclosure is defined as revealing information about oneself to another individual (Collins & Miller 1994). The importance of self-disclosure was underscored some time ago by Cooley (1902/2003), who maintained, "Everyone, in proportion to his natural vigor, necessarily strives to communicate to others that part of his life which he is trying to unfold in himself. It is a matter of self-preservation, because without expression thought cannot live" (94). But self-disclosure is risky because revealing too much about oneself may make a person feel vulnerable. Further, depending upon the nature of the relationship with the recipient, self-disclosure may not always be appropriate. Perhaps for this reason Cooley (1902/2003) saw companions as playing an especially important role in this respect. More specifically, he argued that a person "needs to express himself, and a companion enables him to do so" (Cooley 1902/2003, 85).

As Aron (2003) observed, research on self-disclosure is one of the oldest topics in the study of social relationships. One of the first discussions of self-disclosure was provided in 1959 by Jourard. He argued, "It is through self-disclosure that an individual reveals himself to the other party just exactly who, what, and where is he. Just as thermometers, sphygmomanometers, etc. disclose information about the real state of the body, self-disclosure reveals the real nature of the soul of the self....You cannot love your spouse, your child, or your friend unless he has permitted you to know him and to know what he needs to move toward greater health and well-being" (505). Then, in the same seminal paper, Jourard made what was at the time a rather bold assertion: "I believe in the effort to avoid becoming known a person provides himself a cancerous kind of stress which is subtle and unrecognized but nonetheless effective in producing not only...assorted patterns of unhealthy personality...but also... [a] wide array of physical ills" (502–4).

Since the publication of Jourard's (1959) paper, a number of studies have appeared that examine the relationship between self-disclosure, health, and well-being. This research has been conducted in at least two different ways. First, some investigators focus specifically on the value of self-disclosure in psychotherapeutic sessions (e.g., Pennebaker 1995). In contrast, other researchers study self-disclosure in the wider arena of informal social interaction. The concern in the current chapter is with the second body of work. These studies reveal, for example, that greater self-concealment is associated with more symptoms of physical as well as psychological illness (Larson & Chastain 1990). A number of studies also link self-disclosure with hypertension and heart disease. For example, research by Tardy (2000) reveals that high self-disclosure subjects had lower blood pressure while resting or talking about a variety of topics than low self-disclosure study participants.

Everyone wants to be understood, and everyone wants to share the things that happen in their lives with others. Moreover, the opportunity to share plans, hopes, dreams, and ambitions with a close trusted other generates a flood of positive emotions. This is important because research reveals that the positive emotions that arise from interacting with close others can have a direct and beneficial effect on the body through mechanisms like enhanced immune functioning (Koenig & Cohen 2002a; see also Ryff & Singer 1998).

Self-Expression

In the last book he wrote (*Life and the Student,* 1927), Cooley boldly asserted that he had identified the most essential element in life: "I can only say that I have found self-expression to be in fact, as it is in principle, the heart of life" (1927, 47–48). In using the term "self-expression," Cooley (1927) did not mean the ability to convey thoughts and feelings in an articulate manner. Instead, he was referring to the expression of talents and abilities. Little attention has been given to self-expression in the gerontological literature. Some investigators have focused on creativity in late life (see Sternberg & Lubart 2001, for a review of this research), but the notion of creativity is used in a precise and rather narrow way in this research. More specifically, creativity is viewed as the ability to produce high-quality work that is novel (Sternberg & Lubart 2001). Although talent is clearly involved in the creative process, the notion of creativity is more circumscribed than self-expression because creativity involves products that are innovative and valued highly by members of society. Perhaps this is one reason that studies of creativity often involve highly trained professionals, such as scholars, scientists, and artists (e.g., Reed 2005). As a result, creativity may not be something that is accessible to everyone.

In contrast, self-expression is something that a wider circle of older people can enjoy. The definitive characteristic is that individuals have found an outlet for whatever level of talent they possess, regardless of whether the exercise of these abilities results in something that is novel or of high quality. Instead, people pursue activities that engage their talents because of the innate pleasure they provide, as well as the sense of satisfaction and purpose these activities promote. Even though some people may possess relatively modest talents, they may, nevertheless, experience significant satisfaction in exercising them.

As discussed earlier in this chapter, sharing interests and hobbies is a hallmark of close companion friendships (Rook 1987). This suggests that companion friends help bring out the best in each other by encouraging the expression of talents and abilities. This may, in turn, enhance their sense of psychological well-being. Ultimately, the process of utilizing and cultivating talents helps people discover things that are relatively unique about themselves, and expressing this uniqueness provides the basis for demonstrating their individuality to others. In essence, exploiting talents and abilities represents one way of discovering and constructing a positive sense of self. This is important because, as discussed in chapter 2, a vast number of studies suggest that those who have a well-developed sense of self tend to enjoy significant mental health benefits (e.g., Ryff & Singer 1998). Further evidence of the ways in which self-expression may enhance mental health may be found in the work of Bettencourt and Sheldon (2001). These investigators conducted five studies to examine the interface between self-expression and psychological well-being. Their data suggest that greater self-expressiveness is associated with a more positive affect, greater life satisfaction, and diminished negative affect scores.

There appears to be only one study in the literature that examines the interface between self-expressiveness and well-being specifically among older adults. This study, conducted by Krause (2008), reveals that greater self-expression is associated with fewer symptoms of depression in late life. However, this study was done in a secular setting, and the influence of social relationships was not taken into consideration. As a result, it is not possible to tell if self-expressiveness that is fostered by church-based companion friends has a more beneficial effect on health and well-being than self-expressiveness that is promoted by friends, neighbors, and family members who are not part of an older person's congregation. Examining this issue should be a high priority in future research on church-based social ties in late life.

Trust

Unfortunately, there is considerable debate in the literature over the nature and meaning of trust. In fact, as Das and Teng (2004) point out, "Trust is one of the more frequently used and yet least understood of the significant concepts in the social sciences" (86). This is clearly not the place to resolve long-standing issues in the literature on trust. Instead, for the purposes of this chapter, trust will be defined as "the mutual confidence that one's vulnerability will not be exploited in an exchange" (Barney & Hansen 1994, 177).

As discussed earlier, one of the key characteristics of companion friendships is trust (Thomas, 1987). This sense of trust makes it possible for companion friends to share information about themselves that they would not be willing to reveal to others (Thomas 1987). As a sense of trust in a specific relationship grows, there is some evidence that it may be generalized to relationships with all people in general (Bierhoff 1992). This finding is noteworthy because it suggests that the reach of companion friendships may extend far beyond the immediate dyad, and the benefits that are gained through this relationship may nurture better relations with a wider circle of people as well.

But trust that arises between close companion friends may do much more than improve the nature of their relationship with each other; it may also have beneficial effects on their health. The relationship between trust and health was highlighted in a study by Barefoot, Maynard, Beckham, Brummett, Hooker, and Siegler (1998). The findings from this fourteen-year longitudinal study reveal that greater trust is associated with better physical functioning over time. But perhaps even more important, the data suggest that study participants with high levels of trust tended to live longer than study participants with low levels of trust.

Recently, Welch, Sikkink, Sartain, and Bond (2004) studied the ways in which trust is fostered in religious settings. They conclude that religion plays a major role in the development of trust in other people and that interpersonal ties in a congregation have a lot to do with it. But because there are many different kinds of relationships in congregations, it is not clear which types of social relationship perform this vitally important function. If the rationale provided in the current chapter is valid, then church-based companion friends may play a key role in this respect.

In the process of studying trust in religious settings, another intriguing finding emerged from the study by Welch et al. (2004) that is especially relevant for the current chapter. More specifically, its work re-veals that trust in other people increases with age. If close companion friends at church promote a sense of trust in other people, and trust increases with age, then the health-related benefits of trust should be especially evident in the close companion friends that older people maintain at church.

Self-Absorption

Entering into and maintaining a relationship with a close companion friend tends to draw older persons' focus away from the self. Instead of becoming preoccupied with their own concerns, their attention is focused on their companion friend and issues involved in their relationship with them. The benefits of being distracted from the self were recognized long ago by Adam Smith (1759/2002). He maintained, "In solitude we are apt to feel too strongly whatever relates to ourselves: we are apt to over-rate good offices we may have done, and the injuries we have suffered: we are apt to be too much elated by our own good, and too much dejected by our own bad fortune" (Smith 1759/2002, 178).

The notion of self-absorption is important because there is some evidence that excessive preoccupation with the self is associated with mental health problems. For example, Woodruff-Bordon, Brothers, and Lister (2001) report that greater self-absorption is associated with more depression, more anxiety, greater general psychopathology, and more difficulty in problem solving. In fact, a literature review by Ingram (1990) suggests that self-focused attention, a construct that is closely akin to self-absorption, is related to virtually all forms of psychopathology (but see Pyszczynski, Greenberg, Hamilton, & Nix 1991).

There are two reasons why it may be especially important to examine the relationships among companion friends, self-absorption, religion, and health in late life. First, religion plays an important role in shifting the focus away from the self. Evidence of this may be found in the famous study of American society by Tocqueville (1835/1960), who observed that there is no religion that "does not impose on man some duties towards his kind and thus draw him at times from the contemplation of himself" (23). Second, although self-absorption has not been studied extensively in social and behavioral gerontology, there is some evidence that it may increase with advancing age. More specifically, in summarizing her work on personality change in late life, Neugarten (1965/1996) reports, "Although there are important differences between men and women as they age, in both sexes the older individuals seemed to move toward more eccentric self-preoccupied positions" (258).

Close Companion Friends in Late Life

Although having a close companion friend is likely to benefit people of all ages, it may be especially important to have a close companion friend in late life. Evidence of this may be found in the work of two developmental theorists. The first is Carstensen (1992). According to her theory of socioemotional selectivity, as people go through late life, they become increasingly aware they have relatively little time left to live. This awareness promotes a reevaluation of their social relationships. As Carstensen points out, older people begin to place a greater emphasis on relationships that are emotionally close, while disengaging from more peripheral social ties.

Similar views may be found in Tornstam's (2005) theory of gerontranscendence. He maintains that as people enter late life, they experience a shift in their worldview. Instead of being preoccupied with material things and other worldly issues, they become increasingly concerned with the cosmic dimension, which involves wider existential concerns. But it is especially important to point out that Tornstam (2005) specifies that part of this shift involves changes in the way social relationships are viewed and maintained. More specifically, he argues that older people become more selective in the types of relationships they sustain and that they have a greater preference for deeper, more personal relationships with a smaller circle of individuals. Although neither Carstensen (1992) nor Tornstam (2005) specifically cast their work in the context of close companion friends, the similarity between their views of social ties in late life and close companion friends is striking because close companion friendships are the paragon of intimacy and closeness. It follows from this that if close companion friendships become more important with age, then the health-related benefits of maintaining this type of social tie should be especially evident among older people.

Close Companion Friends and Health: A Preliminary Empirical Examination

In order to further underscore the importance of the association between close companion friends at church and health-related outcomes, a series of preliminary analyses were conducted using data from the third wave of interviews with participants in the RAH Survey (Krause 2002a). Unfortunately, measures of all the intervening linkages identified in this chapter were not available in this data set. Nevertheless, indicators of several key constructs were included in the Wave 3 survey, making it possible to see if at least some of the linkages discussed above merit further consideration. The items shown in Table 3-1 make it possible to explore two sets of research questions. As noted earlier, the first set is concerned solely with the first item, which asks study participants whether they have a close companion friend in the place where they worship. The analyses involving this indicator focus on whether having a close companion friend at church, regardless of the precise nature of this relationship, is associated with select health-related outcomes. The second set of analyses use the remaining items, which were administered only to those who said they had a close companion friend at church. These indicators make it possible to see if the nature of the relationship and the degree of closeness among companion friends is a critical factor. This issue was investigated by summing the indicators used in the confirmatory factor analysis (see Table 3-2) to form a single composite measure that captures the nature and functioning of close companion friendships. Each set of analyses was conducted with the Wave 3 data only. Except where noted otherwise, the analyses were performed using ordinary least squares (OLS) multiple regression analysis. The analyses were performed after the effects of age, sex, education, marital status, race, the frequency of church attendance, and the frequency of private prayer were controlled statistically.

Does Having a Close Companion Friend Make a Difference?

Earlier, it was proposed that having a companion friend at church is more likely to make an older person feel that he or she belongs in a congregation. A simply binary variable was created that contrasts older study participants who have a close companion friend at church with those who do not maintain this kind of relationship with a fellow church member. A new index was created for the Wave 3 RAH Survey to assess belonging. The following indicators were part of this six-item index: "I feel like I really belong in my congregation," "I feel welcomed in my congregation," and "I feel I am accepted by the people in my congregation." Consistent with the theoretical rationale provided earlier, the data suggest that older people who have a close companion friend where they worship are more likely to feel they belong in their congregation than older adults who do not have a close companion friend at church (Beta = .147; $p < .001$).

The next analysis was designed to see if having a close companion friend is related to one specific type of health behavior: ever drinking alcohol. A simply binary outcome measure was created that contrasts older adults who ever drink with older people who say they never consume alcoholic beverages. Then, a logistic regression analysis was conducted to see if older people who do not consume alcohol are more likely to have a close companion friend in their congregation. The data failed to provide support for this hypothesis. More specifically, having a close companion friend was not significantly associated with ever drinking alcohol ($b = -.088$; ns).

The final analysis was designed to see if having a close companion friend at church is related to a core measure of psychological well-being in late life: life satisfaction (George 1981). Analysis with this outcome revealed that older people who have a close companion friend in their congregation do not tend to be more satisfied with their lives than older adults who do not have a close companion friend at church (Beta = .034; ns).

Taken as a whole, the findings presented in this section do not provide strong, consistent support for the notion that having a close companion friend at church is associated with select health-related outcomes. However, as the data in the next section reveal, a different picture emerges when the nature and function of close companion friends is taken into account.

Does the Nature of the Relationship Matter?

The second main set of analyses were designed to see if the nature and functions of close companion friendships at church are associated with the three outcomes examined in the previous section (i.e., belonging, ever consuming alcohol, and life satisfaction). Consistent with the theoretical rationale that was developed in this chapter, the data suggest that older people who are more deeply involved with a companion friend at church are more likely to feel they belong in their congregation than older people who are not as deeply involved with a companion friend in the place where they worship (Beta = .182; $p < .001$).

Consistent with the approach taken in the previous section, a logistic regression analysis was performed to see if the degree to which an older person is involved with a close companion friend at church is associated with whether they consume alcohol. Consistent with Rook's (1990) views on social control, the data suggest that older people who are more involved with a close companion friend at church are not as likely to have ever consumed alcohol as older adults who are not as involved with a close companion friend at church ($b = -.050$; $p < .01$; odds ratio = .951).

The third analysis had to do with assessing the relationship between involvement with a close companion friend at church and life satisfaction. The findings reveal that older people who are more deeply involved with a companion friend at church tend to be more satisfied with their lives than older adults who are less involved with companion friendships in the place where they worship (Beta = .132; $p < .05$).

When all the analyses involving close companion friends are taken together, the data suggest that merely knowing that an older person has a companion friend at church is not sufficient and that deeper insight into this key type of church-based social relationship may be found by exploring the nature and depth of involvement that an older person has with this close significant other. The difference between the two sets of analyses may arise from the fact that older study participants do not define close companion friendships in the same way; and in order to get a better perspective on health-related benefits of these social ties, it is important to move beyond assessing the presence of such a relationship to the measurement of what actually transpires in it.

In addition to providing evidence that closer involvement with companion friends at church is associated with health-related outcomes, the analyses provide preliminary evidence of the validity of the newly devised multiple-item church-based companionship measures. One widely used type of validity is called construct validity (Nunnally & Bernstein 1994). Construct validity is concerned about the extent to which a newly developed measure is related to different constructs in a theoretically meaningful way. Construct validity is never determined conclusively in a single study, and it can arise only over the course of repeated assessments in different samples. Nevertheless, the findings reported above provide at least some preliminary evidence that the measures of the nature and functioning of church-based companion friends that have been devised for the RAH Survey are valid as well as reliable.

Clearly, a good deal of research remains to be done on companion friends at church and health-related outcomes. There are at least two ways to move the field forward. First, only a limited range of outcomes were examined in this section. Research is needed on a range of physical and mental health outcomes. Second, as the confirmatory factor analysis in Table 3-2 reveals, the measure of the nature and functioning of close companion friends comprises three factors. Research is needed to see if the three factors exert a differential impact on health and well-being. This point is especially important given the relatively low correlation between the factor assessing self-enhancement and the factor that evaluates openness ($r = .233$).

Conceptual and Methodological Challenges

In the process of evaluating the issues discussed above, researchers must keep at least five methodological and conceptual challenges in mind as they pursue work on church-based companion friendships and health in late life. Each of these issues is examined briefly below.

Companion Friendships and Social Support

First, more studies are needed on the interface between close companion friendships and social support that is provided during stressful times. Depending upon the nature of the stressor that is present, an older person may be especially likely to turn to a companion friend for assistance because the trust and intimacy that have developed between them should greatly facilitate the sharing of information about the event and should provide an environment in which frank recommendations for the resolution of the problem can be offered. But when this happens, the conceptual boundaries between social support and companion friendships become harder to determine. Put another way, the correlation between measures of companion friendships and social support may be substantial. Moreover, as the theoretical perspectives devised by Carstensen (1992) and Tornstam (2005) suggest, this correlation may be especially large in studies of older adults because close companion friends are likely to constitute an increasingly larger part of an older person's social network. If the correlation between companion friends and social support is sufficiently large, researchers may encounter data analytic problems. Fortunately, it is possible to obtain some preliminary insight into the extent of this potential problem with the data from the RAH Survey. An analysis was conducted by estimating the correlations among having a close companion friend at church, the nature and functioning of close companion friendships, and emotional support from fellow church members. The results reveal that the bivariate correlation between having a close companion friend at church and emotional support from fellow church members is .283 ($p < .01$). In addition, the data suggest that the correlation between church-based emotional support and the nature and function of a close companion friend is (r = .359; $p < .01$). Although there is some overlap between these indicators, the size of this correlation suggests it is not prohibitively large. This conclusion may be brought into sharper focus by probing the second and larger of the two correlations (i.e., the correlation between church-based emotional support and the nature and functioning of close companion friends in a congregation). Squaring this correlation coefficient suggests that only 12.9 percent of the variance in these measures is shared variance, whereas the remainder (87.1 percent) reveals that these constructs are measuring something different (i.e., most of the variance is unique variance). Viewed more broadly, these preliminary analyses suggest that the correlation between companion friendships and emotional support from fellow church members is not too large, and the two types of relationships may therefore assess two distinct domains of church-based social relationships in late life.

But the analyses presented here should be viewed with caution because they do not provide a full evaluation of the relationship between church-based emotional support and companion friendships. Recall that the measure of church-based emotional support was designed to capture how often a respondent receives emotional assistance from *all* the members of his or her congregation taken as a whole (see Table 2-1), whereas the indicators that assess companion friendships in church refer to one specific individual. The difference in the focus of the measures of these two constructs may well produce some slippage in estimates of the correlation between them.

The best way to resolve conclusively the issue of measurement overlap between church-based social support and church-based companion friends is to turn to a social network analysis in which study participants are asked to name the specific person who provided the most emotional support to them during a recent stressful experience as well as the specific individual who is their close companion friend. If the same significant other is not identified in both instances, then it would be clear that measures of close companion friendships are not confounded with indicators of church-based emotional support. But if this proves to be the case, then additional research questions come to the foreground. More specifically, researchers need to learn more about why close companion friends are not key sources of emotional support during difficult times. Perhaps the nature of the stressor that confronts an older person may come into play here. More specifically, if an older adult is the architect of his or her own misfortune, he or she may be reluctant to bring the problem to a companion friend because of the possibility that this important significant other would think any less of him or her. In contrast, if research reveals that the same church member is both a close companion friend and a significant source of emotional support during stressful times, then researchers need to know how the characteristics of one type of social relationship influence the other. For example, does the degree of openness in close companion friendships facilitate full disclosure of problems and concerns that arise over a stressor, and does this full disclosure, in turn, lead to the delivery of more effective emotional assistance?

Moving beyond Companionship in Dyads

The second challenge involving the study of close companion friendships at church arises from the way this type of social relationship has been discussed in the current chapter. More specifically, companion friends were viewed primarily in terms of dyads, but there is no reason why companion friendships cannot involve more than two people. And if they do, then it is important to determine if the inclusion of three or more individuals changes the nature and functioning of companion friendships. For example, are secrets shared with everyone, or only one member of the group? And if secrets are not shared with everyone, does this differential self-disclosure produce variations in closeness among members of the group, and might it ultimately produce conflict among close companion friends over time?

Studying the Development of Close Companion Friendships

Third, research is needed to study how companion friendships are formed in the first place. Undoubtedly, a number of factors are likely to be involved. However, social skills are likely to be an important prerequisite for the formation of close companion friendships at church. As Krause (2006a) points out, social skills are interpersonal abilities that promote successful and beneficial relationships with others. Although a wide range of skills are clearly needed for successful social interaction, a key social skill involves the ability to take the role of other. As Cooley (1902/2003) put it, this involves the ability to enter into the mind of another sympathetically. In fact, Schlenker (2003) argues, "The ability to put oneself in the place of others and imagine how they are likely to interpret and respond to information is the basis for effective communication" (502–503). That is, in order to interact effectively with others and build strong relationships with them, an individual must be able to put themselves in the place of others, carefully taking into account their knowledge and value systems, and packaging information using examples, ideas, and evidence that makes sense to them (Schlenker 2003).

Unfortunately, very little research has been done on social skills in social and behavioral gerontology (for notable exceptions, see Hansson & Carpenter 1990, as well as Hogg & Heller 1990). And no one has investigated the potentially important influence of social skills on the development of close companion friends at church, which is regrettable because shared religious values, beliefs, and practices may make it easier to take the role of the other and enter into the mind of the other sympathetically. More is said in the next chapter (chap. 4) about other social factors that may shape the development of close companion friends in the church.

Change in Close Companion Friendships over Time

The fourth challenge that arises in the study of close companion friendships at church involves determining how these key social ties change over time. One potentially important issue involves the sheer length of time that two older people have been close companion friends. Some older people have been members of the same congregation for decades, and the companion friendships they may have developed may therefore have been in place for a long time. This point is important because a long shared history may change the nature and functioning of the relationship. For example, Wuthnow (1999) discussed the important role that religious ceremonies (e.g., baptisms, confirmations, weddings, and funerals) play in marking key passages in life and deepening religious faith. Perhaps taking part in these ceremonies with close companion friends serves to enhance, enrich, and more tightly bind the relationship between them. This may be especially likely to occur among close companion friends because the intimate nature of the relationship between them may provide a critically important forum for sharing the powerful emotions that ceremonies, such as funerals, typically invoke.

The accumulated history shared by long-standing companion friends may also affect the way routine aspects of social relationships are handled. For example, consistent with Antonucci's (1985) notion of the support bank, two church members who have been companion friends for so long that they do not feel pressured to return favors immediately may be more likely to forgive or overlook interpersonal transgressions should they arise.

Limits to the Closeness of Companion Friends

The fifth way to improve research on church-based companion friends is at once a theoretical and data analytic issue. By definition, church-based companion friendships are close relationships. But this notion of closeness raises the possibility that relationships may become too close, and people may feel smothered by another and wish for a greater degree of distance and personal space. This is hardly a new issue. As a character in Euripides' play, *Hippolytus*, proclaims, "Friendship between mortals should be taken in moderation. Don't let it get down into the marrow of the soul. Bonds of affection ought to be elastic, for letting apart or drawing together" (Euripides 1960, 72). Contemporary researchers have investigated the ancient insights of Euripides. For example, Hodges, Finnegan, and Perry (1999) discuss the impact of excessive closeness in relationships formed by children and adolescents. These researchers point out that excessive closeness can threaten feelings of autonomy and lead to avoidance behavior. However, there do not appear to be any studies in the literature that examine this issue among older adults. Doing so should be a high priority because a number of investigators have pointed out that older adults value their independence highly (e.g., Lee 1985).

The notion that social relationships may become too close suggests that older people may have a comfort zone when it comes to companion friends at church, where some degree of closeness is welcomed, but too much closeness fosters discomfort. This scenario calls for the estimation of a nonlinear relationship between close companion friendships at church and well-being, whereby initial levels of involvement are associated with health benefits, but beyond a certain threshold, additional degrees of involvement or closeness are associated with a decline in well-being.

Informal Companion Friendships with the Clergy

So far, the discussion throughout this chapter has focused on the nature, development, and health-related effects of close companion friendships that arise between rank-and-file church members. But researchers also need to know more about close companion friendships that may form between members of the clergy and rank-and-file congregants. Formal aspects of relationships with the clergy are discussed in the next chapter, and the discussion reveals a good deal of research on this issue. However, few empirical studies have been conducted on informal close companion friendships between rank-and-file church members and the clergy. One of the few studies to examine this issue was conducted by Blackbird and Wright (1985), who gathered data from pastors and rank-and-file church members. Blackbird and Wright (1985) used this data to examine a phenomena they call the pedestal effect. According to this perspective, close personal relationships between the clergy and church members are discouraged by norms of propriety, anti-fraternization norms, and the guarded and defensive way in which a church member presumably relates to his or her pastor. Nevertheless, Blackbird and Wright (1985) report that norms and behaviors that constitute the pedestal effect were not widespread in the typical congregation. However, their study further reveals that if parishioners subscribe to these norms and behaviors, then they were less likely to develop a close friendship with their pastor.

Unfortunately, Blackbird and Wright (1985) did not examine the relationship between close friendships with the clergy and health or well-being. It is important to know if close companion friendships with rank-and-file church members have a different effect on health and well-being than close companion friendships with a pastor. It is difficult to determine beforehand which would be most advantageous. On the one hand, one might argue that the prestige and authority bestowed on the clergy might serve to accentuate the potentially beneficial health-related effects of close companion friendships that are formed with them. But on the other hand, this may depend upon the individual characteristics of the rank-and-file member, including one's attitude toward authority as well as the level of comfort in a relationship in which a status differential is present.

Conclusions

Much has been written about the presumably unique ties of fel-lowship (i.e., communities of faith) that are found in Christian churches (Tillich 1987), yet it is surprising to find so little empirical research on them. This chapter was designed to lay the groundwork for this kind of study by casting research on church-based fellowships in the context of close companion friends. Doing so made it possible to take what is known in the secular literature and extend and elaborate upon it to pro-vide new insight into the way close companion friendships are manifest in the church and how they may influence the health and well-being of older people. Throughout, the goal was to derive propositions that can be evaluated empirically, thereby providing a way to move the field for-ward. Two critical issues were explored in detail. The first involved what companion friends provide (i.e., the functions they perform), whereas the second had to do with ways in which close companion friends at church may influence health and well-being in late life. Constructs like self-disclosure, trust, the sharing of interests and things that are valued highly, as well as the emulation of close others and the development of an ideal religious self were introduced in an effort to provide a well-articulated theoretical foundation for conducting this kind of research. But sound conceptualization does not go far enough. Consistent with the overall strategy that is taken throughout this volume, an effort was made to bridge these theoretical insights with issues in the measurement of close companion friendships at church as well.

Some investigators may disagree with the intervening constructs that were evoked to link close companion friends at church with health and well-being, or they may not concur with the way these constructs were defined and measured. Such disagreements should not only be expected in an underdeveloped field, but they should also be welcomed. Embrac-ing this kind of debate is crucial because it provides the basis for the development of sound mid-range theories on church-based companion friends and health in late life.

Chapter 4

Social Relationships That Arise
from Formal Roles in the Church

Research indicates that it is important to take the source of support into consideration when evaluating social relationships in the church (e.g., Krause et al. 2001). It makes sense to think about the source of support when studying social ties in the church because religious institutions are complex organizations consisting of people who occupy a number of different formal roles. As a result, the status, norms, and proscriptions associated with these formal roles influence the nature and effectiveness of the relationships that are formed through them. Because the goal of this volume is to provide an in-depth examination of social ties in the church, formal relationships in the church must be taken into consideration. This issue is important because, as the discussion provided below reveals, some studies suggest that formal relationships in the church may have a significant effect on the health and well-being of older church members. Four types of formal social relationships in the church are examined in this chapter: (1) formal social ties with the clergy (i.e., pastoral counseling), (2) relationships that arise in formal church groups (i.e., Bible study and prayer groups), (3) relationships that emerge in formal volunteer programs in the church, and (4) social relationships that take place in formal outreach programs maintained by the church to minister to older members who are homebound.

Formal Relationships with the Clergy

Of all the formal roles in the church, the role of pastor is the most authoritative and prestigious position in the congregational hierarchy. As Stark and Bainbridge (1987) point out, because members of the clergy occupy a highly prestigious position in the church, they "share in the psychic rewards offered to the gods, for example: Deference, honor and adoration" (101). In addition, researchers have recognized for some time that the minister, more than any other church member, is supposed to embody and practice the core tenets of the faith (Lenski, 1961). Among these core tenets are the expression of empathy and concern for others as well as being deeply committed to assisting church members who are in need. This is important because, as Reis and Collins (2000) argue, social support is more likely to be effective when it is delivered in relationships that are characterized by high levels of trust, commitment, and respect.

Although members of the clergy interact with fellow congregants in a number of ways, one of the most important involves providing formal counseling to those who are experiencing stressful life events or who are suffering from mental health problems. Research indicates that the clergy spend a significant amount of time in the counseling role. For example, research reviewed by Hohmann and Larson (1993) suggests that pastors report spending, on average, between 10 percent and 20 percent of their time (i.e., six to eight hours) per week providing counseling services. This is consistent with estimates provided by Oppenheimer, Flannelly, and Weaver (2004), who report that members of the clergy spend an average of 15 percent of their working time providing pastoral counseling. In fact, counseling has become so central to the pastoral role that a number of journals are devoted specifically to this function (e.g., the *Journal of Pastoral Counseling, Journal of Pastoral Care,* and *Pastoral Psychology*). Because research conducted in secular settings suggests that relationships that arise in therapeutic settings can be quite intimate, emotionally charged, and especially consequential for the mental health of the client (Frank 1961; Kirschenbaum & Henderson 1989), it is essential to see if the same health-related consequences emerge from the pastoral counseling process.

The discussion that follows is divided into three sections. First, research is reviewed on the extent to which rank-and-file church members seek out formal counseling from their pastor or priest. As these data reveal, church members make frequent use of pastoral counseling services. Consequently, the reasons for these high rates of utilization are examined at this juncture as well. Second, it would be difficult to cover all the ways that pastoral counseling may benefit older church members in a single chapter. As a result, three ways in which pastoral counseling may be especially likely to restore and enhance the mental health of older church members are explored in detail. Third, methodological and conceptual challenges in the study of pastoral counseling are identified and discussed.

The Use of Pastoral Counseling Services

According to the widely cited study by Veroff, Douvan, and Kulka (1981), 39 percent of Americans who have a serious problem seek help from a member of the clergy. Moreover, the findings from this study reveal that people are more likely to request assistance from members of the clergy than any other kind of mental health professional, including psychiatrists, psychologists, and social workers (see also Chalfant, Roberts, Heller, Briones, Aguirre-Hochbaum, & Farr 1990; Neighbors, Musick, & Williams 1998). It is especially important for the purposes of the current volume to point out that Veroff et al. (1981) report that older women are more likely than either older men or younger people to turn to the clergy for help with personal problems.

The findings reported by Veroff et al. (1981) have been replicated and extended by three studies. The first study was conducted by Hohmann and Larson (1993). These investigators analyzed data from the widely known Epidemiological Catchment Area (ECA) Study. The ECA Study represents one of the first efforts to assess clinical mental disorders systematically across the nation. This extensive survey involved interviews with 18,572 people in five sites across the United States. Three findings from this research are especially noteworthy. First, Hohmann and Larson (1993) report that women, people who are widowed, and individuals aged sixty-five and older are more likely to seek help for mental health problems from the clergy than from other mental health specialists. Second, these investigators found that the type and severity of mental disorder were not significantly related to the source of help. Put another way, members of the clergy were just as likely as mental health professionals to counsel individuals who were suffering from severe types of mental disorder. Third, the fact that members of the clergy refer fewer than 10 percent of the people they counsel to mental health professionals speaks directly to their role as front-line mental health workers (Hohmann & Larson 1993).

The second study to provide data on pastoral counseling for mental health problems was conducted by Wang, Berglund, and Kessler (2003). These investigators analyzed data from the widely known National Comorbidity Survey. Like the ECA Study, the National Comorbidity survey was designed to provide prevalence data on psychiatric disorders in the American adult population. But unlike the ECA Study, the National

Comorbidity Survey was based on a random probability sample. Three important findings emerged from this work. First, the results suggest that nearly one in four adults who ever sought treatment for a clinical mental disorder did so from a member of the clergy. Second, of those who sought help from a pastor, approximately one in four had a serious type of mental disorder. Third, the majority of people who sought help from the clergy for mental health problems did not receive mental health services from other mental health professionals.

The third study to assess the use of pastoral counseling for mental health–related problems was conducted recently by Ellison, Flannelly, and Weaver (2006). Based on data from the 1996 General Social Survey, these investigators studied responses to a number of vignettes about people who were experiencing symptoms of a range of mental health problems. Study participants were asked where the individual who was described in the vignette should go for help. Overall, the data suggest that approximately one in three study participants indicated that a member of the clergy would be the first or second choice for getting help for the mental health problem. It is especially important to note that, like Hohmann and Larson (1993), Ellison et al. (2006) report that older individuals (i.e., those aged sixty and older) were much more likely to recommend that the person in the vignette seek help from a member of the clergy for their mental health problem.

A number of reasons have been identified in the literature for the high use of pastoral counseling services. Five are especially important because they involve issues that speak directly to the situation of older people. First, as Taylor, Ellison, Chatters, Levin, and Lincoln (2000) maintain, one of the primary factors for seeking pastoral counseling is financial. More specifically, these investigators argue that members of the clergy do not charge fees for their services, nor do they require co-payments or the completion of lengthy intake forms. These considerations are important because many people do not have insurance that covers mental health care. In fact, this issue may help explain why women, the elderly, and widows are especially likely to seek out pastoral counseling services. More specifically, as Schulz (2001) reports, older women who are not married are especially likely to be either poor or near-poor (i.e., have incomes that are within 125 percent of the poverty level).

Second, as Taylor et al. (2000) maintain, older church members are likely to use pastoral counseling services because they often have developed a long-standing relationship with the clergy care provider. As a result, these long-standing relationships make it possible for the clergy to observe changes in behavior that signal early signs of mental health problems (Oppenheimer et al. 2004).

Third, research by Robb, Haley, Becker, Polivka, and Chwa (2003) reveals that older people are less confident about their knowledge of mental health care and appropriate treatment than younger adults. Perhaps this is one reason that the older respondents in their study were just as likely to report that they feel more comfortable discussing mental health problems with a member of the clergy than with any other type of mental health professional.

Fourth, as Kelcourse (2002) points out, mental health professionals are sometimes viewed with suspicion because they provide services that are based on a secular belief system that may not be in keeping with or adhere to the religious principles that are valued highly by an older person who is in need. More specifically, some older adults elect to frame their problems in religious terms. For example, Burton (2003) discusses how problems such as disordered relationships, anger, and depression are viewed by some individuals in terms of spiritual pain (see also Bartel's [2004] discussion of spiritual suffering). If people interpret stressors and subsequent psychological distress in religious terms, then they will be more inclined to seek religious explanations for the origins of these difficulties, and they will be more likely to prefer religious solutions to them. This consideration is important when studying older people because, as discussed in chapter 1, research indicates that the current cohort of older adults is more deeply involved in religion than the current cohort of younger people (Barna 2002).

Fifth, as discussed in chapter 1, Eckenrode and Wethington (1990) point out that people sometimes feel uneasy about asking for support from informal social network members because they fear their request for assistance may be rejected or they believe that asking for help may expose their weaknesses and inability to deal with problems on their own. Seeking help from formal sources (e.g., members of the clergy) who are officially charged with providing assistance may go a long way toward alleviating these concerns.

The Health-Related Benefits of Pastoral Counseling

As Gordon and Mitchell (2004) recently pointed out, there is no recognized or agreed-upon definition of religious or spiritual care, nor is there a valid survey instrument to assess the effectiveness of pastoral counseling services. In addition, a range of beneficial effects have been identified in a number of books written on pastoral counseling.

Given the plethora of views and perspectives, reviewing all the ways in which pastoral counseling may improve the mental health of older adults would be difficult. Instead, a more circumscribed approach is taken below that is consistent with the overall thrust of the current volume. In particular, an effort is made to develop viable mid-range theories of three common pastoral counseling issues that can be evaluated empirically: the first has to do with the alleviation of guilt, the second involves counseling those who are near death and the significant others whom they eventually leave behind, and the third is concerned with recent extensions of attachment theory to the study of religion.

Alleviation of Guilt. Guilt and feelings of sinfulness are seen frequently in pastoral counseling sessions (Oates 1997). In the discussion that follows, this issue is embedded in a web of religious and secular constructs in an effort to depict one way in which pastoral counseling may help older people who are in need. Forgiveness figures prominently in this conceptual framework. More specifically, this mid-range conceptual model contains the following theoretical linkages:

1. Older people with mental health problems who seek pastoral counseling often suffer from feelings of guilt and are unable to forgive themselves for things they have done.
2. However, older adults will be more likely to forgive themselves if they feel they are forgiven by God.
3. Elderly people who feel forgiven by God are subsequently more likely to feel they have a close personal relationship with God.
4. Older people who have a close personal relationship with God will have a greater sense of hope and optimism.
5. Older adults with a strong sense of optimism will tend to enjoy better mental and physical health.

The ways in which a pastor may influence each of these key linkages is examined in detail below.

As Oates (1997) maintains, a common complaint that arises in pastoral counseling sessions among people who are suffering from mental health problems is the feeling that they have committed an unpardonable sin or that they are about to do so. Oates (1997) goes on to argue that beneath the feelings of guilt, shame, and hurt that are associated with these sins "lie the need to forgive or be forgiven" (526). Of the two, self-forgiveness may be the most important because, as Oates (1997) points out, the client is the one who has often committed the troublesome act (i.e., the unpardonable sin). Unfortunately, the literature on self-forgiveness is not well developed. In fact, Hall and Fincham (2005) refer to self-forgiveness as "the stepchild of forgiveness research" (621). Enright (1996) defines self-forgiveness as "a willingness to abandon self-resentment in the face of one's own acknowledged wrong, while fostering compassion, generosity, and love toward oneself" (115).

A key issue that arises at this juncture is how pastors help troubled church members find self-forgiveness. Although this may be accomplished in a number of different ways, one potentially important mechanism is identified by Hall and Fincham (2005). More specifically, these investigators argue that people who believe they have been forgiven by God are more likely to forgive themselves for the things they have done wrong, thus suggesting that one goal of the pastoral counseling process is to help older clients find God's forgiveness. As Rost (2003) points out, this may be accomplished, in part, by helping older church members rediscover a sense of God's grace. This point is important because, as Rost (2003) maintains, grace involves a number of factors, including "God's overflowing, undeserved forgiveness of sinful humanity" (239).

Some preliminary empirical evidence that forgiveness by God is a prerequisite for forgiveness of oneself may be found in unpublished data from the RAH Survey (Krause 2002a). These analyses involved assessing the relationship between forgiveness by God ("I believe God forgives me for the things I have done wrong") and change in self-forgiveness over time ("I forgive myself for the things I have done wrong"). Controlling for the effects of the frequency of church attendance and private prayer, as well as a number of demographic variables, the data suggest that older people who believe they are forgiven by God are more likely to report an enhanced sense of self-forgiveness over time (Beta = .104; $p < .005$). Unfortunately, data on the role the pastor may play in this process were not available in this survey. However, if Rost (2003) and others are correct, members of the clergy may play an indispensable part by promoting a sense of self-forgiveness through renewed awareness of the grace (i.e., forgiveness) of God.

Although findings of self-forgiveness are illuminating, it is important to discuss how self-forgiveness is, in turn, associated with better mental health. As identified above, one possibility is that people who feel they are able to forgive themselves tend to develop a closer relationship with God. This feeling of closeness may arise from a number of factors, including feelings of gratitude toward God for the forgiveness of sins. Once again, empirical support for this hypothesis may be found in unpublished research from the RAH Survey. After controlling for the effects of the frequency of church attendance and private prayer, as well as a range of demographic indicators, the data suggest that older people who feel that God has forgiven them for the things they have done wrong are more likely to feel they have developed a closer relationship with God (e.g., "I have a close personal relationship with God") (Beta = .189; $p < .001$).

Finally, as noted in chapter 2, published research by Krause (2002c) reveals that older people who have a close personal relationship with God are more likely to be optimistic, and people who have a greater sense of hope and optimism are, in turn, more likely to enjoy better health. Although mental health–related outcomes were not evaluated in the study by Krause (2002c), further unpublished analyses from the RAH Survey reveal that older people with a greater sense of hope are also less likely to report experiencing symptoms of depression (Beta = $-.239$; $p < .001$).

The role of hope in this conceptual scheme is intriguing because it fits nicely with ongoing debates about secular psychotherapeutic effectiveness. Researchers have recognized for decades that even though there are many different psychotherapeutic schools of thought, the various types of therapy appear to have roughly the same degree of effectiveness (Hubble, Duncan, & Miller 1999). This work was prompted, in part, by the pioneering research of Jerome Frank (1961), who strove to identify the common elements shared by all types of therapy that are responsible for their comparable levels of success. It is especially important to point out that in the process of identifying the common elements that all types of therapy share, Frank (1961) mentioned hope. More specifically, Frank argued that people do not seek help immediately after they encounter a psychological problem; instead, they seek assistance only after they have become demoralized over their own ineffective problem-solving efforts. Frank and Frank (1991) went on to maintain that the presence of an emotional, confiding relationship with a therapist who is hopeful, as well as determined to help, serves to offset this initial sense of demoralization. This is one reason why Snyder, Michael, and Cheavens (1999) argue that this essential sense of hope is what lies behind a good deal of psychotherapeutic success. In fact, they maintain that the sense of hope fostered by a mental health professional is one reason why anywhere from 40 percent to 66 percent of clients report experiencing improvement with their problems even before they attend the first therapeutic session. The observations of Snyder et al. (1999) are important because one of the core beliefs in the Christian faith focuses on hope through forgiveness, grace, and salvation. As C. S. Lewis (1942/2001) wrote, "Hope is one of the theological virtues" (134). In fact, Lewis (1942/2001) devoted an entire chapter to hope in this widely cited volume. Given the central role of hope in Christian theology, it is not hard to see why the restoration and promotion of hope may occupy a central place in the pastoral counseling process.

Viewed broadly, the simple conceptual model developed in this section suggests that one way pastoral counseling may improve the mental health of older adults is through the reassurance of God's forgiveness and the benefits associated with having a close relationship with God. Clearly, much more work remains to be done on this and other models that document the different ways that pastoral counseling may improve the mental health of older church members who are in need. Nevertheless, conceptual schemes, such as the one presented here, provide a template for how more sophisticated models of pastoral counseling effectiveness can be developed.

Ministering to Those Who Are Near Death. One of the most important and sensitive functions of pastoral counseling involves ministering to those who are near death as well as tending to the needs of family members and close friends of the dying. A poll conducted by the George H. Gallup International Institute (1997) of twelve hundred American adults reported that half the study participants anticipate a need for companionship and spiritual support when they are close to death. Moreover, 36 percent of the respondents in this survey specifically mentioned they would like to receive this support from a member of the clergy.

Although a pastor may help those who are near death in a number of ways, one way that may be especially important has to do with helping the dying find a sense of meaning in life. Evidence of this may be found in a study by Moadel, Morgan, Fatone, Grennan, Carter, and Laruffa (1999) of 248 cancer outpatients. They found that 40 percent of the participants reported that they needed help in finding a sense of meaning in life. This finding is replicated by a qualitative study by McGrath (2002) with twelve survivors of hematological malignancies. McGrath (2002) reports that the struggle to find a sense of meaning in the face of these debilitating physical health problems was a key source of existential pain and suffering.

Meaning in life was discussed in chapter 2 as an important resource for coping with the effects of stress. Therefore, it makes sense to return to meaning in life when examining how older people cope with one of the greatest stressors in life: dying. However, when meaning was reviewed in chapter 2, a full sense of the vast nature of the conceptual domain of this complex construct was not developed fully. Research conducted in secular settings by Krause (2004a) suggests that meaning may encompass at least four key dimensions: having (1) a sense of values, (2) a purpose in life, (3) goals, and (4) the ability to reflect on things that have happened in the past. Reflecting on the past may be the most important of these factors when ministering to those who are dying. Evidence of this may be found in the work of Paulson (2004), who points out in his discussion of pastoral counseling in the near death process that it is helpful to have clients "recall people, events, and things that have occurred in their lives, and...realize they experienced these things in the context of the Mystery. This authentic inquiry of thought and experience can generally be integrated by clients to greatly increase their meaning in life" (350). As this observation reveals, this therapeutic technique involves reminiscing about the past, but in a way that ties memories and events specifically with religious themes (i.e., the Mystery).The more general use of reminiscence as a form of therapy has been investigated widely in the secular literature. In fact, entire volumes have been devoted to this issue (e.g., Haight & Webster 1995; Sherman 1991). But more importantly, several interventions have been devised to help people who are dying find a sense of meaning in life (e.g., Chochinov & Cann 2005). For example, Chockinov and Cann (2005) report that 67 percent of the terminally ill participants in their intervention reported obtaining a heightened sense of meaning in life. Unfortunately, there do not appear to be any studies that provide empirical evidence of the effectiveness of reminiscence therapy in pastoral counseling with older people who are near death. It is time for researchers to turn to this issue.

Initially, it may seem that helping the dying think about the afterlife may be a useful therapeutic tool as well. After all, it seems reasonable to assume that individuals who are about to leave this life may have concerns about whether they will continue to exist, and if they do, what this existence is like. However, as Paulson (2004) points out in his review of pastoral counseling with those who are dying, knowledge of the afterlife "does little to prevent the physical and emotional suffering of the client" (344). Although this may be true, some evidence exists that beliefs about the afterlife may help close friends and family members of those who have died cope more successfully with the grieving process. For example, Hill (2002) provides a comprehensive list of pastoral counseling tactics to help mothers deal with the death of a child.

Among them are recommended scriptural passages to read, including some that emphasize the promise of heaven and a good afterlife.

In order to see why beliefs about the afterlife may ease the pain associated with grieving, it is important to examine four issues. First, existing ties with those who have passed away have obviously been severed. As a result, people who were once an important source of social support and companionship are no longer accessible. Believing there is an afterlife holds out the prospect of seeing the deceased again and speaks directly to resuming ties with them following one's own death. Second, for many, death is an uncertain outcome. No one has direct knowledge about what happens after death, and if there is an afterlife, no one is certain about what it is like. Consequently, when a significant other dies, those who are left behind may worry about what has happened to the departed loved one. More specifically, concerns may arise about whether the deceased continues to exist at all, and if they do, whether they are safe, cared for, and content. Third, the death of a significant other clearly brings thoughts about one's own mortality to the foreground (Wuthnow, Christiano, & Kuzlowski 1980). Believing there is no life after death, or believing the dead may face a precarious existence in the next life may be a source of significant distress for those who are left behind. Finally, as research reviewed by Benore and Park (2004) reveals, belief in an afterlife may go a long way toward helping those who are grieving find a sense of meaning in their own lives. Clearly, empirical research on pastoral counseling with the grieving process may benefit from exploring the ways in which belief in the afterlife may help the bereaved deal more effectively with the loss of a loved one.

Extensions of Attachment Theory. Recently, Kirkpatrick (2005) developed a fascinating adaptation of attachment theory to the study of religion. It is not possible to summarize the vast literature on attachment theory here. However, reviewing a few basic postulates helps convey a general sense of the core theoretical thrust of this conceptual framework. According to Bowlby (1969, 1973, 1980), the nature of the relationship that a child forms early in life with a key caregiver (typically the mother) serves as a prototype for the kind of relationships he or she will develop later in adult life. When a relationship with an early caregiver develops in a positive manner, the caregiver will be viewed as a safe and secure haven in times of threat and difficulty. Later in life, the person who has successfully formed a positive relationship with the early caregiver will develop relationships that are secure, comfortable, and intimate. But if the early attachment relationship fails to develop in a

positive manner, subsequent social ties in adult life will be characterized by fear, anxiety, and insecurity. Five key characteristics distinguish
between successful attachment relationships and other close social ties
(Ainsworth 1985):

1. The individual makes an effort to be close to the caregiver, especially when he or she is frightened or alarmed.
2. The caregiver provides care and attention to the attached person,
   creating a safe haven.
3. The caregiver also promotes a sense of security.
4. The threat of being separated from the caregiver causes the
   attached person to feel anxious.
5. Loss of the caregiver causes the attached person to experience a
   sense of grief.

The ability to form positive attachment relationships is important because research reviewed by Kirkpatrick (2005) suggests that people who
fail to develop such ties are more likely to experience a number of mental health problems, including depression and anxiety.

Kirkpatrick (2005) argues that many religious beliefs and behaviors
can be explained by the fact that a significant number of people tend to
view God as an attachment figure. But it is especially important for the
purposes of the current chapter to point out that Kirkpatrick (2005) also
considers whether attachment relationships can be formed with other
religious figures, especially members of the clergy: "Whether these leaders also function as a secure base in the true manner of an attachment
figure is a more difficult question, but it surely seems possible" (Kirkpatrick 2005, 93). This is a difficult issue because, as Kirkpatrick (2005)
points out, a member of the clergy does not necessarily act as an attachment figure simply because he or she occupies a prestigious and authoritative role in the church. Instead, a clergy member must be accessible,
and responsive, and meet the criteria identified by Ainsworth (1985) that
are provided above. Because all members of the clergy clearly do not serve
as attachment figures for all the members in their congregations, a key
issue involves identifying when such a relationship is likely to emerge.
A key premise in the current chapter is that an attachment relationship
with a member of the clergy is especially likely to arise in the pastoral counseling setting. More specifically, it not difficult to see why rank-
and-file church members would seek pastoral counseling when they feel
threatened, frightened, or alarmed. Moreover, if pastoral counseling is
provided effectively, the rank-and-file church member is likely to develop

a relationship with the pastor in which he or she feels safe and secure. This rationale is bolstered by the fact that a number of investigators have identified the ways in which secular therapists may serve as attachment figures (see Bachelor & Horvath 1999 for a review of this research). If the argument developed here is valid, then it opens the door to a vast array of principles and measures that may fruitfully be applied to the assessment of the pastoral counseling process. Unfortunately, there do not appear to be any investigators who have taken advantage of the literature on attachment theory to conduct empirical studies of pastoral counseling with older adults. Perhaps it is time they did so.

Conceptual and Methodological Challenges

Although a number of methodological and conceptual issues face investigators who wish to study the pastoral counseling process, three that may be especially important are reviewed in this section. First, Hubble, Duncan, and Miller (1999) published an important edited volume on the factors that make psychotherapy successful. Although a range of factors may contribute to the beneficial outcome of therapy, a major component was identified in the chapter that Tallman and Bohart (1999) wrote for this volume. These investigators identified studies showing that "the client is responsible for 70% or more of the outcome variance" (95). Included among the reasons for this remarkable figure is the willingness for change that the client brings to the therapeutic relationship. Researchers need to learn more about the uniquely religious factors that a client may bring to pastoral counseling sessions that enhance the quality of the assistance they receive. One relatively straightforward client-based factor that is unique to religious settings may be especially important: the extent to which an older person is committed to his or her faith. Not everyone in a congregation has the same level of dedication and commitment to his or her faith. If a good deal of pastoral counseling involves the provision of religiously based explanations and solutions to the problems that congregants face, then it follows that the deeper the religious convictions of the client, the more likely that religious explanations and solutions are to be effective. This relationship can be evaluated by testing for a statistical interaction effect between religious commitment and participation in pastoral counseling on mental health–related outcomes.

The issue of commitment to one's faith reaches far beyond pastoral counseling issues. More specifically, the relationship between many religious constructs and health-related outcomes may depend upon the degree to which a study participant is committed to his or her faith. For example, the effect of informal support from fellow church members on health may also depend upon the support recipient's degree of religious commitment; and the effectiveness of basic religious practices, such as prayer, may be determined in part by how deeply committed a person is to his or her faith. Given the straightforward nature of this issue, it is surprising to find that it has been largely overlooked in the literature on religion, aging, and health.

Second, as discussed in chapter 2, rank-and-file church members may also be an important source of support when difficult times arise, which raises a number of questions that have to do with the interface between informal help from fellow church members and formal pastoral counseling. For example, researchers need to identify the circumstances under which older people seek help from fellow church members and when are they more likely to request formal counseling from their pastor. Perhaps the sensitivity of the presenting problem may have something to do with this issue. Maybe older people are more inclined to take more delicate and sensitive problems to their pastor instead of their fellow rank-and-file church members. This inclination may be due, in part, to concerns about confidentiality. In the process of conducting the detailed qualitative research for his study on religion and health, Krause (2002a) presented study participants with an open-ended question that focused on how formal support from the pastor may differ from assistance provided by rank-and-file church members. One older black woman succinctly captured the issue of confidentiality when she said, "And there is the issue of confidentiality too. When you talk to your friends (at church), you don't know where the information is going to go from there...but the minister, he's bound by confidentiality."

But confidentiality may be only one of several issues that are involved in the study of the interface between formal and informal assistance in the church. For example, instead of preferring one source of assistance over the other, older adults may use both in sequence. More specifically, they may first seek help from fellow congregants and then subsequently request pastoral counseling if the informal assistance provided by a rank-and-file church member fails to be effective. Alternatively, older people may rely on both sources at once by turning to fellow church members at the same time they seek formal counseling from the pastor. And if older church members turn to both formal and informal sources for assistance, researchers need to know if the combined effect of both is greater than the effect of either source of assistance taken separately. As this brief overview reveals, there are a number of ways in which to approach the use of formal and informal helping in the church. Researchers need to know which of these scenarios is pursued most often and which has the most beneficial effects on mental health.

A third issue involves how researchers should specify the models they develop to study the use of informal church-based social relationships to handle the stressful events that arise in the lives of older congregants. More specifically, it is important that these models contain measures of formal counseling from the clergy as well as assistance from fellow rank-and-file church members. The dangers of ignoring formal support from the clergy are straightforward. Assume an older church member has a personal problem of a highly sensitive nature. Assume further that he or she elects to discuss this problem with his or her pastor, but not with fellow church members. Finally, assume that counseling provided by the pastor is effective, thereby alleviating the psychological distress the older church member was experiencing. If a researcher were to focus solely on informal support provided by fellow church members under these circumstances, then the resulting analyses would be misleading because the older person in this example would report that he or she received no informal support for his or her problem, yet the stressor would have no impact on their mental health. However, in this case, the lack of association between informal support and mental health would be explained by the fact that the older person's mental health problems were alleviated by the unmeasured assistance of his or her pastor. As this simple example reveals, it is important to take all forms of church-based assistance into account when studying the effects of stressors that arise in the lives of older church members.

Bible Study Groups and Prayer Groups

Bible study groups and prayer groups provide another important forum for formal social relationships to develop within the church. Although there is no agreed-upon definition of "Bible study groups," they are defined here as formal groups in the church that meet on a regular basis outside of formal worship services so that group members may discuss the Bible, arrive at a better understanding of it, and learn how to apply biblical teachings in their daily lives. In addition to the direct study of biblical passages and stories, Bible study group members may also read and discuss other works and commentaries related to the Bible. "Prayer groups" are defined as formal groups in the church that meet on a regular basis outside of formal worship services to pray and to discuss issues related to prayer. Bible study groups and prayer groups may meet either in the church edifice or in the homes of group members.

It is difficult to find nationally representative data on the rates of attendance in Bible study groups and prayer groups among older people. However, unpublished data from the RAH Survey provide some insight into this issue. More specifically, the data from this study suggest that slightly over half (50.9 percent) of older adults say they attended Bible study groups at least once in the year prior to the survey. Moreover, about 33.5 percent say they attended Bible study groups about once a month or more during this time. In contrast, the findings from this study further indicate that older adults do not attend prayer groups as often. More specifically, approximately one-third of the older study participants (i.e., 36.7 percent) indicated they had attended formal prayer groups at least once in the past year, and only 18.4 percent report they attended prayer groups once a month or more often.

The discussion that follows is divided into two main sections. First, the relationships among participation in Bible study groups, prayer groups, and health-related outcomes are examined. Unfortunately, there do not appear to be any studies in the literature that empirically evaluate the relationships among these constructs with nationwide data that have been provided specifically by older people. Consequently, research on adults of all ages is used as a point of departure in order to provide some insights into the ways in which participation in these groups may affect health and well-being in late life. Second, a series of conceptual and methodological challenges that face investigators who wish to study Bible study groups, prayer groups, and health will be provided.

Bible Study Groups, Prayer Groups, and Health-Related Outcomes

Perhaps no one has contributed more to the study of Bible study groups and prayer groups than Robert Wuthnow (1994, 2000). His nationwide surveys have shed light on a number of benefits that participation in these formal groups provide for adults of all ages. Although Wuthnow (1994, 2000) does not explicitly assess whether attendance at Bible study groups and prayer groups improves health, he examines a number of factors that may mediate the effects of participation in these formal groups on health and well-being. Even though it is not possible to review here all the intervening mechanisms that Wuthnow (1994) discusses, some are especially important because they are consistent with a number of factors discussed elsewhere in the current volume. For example, Wuthnow (1994) reports that people who attend Bible study groups and prayer groups report having better relationships with others, and they are more likely to forgive others for things they may have done wrong (see especially Wuthnow 2000). These benefits are important because, as discussed in chapters 2 and 3, they are associated with better health and well-being in late life. In addition, Wuthnow (1994) further reports that people who attend these formal groups also report having a closer relationship with God, and some participants feel it is important to "sit back and let God work things out" (234). The potential health-related aspects of this notion of God-mediated control were also discussed in chapter 2. Finally, Wuthnow (1994) indicates that the participants in his study felt like participation in Bible study groups and prayer groups deepened their faith significantly. The potential health-related benefits of experiencing a deeper faith are reviewed later in this chapter when programs for the homebound are discussed.

In order to arrive at a deeper appreciation for the ways in which participation in Bible study groups and prayer groups may improve the health and well-being of older people, an effort is made below to extend the valuable sights provided by Wuthnow (1994) in three key areas: beliefs about the answers to prayers, forgiveness, and beliefs about the benefits of praying for others. Following this, a straightforward way in which prayer groups may influence health is examined; simply put, prayer groups may be associated with health because group members offer prayers that specifically request divine healing.

Beliefs about Answers to Prayers. Wuthnow (1994) reports that people who participate in Bible study groups and prayer groups tend to believe that forming a close relationship with God helps them get answers to their prayers. This observation ties in nicely with findings from research by Krause and his colleagues. As discussed in chapter 1, a series of focus groups were conducted in order to develop closed-ended survey questions for his nationwide survey. The findings involving prayer that emerged from these focus groups were published by Krause, Chatters, Meltzer, and Morgan (2000a). This qualitative work reveals that although most study participants felt their prayers were answered, they also believed that the best answers are more likely to come under certain circumstances. More specifically, the older focus group participants indicated that it is best to be patient when waiting for an answer to a prayer, and that God provides the answer precisely at the right time—not too early or not too late. In addition, a number of the focus groups' participants indicated that many times they did not get exactly what they prayed for, but when they took time to think about it, they found the answer they received was precisely what they needed the most. Viewed more generally, these beliefs about the way prayers are answered may be construed as prayer expectancies (Olson, Roese, & Zanna 1996). Expectancies are beliefs about what may happen in the future, and they are important because they allow individuals to know what to expect, thereby serving as a guide that shapes their subsequent actions and reactions. However, expectancies differ with respect to prayer because in this instance they involve beliefs about what God will do next.

A set of unpublished analyses of the RAH Survey data were performed to see if people who attend Bible study groups and prayer groups are more likely to endorse these prayer expectancies and whether these prayer expectancies are, in turn, associated with better health. A two-item prayer expectancy measure (i.e., "Learning to wait for God's answer to my prayers is an important part of my faith," and "When I pray, God does not always give me what I ask for because only He knows what is best") was regressed on the frequency of attendance at Bible study groups, prayer groups, formal worship services, private prayer, and a number of demographic control variables. The data suggest that the more often people attend Bible study groups, the more likely they are to endorse these prayer expectancies (Beta = .126; $p < .001$). But surprisingly, the frequency of attendance at prayer groups was not significantly associated with prayer expectancies (Beta = .040; ns). Although it is hard to determine why Bible study groups emerged as being more important in this respect, it could be that instead of arising from informal conversation with others in prayer groups, expectancies about prayer are more likely to be fostered in Bible study groups by the discussion of explicit biblical passages and stories related to prayer.

The impact of the prayer expectancies identified above on well-being in late life were explored in a published study by Krause (2004b). The findings suggest that feelings of self-worth are higher among older adults who believe that only God knows when it is best to answer a prayer and when they believe that only God knows the best way to answer them.

Forgiveness. Wuthnow (1994) reports that adults of all ages who attend Bible study groups and prayer groups are more likely to forgive others than individuals who are not associated with these formal church groups. This finding was replicated in an unpublished analysis of the RAH Survey data. Forgiveness of others ("How often do you forgive others for the things they have done to you?") was regressed on the frequency of attendance at Bible study groups, prayer groups, formal worship services, private prayer, and a number of demographic control variables. The data reveal that older adults who attend prayer group meetings more often are slightly more likely to forgive others than older people who do not go to prayer group meetings as frequently (Beta = .074; $p < .05$). In contrast, attendance at Bible study groups was not associated with forgiving others (Beta = $-.019$; ns).

But recall from the discussion of forgiveness in chapter 1 that the key issue may not be whether an older person forgives someone else; instead, it might be how they go about doing so. More specifically, as the findings from the study by Krause and Ellison (2003) reveal, older adults who forgive others unconditionally tend to experience fewer symptoms of depression and death anxiety, and they report having greater life satisfaction than older people who require others to perform acts of contrition (e.g., apologize, provide restitution whenever possible).

A set of unpublished analyses from RAH Survey data reveals that attendance at formal group meetings in the church has a bearing on whether older people require transgressors to perform acts of contrition, but the findings are complex. When the data from the first wave of the RAH Survey were assessed, neither the frequency of attendance at prayer groups (Beta = $-.015$; ns) nor the frequency of attendance at Bible study groups (Beta = $-.047$; ns) were associated with the number of acts of attrition that a transgressor is required to perform. However, a different picture emerged when the data from Waves 1 and 2 were evaluated. More specifically, the number of acts of contrition at Wave 2 was regressed on the Wave 1 measures of frequency of attendance at Bible study groups, prayer groups, formal worship services, private prayer, a number of demographic control variables, and the baseline measure of the number of acts of contrition. The data suggest that older people who attend Bible study groups often are likely to require transgressors to perform fewer acts of contrition over time (Beta = $-.119$; $p < .01$), but significant findings failed to emerge with respect to prayer groups (Beta = $-.055$; ns). It may be helpful to reflect on why it took some time for the effects of attendance at Bible study groups to become manifest (i.e., why lagged effects emerged from the data). Perhaps this finding has to do with the fact that forgiving others is often a difficult task, and that it may take time before older people are ready to forgive without requiring the person who hurt them to perform acts of contrition.

Praying for Others. Wuthnow (1994) reports that an important part of participating in prayer groups involves praying for the needs of others. More specifically, he reports, "Members uniformly asserted that they felt cared for and supported because other people were praying for them" (Wuthnow, 1994, 240). Although having others pray for oneself has important health-related benefits (e.g., Harris, Gowda, Kolb, Strychacz, Bacek, Jones, Forker, O'Keefe, & McCallister 1999), the study by Krause (2003c), mentioned briefly in chapter 2, reveals that the person who offers the prayer may benefit as well. More specifically, the finding from this study suggests that the deleterious effects of chronic financial problems on the physical health status of older adults are reduced significantly when they pray often for others. However, the measure of prayer used in this study focused solely on the frequency of private prayer. Unfortunately, measures of how often someone prays for others in Bible study or prayer groups were not available in the RAH Survey. Nevertheless, it seems likely that if such data were available, effects similar to those reported by Krause (2003c) would be found. Viewed more generally, this suggests that prayer providers as well as prayer recipients may both enjoy the health-related benefits of prayer.

Requests for Divine Healing. Up to this point, several somewhat complex ways in which participation in Bible study groups and prayer groups may affect health and well-being have been reviewed. However, there is another straightforward mechanism that is especially likely to emerge in prayer groups. More specifically, participation in prayer groups may be associated with better health simply because group members offer prayers that explicitly request divine healing. Evidence of this may be found, for example, in the extensive qualitative study by McKay and Musil (2005) of ninety-six United Churches of Christ. They report that many of the congregations in their sample have formal lay intercessory prayer groups and that group members often pray for either their own health or the health of others. This point is important because a number of controlled trials indicate that intercessory prayer may actually improve the health of the individual who is being prayed for (Byrd 1988; Harris et al. 1999).

Conceptual and Methodological Challenges

Clearly, the biggest problem facing research on Bible study groups, prayer groups, and health is the lack of work that has been done so far. Much more research is needed before investigators can determine if participation in these formal church groups is related to health, and if it is, how these health-related benefits arise. In the process, it would be helpful to explore four more specific methodological and conceptual issues that are discussed briefly below.

First, participation in Bible study groups and prayer groups was measured with a single-item indicator in the RAH Survey. Investigators need to move beyond this simple measurement strategy by developing multiple-item batteries that assess precisely what transpires in these potentially important formal church groups. Wuthnow (1994) collected data along these lines, but a number of questions remain unanswered. For example, it is quite likely that prayer is used in Bible study groups as well as prayer groups. Researchers need to know more about the nature and content of prayers in Bible study groups to make sure that the effects of participation in Bible study groups does not become confounded with participation in prayer groups.

Second, research discussed above suggests that private prayer may have a beneficial effect on health (Harris et al. 1999). Presumably, group prayers that are offered in formal prayer groups have potentially important health-related effects as well. It is important to know if group prayer is more efficacious than private prayer or whether both modes of praying have an equally important influence on health and well-being in late life. This issue was explored in the qualitative study by Krause et al. (2000). Some of the participants in their focus groups felt that private prayer and group prayer worked equally as well, but others reported that group prayers have more important effects. As one older woman in this study put it, "You have a feeling that it's going to make a difference because you have all these forces coming together and unified and it's a sense of power" (Krause et al. 2000, 204). But disentangling the effects of group prayer and individual prayer is not likely to be easy, because the participants in the study by Krause et al. (2000) indicated that group prayers and private prayers are not always used for the same problems or issues. More specifically, some focus group members claimed that group prayers were reserved for more serious issues while others reported that group prayers typically are used for common concerns in the group or congregation, whereas more personal or individual concerns are more likely to be expressed in private prayer.

Third, some of the analyses presented in the previous section reveal that Bible study groups and prayer groups do not always have the same effects on health-related outcomes. However, some people attend Bible study groups and prayer groups at church. In fact, unpublished data from the RAH Survey reveals that the bivariate correlation between the measure of attendance at Bible study groups and attendance at prayer groups is .550 ($p < .001$), which raises several important research issues. To begin with, if a person attends Bible study groups and prayer groups, it may be difficult to determine the independent contribution that each might make on health. But some advantages may also accrue to having some overlap between participation in the two types of formal church groups. More specifically, having this type of data makes it possible to see whether participation in both Bible study groups and prayer groups conveys health-related benefits that are greater than the benefits that arise from taking part in either one alone. Stated in more technical terms, it would be important to know if there is a statistical interaction effect between participation in Bible study groups and participation in prayer groups on health and well-being in late life.

Fourth, older people who attend Bible study groups or prayer groups are more likely to be deeply committed to their faith than people who decide not to take part in these formal groups. If more general measures of religious involvement and commitment are not included in the model, then the beneficial effect of Bible study group or prayer group participation on health that emerge from a study may reflect the influence of these unmeasured selection factors rather than the effects of Bible study group or prayer group participation per se. As this simple example reveals, models that are designed to study the influence of Bible study groups and prayer groups on health must be constructed with great care.

Formal Relationships in Church Volunteer Programs

Researchers have wrestled with deriving a good definition of volunteering for some time. Wilson (2000) defines volunteering as "any activity in which time is given freely to benefit another person, group, or organization" (215). He goes on to point out, but does not necessarily agree with the notion, that some researchers maintain that efforts to help others may still be considered volunteering even if the volunteer is compensated for his or her efforts. There are, however, at least two problems with this definition. First, if volunteering involves any activity that benefits another person, then it becomes impossible to distinguish between volunteer work and informal social support even though the two are clearly not the same. Second, the notion that a person may be compensated for his or her efforts seems to violate the underlying spirit or essence of volunteering; it should, as Wilson (2000) points out, be given freely. In fact, as discussed later in this section, the fact that volunteer work is given freely may be one reason why older people derive health-related benefits from performing volunteer activities. Recognizing that a perfect definition does not exist, two factors are used in the current chapter to define volunteering in the church: (1) first, it is the provision of assistance to others through formal programs that are operated by the church, and (2) this assistance is given freely, without the receipt of monetary or other material compensation for such efforts.

The discussion that follows is divided into four main sections. First, data are presented on how often older people perform volunteer work and how often they do so in religious institutions. Second, research is examined that focuses on the relationship between performing volunteer activities and physical as well as mental health. Third, efforts to explain the potentially beneficial relationship between volunteering and health are reviewed. Fourth, a series of methodological and conceptual challenges is identified in an effort to set the agenda for further research in this field.

Engaging in Volunteer Activities during Late Life

Data from two studies suggest that older people are deeply involved in volunteer activities and that a good deal of this work is likely to take place in religious institutions. The first study was done by investigators in the Department of Labor (2002). However, the findings from this study suggest that determining whether older people are more likely to volunteer than younger people is not as simple as it may seem initially. More specifically, different conclusions about age differences in volunteering emerge depending upon how volunteer work is operationally defined. If volunteer work is measured solely in terms of whether a person is involved in it or not, then the data suggest that most volunteer work appears to be done by people aged thirty-five to forty-four (i.e., 34.4 percent of the people in this age group perform volunteer activities), whereas people who are aged sixty-five and older are among the least likely to volunteer (22.7 percent). In fact, only people between the ages of twenty and twenty-four have lower rates of volunteering (18.2 percent).

But a different picture emerges when volunteering is defined in terms of the total number of hours spent helping others. When operationalized in this manner, people aged sixty-five and older appear to be the most involved in helping others. More specifically, the data suggest that people in this age group spend approximately ninety-six hours per year volunteering. People in the next closest age group (those who are between fifty-five and sixty-four years of age) spend significantly less time helping others (about sixty hours per year).

Taken as a whole, the data on age differences in volunteering provided by the Department of Labor (2002) suggest that older people may be less likely than younger people to become involved in volunteer work. However, if older adults decide to volunteer, then they spend more time helping others than individuals in any other age group.

If the participants in the Department of Labor (2002) survey indicated that they performed volunteer work, they were asked to identify where these activities were performed. Data were provided on age differences in eight different types of organizations ranging from civic organizations to hospitals, secular community service organizations, and religious institutions. The pattern of findings is intriguing. The data reveal that if older people engage in volunteer work, they are especially likely to do so within the context of a religious institution. More specifically, the findings suggest that 45.2 percent of all volunteers aged sixty-five and over helped others through religious institutions. The second most frequent setting for people in this age group was secular community service organizations (17.6 percent).

Data on volunteer work were recently updated in a report issued by the Corporation for National and Community Service (2006). The investigators in this organization used data from the 1974, 1989, and 2005 Current Population Surveys (CPS) that were administered by the U.S. Census Bureau. Because data were available at multiple points in time, these researchers were able to chart trends in volunteering over time. They report that rates of volunteering declined overall from 1974 to 1989, but then rose sharply by 2005. In fact, as of 2005, the rate of volunteering reached an all-time high. Some interesting age differences emerged in these overall trends as well. The data suggest that even though the overall rate of volunteering declined from 1974 to 1989, the volunteer rate for people aged sixty-five and over actually increased during this time. In fact, these investigators report that the rate of volunteering among older adults has been on an upward trajectory through the past three decades, growing from 14.3 percent in 1974 to 23.5 percent in 2005.

Two additional findings from the survey by the Corporation for National and Community Service (2006) are important because they replicate and extend those reported by the Department of Labor (2002). First, when defined in terms of hours of volunteer service provided per year, older adults in 2005 are more likely to perform one hundred hours of volunteer work annually than individuals in any other age group. In addition, the proportion of people of all ages who performed volunteer work in religious institutions has declined over time, but the proportion of older adults volunteering through religious institutions has held steady. In fact, 45.5 percent of older people who performed volunteer work in 2005 did so through a religious organization. This figure is remarkably close to the 45.2 percent figure reported by the Department of Labor (2002).

The fact that older adults are especially likely to perform volunteer work through religious institutions makes sense for three reasons. First, as discussed in chapter 1, research consistently shows that people who are currently older are more involved in religion than people who are presently young (Barna 2002). Second, virtually all the major world religions (especially Christianity) place a heavy emphasis on helping others (Princeton Religion Research Center 1994). Third, religious institutions frequently have a range of formal programs in place that are geared specifically toward helping people who are in need (Trinitapoli 2005). Therefore, if older people are more involved in religion, and religion encourages people to help others, and places of worship provide the opportunity to become involved in a range of volunteer programs, it is not surprising to find that older people are especially inclined to perform volunteer work within the context of a religious institution.

Earlier, when age differences in religion were discussed in chapter 1, the problem of distinguishing between age and cohort effects was examined. The report by the Corporation for National and Community Service (2006) provides some interesting findings with respect to age versus cohort differences in volunteering. Previous research cited in this report indicates that people born between 1910 and 1930 (i.e., members of the so-called Greatest Generation) were more likely than members of previous generations to volunteer once they reached age sixty-five. However, the youngest members of the Greatest Generation are now seventy-five years old, and due to increasing health problems, their involvement in volunteer work has declined. Even so, rates of volunteering among older adults continue to grow. This suggests that members of succeeding generations (i.e., those born between 1931 and 1945—the so-called Silent Generation) have continued to volunteer at a rate comparable to that of the Greatest Generation when members of this cohort were at their peak. Viewed broadly, these findings provide some preliminary evidence that age differences in volunteer work may represent an age rather than a cohort effect. Even so, distinguishing between age and cohort effects is a difficult task; as a result, a considerable amount of work needs to be done to resolve this issue conclusively.

Volunteer Work, Health, and Well-Being in Late Life

A number of studies have been conducted to examine the relationship between engaging in volunteer activities, health, and well-being. However, not all of this research has focused on volunteering through the church, and many studies do not focus specifically on older adults. Nevertheless, a preliminary sense of whether volunteering at church may have health-related benefits for older people may be gleaned by selectively reviewing some of this extant literature.

Some of the better research on volunteering comes from Musick and Wilson (2003). Three findings from their study are especially important. First, these investigators report that performing volunteer work at the baseline survey was associated with fewer symptoms of depression at the Wave 3 follow-up. However, these findings emerged only among people age sixty-five and older. Second, their results reveal that performing volunteer work in religious institutions was more strongly associated with a decline in depressive symptoms than volunteer work that was performed in secular organizations. But once again, this effect was observed only among individuals who were at least sixty-five years of age. Finally, Musick and Wilson (2003) examined the relationship between sustained volunteer activities and depressive symptoms. A measure of sustained volunteer work was devised by taking a simple count of whether a respondent reported performing volunteer work at the Wave 1, 2, and 3 interviews. The findings reveal that sustained volunteer work benefits individuals in all age groups, but the effects were significantly greater for people age sixty-five and over.

The finding that older adults may enjoy greater health-related benefits from volunteering than younger people is supported by a longitudinal study by Van Willigen (2000). The data from this study suggests that compared to younger adults, older people who perform volunteer work are more likely to report a greater increase in life satisfaction over time.

Consistent with the findings that have been reviewed so far, research by Thoits and Hewitt (2001) reveals that volunteering exerts a potentially beneficial influence on depressive symptoms, happiness, and life satisfaction. However, their research further reveals that people with an initially greater sense of well-being were more likely subsequently to perform more hours of volunteer work than individuals who had a diminished sense of psychological well-being at the baseline survey. Thoits and Hewitt (2001) went on to argue that a self-selection bias may be at work whereby people with initially good mental health are more likely to become involved in volunteer work in the first place. However, Wilson (2000) provides another way to look at findings such as these. He argues that potential causal effects, such as those reported by Musick and Wilson (2003), and self-selection effects, such as those observed by Thoits and Hewitt (2001), are not necessarily mutually exclusive and that they may instead be mutually reinforcing. In particular, Wilson (2000) suggests, "Volunteering improves health, but it is also most likely that healthier people are more likely to volunteer. Good health is preserved by volunteering; it keeps healthy volunteers healthy" (232). The notion that various facets of religion may do more than merely help people avoid developing new physical and mental health problems is examined in greater detail later in this chapter, when discussing programs for the homebound.

In addition to promoting better mental health, some evidence exists that performing volunteer work may also exert a positive influence on physical health. For example, a longitudinal study by Luoh and Herzog (2002) with older adults reveals that older people who performed at least one hundred hours of volunteer work annually tend to rate their health more favorably over time and experience fewer problems with physical functioning over time than older adults who do not volunteer as often.

But perhaps the most convincing evidence of the impact of volunteering on health may be found in two studies that examined the relationship between volunteering and mortality. The first study was conducted by Musick, Herzog, and House (1999). Two important findings emerged from this work. First, the data suggest that older people (i.e., those age sixty-five and over) who do volunteer work were less likely to die over the eight-year study follow-up period than older adults who did not engage in volunteer activities. Second, the findings reveal that the benefits of volunteering were most evident among older people who had relatively little informal contact with others, suggesting that volunteering may perform a compensatory function whereby it tends to offset the otherwise noxious effects of social isolation.

The second study on volunteering and mortality was conducted by Oman, Thoresen, and McMahon (1999). Like Musick et al. (1999), Oman and his colleagues found that people age fifty-five and older who do volunteer work tend to live longer than individuals who do not help others in this way. However, it is especially important for the purposes of the current chapter to note that the work of Oman et al. (1999) further

reveals that the beneficial effects of volunteering on mortality are especially evident among people who are more deeply involved in religion
(see also Luoh & Herzog 2002).

Explaining the Link between Volunteering in the Church and Health

The research that has been reviewed up to this point suggests
that older people are more likely to spend more time performing volunteer work than younger people, and older adults are more likely to volunteer in programs that are operated by the church. Moreover, there is
some evidence that older people who perform volunteer work are likely
to enjoy better mental and physical health, and they are less likely to die
than individuals who are not involved in volunteer programs. Although
much more research is needed, it is important to reflect on how the
potential health-related benefits of doing volunteer work in the church
may arise. Earlier, the work of Reissman (1965) was evoked to explain
the health-related benefits of providing informal support to others (see
chap. 2). The factors discussed by Reissman (1965) (e.g., an enhanced
sense of self-esteem) may also help explain how volunteer work provides
health-related benefits; however, no effort is made to review the work of
Reissman (1965) again. Instead, five potentially important mechanisms
that have not been discussed up to this point are examined here.

First, people encounter a number of role losses when they enter late
life. For example, many people retire by age sixty-five, their children
reach adulthood and move out of the home, and many older people
experience the death of a family member (especially a spouse) or close
friend. Volunteer work helps fill the social void created by these late-
life role exits. In fact, this function is consistent with the basic tenets of
one of the long-standing theoretical perspectives in social gerontology:
activity theory (Havighurst, Neugarten, & Tobin 1968). According to
this perspective, most people do not want to disengage from society as
they grow older. Instead, they prefer to remain active, and they do so by
finding activities that substitute for the ones they have given up either
through role loss or declining health. As Wilson (2000) puts it, volunteer work helps "inoculate" older people from the deleterious effects of
role losses and age-related decline.

The second explanation for the link between volunteering and health
may be found in the work of Wilson (2000). Based on the basic principles of exchange theory, Wilson (2000) cites several studies suggesting
that some people volunteer because they feel they have received much

in life, and they want to give back something for all these blessings. The notion of giving back for things one has received in the past is consistent with, and extended by, Erikson's (1959) notion of generativity. This refers to helping, supporting, and developing members of younger generations. According to Erikson (1959), generativity grows in salience and strength through young adulthood and midlife, but then tapers off to a certain extent when people reach late life. However, an empirical study by McAdams, Aubin, and Logan (1993) found no difference in generativity between young, middle-aged, and older adults. Because some church-based volunteer groups are designed to help younger people, they provide an opportunity for older people to engage in generativity, as discussed by Erikson (1959). Focusing on generativity is important because the extensive program of research by Vaillant (2002) reveals it is associated with better mental health in late life (see also Westermeyer 2004).

Third, many older adults do not have direct contact with individuals who are in dire need (e.g., people who are desperately poor or individuals suffering from HIV). Instead, most older people live in relatively comfortable settings (Schulz 2001). Because social networks and congregations tend to be relatively homogenous with respect to social class (McPherson et al. 2001), the informal help that older adults typically give is provided to social network members who are living in relatively comfortable settings as well. Nevertheless, as discussed in chapter 2, older support providers are likely to derive health-related benefits from the informal assistance they provide to people who are like themselves. In contrast, volunteer groups that some churches operate provide a forum in which relatively well-to-do elders can come into contact with and assist individuals who are facing extraordinarily difficult circumstances and are therefore often not like themselves. This is an especially important issue because, as Wilson (2000) points out, highly educated elders more especially likely to volunteer. It is important to see if the benefits of helping those with the greatest needs are enjoyed by people with the greatest advantages or whether those who have relatively little benefit the most from helping individuals who are in need. In the process, it would be important to determine if the health-related benefits that arise from volunteering are commensurate with the needs of the help recipient.

Fourth, as discussed in chapter 2, providing informal assistance to others often requires certain social skills; older support providers must know how to approach someone in need, and they must know how to provide assistance in a way that is sensitive to the needs and perspective of the recipient. Otherwise, help that is offered with the best of intentions may ultimately be ineffective. The structure provided by formal volunteer programs may help older support providers avoid these problems because a clear protocol for contacting and delivering assistance is often firmly in place. Because this protocol is understood by both the support provider and the support recipient, the odds that helping behaviors will go awry are likely to be reduced, which may, in turn, help ensure that the benefits of assisting others will be forthcoming.

Fifth, support that is provided through volunteer programs is often given without any expectation of repayment. In fact, in many instances, repayment is not possible. This point is important because selfless giving (i.e., helping without repayment) is a core tenet of the Christian faith. Complying with this core tenet may provide a number of mental health benefits, such as an increased sense of life satisfaction and an elevated mood.

Conceptual and Methodological Challenges

Although research on volunteering, religion, and health has provided some exciting findings, a great deal of work remains to be done. Six issues that may help move research in this area forward are reviewed briefly below.

First, more research is needed on the relationship between religion and the decision to perform volunteer work, especially when it is provided through the church. So far, many studies that examine the factors that influence volunteering do not differentiate between volunteering in church and volunteering in secular programs (see Wilson 2000, for a review of this research). Moreover, even when investigators examine the factors that influence volunteering in the church, they typically rely on crude measures of religion, such as the frequency of church attendance (e.g., Okun & Michel 2006). As discussed in chapter 1, work on the measurement of religion has moved far beyond simple indicators like the frequency of church attendance. Consequently, it is important to bring other facets of religion to the foreground. For example, Allport (1966) distinguished between extrinsic and intrinsic religious orientations. An extrinsic orientation refers to religious behaviors and beliefs that are motivated by utilitarian motives, such as the acquisition of social status, whereas an intrinsic religious orientation arises from a selfless dedication to basic religious principles. Perhaps older people with an intrinsic religious orientation are more likely to benefit from participating in church-based volunteer programs because they are helping others out of a genuine sense of commitment and concern. Examining this relationship may provide one reason why research reveals that an intrinsic religious orientation is associated with greater psychological well-being (e.g., Genia 1996).

Second, if various facets of religion affect volunteering (which seems highly likely), and these various aspects of religion are related to better health, then researchers need to know if volunteering is a root cause of good health per se or whether volunteering merely reflects the influence of other dimensions of religion. At its base, this is a model specification issue. Researchers need to decide whether the relationship between volunteering in the church and health is best studied by estimating single-equation models that control for the effects of other religious factors, like intrinsic religiousness, or if this issue is best handled within a causal modeling framework, where factors like intrinsic religiousness affect volunteering, and volunteering, in turn, leads to better health. The latter strategy makes more sense because it provides the opportunity to derive explicit estimates of the indirect effects of intrinsic religiousness that operate through volunteering, thereby providing greater insight into how various facets of religion operate together to influence health and well-being in late life.

Third, more research is needed on the relative contribution of providing informal support and volunteer work on the health of older people. Krause, Herzog, and Baker (1992) examined the effects of providing informal support to others and volunteering on depressive symptoms. They report that informal help, but not volunteer work, was associated with fewer symptoms of depression in late life. However, these investigators did not study informal support that was provided specifically in religious settings, nor did they explicitly compare and contrast the effects of secular volunteer programs and volunteer programs that are offered through the church. If it turns out that helping others through formal volunteer programs in the church has the most beneficial effect on health, then researchers will have found the basis for developing more targeted interventions to improve the health and well-being of older people.

Fourth, pitting informal support in the church against volunteer work in the church to see which has the greatest effects on health is not the only, or perhaps not even the best way to approach the study of different venues for helping people who are in need. Perhaps greater insight may be obtained by evaluating the joint effects of engaging in both types of helping behavior. More specifically, researchers need to know if engaging both in volunteer work in church and in providing informal assistance to their fellow congregants has a greater impact on health than either of these factors taken alone. This specification calls for the estimation of a statistical interaction effect between performing volunteer work in the church and providing informal support to fellow church members on health.

Fifth, so far, all of the studies on volunteering focus solely on the behavior of a single individual. However, interesting insights may emerge when volunteering is studied in dyads. So, for example, both an older husband and wife may participate in the same volunteer program at church. Perhaps the shared participation in this activity serves to strengthen the bond between them, which may happen for several reasons. To begin with, because both participate in volunteering, they both obviously value this activity. Therefore, seeing a close other engage in an activity that a focal person values highly should raise the level of respect that the focal person feels toward the other. In addition, because both members of a dyad are involved in the same program, they can serve as a source of encouragement for each other, and they can serve as an informed resource for working out problems that inevitably arise in any formal activity. Working through mutual problems and serving as a source of encouragement and support in the process may serve to strengthen the relationship between them.

Sixth, there are ways to donate time and effort in the church that do not involve volunteering specifically to help people who are in need. For example, older people may assume a number of formal roles that are essential for the smooth functioning of the church, such as deacon or elder, as well as lay minister or chair of key church committees. Because both activities fit the definition of volunteering provided earlier, seeing whether both types of volunteer work have a beneficial effect on health is important. Moreover, it is important to know whether one type of volunteer work conveys greater health benefits than the other. On the one hand, the basic tenets of activity theory suggest that both types of volunteer activity should provide health benefits because they both provided the opportunity for greater social involvement in late life (Havighurst et al. 1968). In contrast, it may turn out that helping people who are specifically in need has a greater effect on health because doing so complies with core tenets of the faith.

Formal Assistance for the Homebound

A number of older adults are unable to participate in formal church activities (e.g., worship services) because they are either too ill to do so or because they are providing care for a family member or friend who is suffering from a physical or mental health problem. Unfortunately, it is hard to find precise estimates of the number of older people who are homebound for these reasons. However, indirect evidence suggests it may be a significant problem. More specifically, the fact that many congregations offer formal services that cater to the needs of homebound church members suggests there is a substantial need. For example, Knapp (2001) conducted a survey of 753 Church of Christ churches to study the nature and extent of the formal services they provide to their older church members. His data suggest that 79 percent of the congregations provide visits to shut-ins and 53 percent provide Communion in the homes of older people. More recently, Trinitapoli (2005) analyzed data from the National Congregations Survey, which gathered data from 1,236 theologically diverse congregations across the United States. Her findings suggest that home visitation is the most frequently provided formal support program for older adults. Further support for the findings provided by Knapp (2001) and Trinitapoli (2005) may be found in unpublished analyses from the RAH Survey. These data suggest that 22.7 percent of the older people in this nationwide survey report that they attended church one or twice a year or less. Moreover, of this group, 33.7 percent reported that they maintained contact with either the pastor or the members of a congregation, and 27.9 percent of those who maintained contact with a congregation indicated that church members came to their home to help them worship. When congregations provide services that attend to the need of homebound elders, the opportunity to form a unique type of formal social relationship arises.

Because providing help to homebound church members may be construed as a particular type of church-based volunteer work, it is important to discuss why a separate section in this chapter was set aside for this type of activity. There are two reasons why providing help to homebound church members was not examined in the previous section where a range of church-based volunteer activities were discussed. First, as the study by Knapp (2001) reveals, church-based programs for shut-ins are often (but not always) provided solely for fellow church members, whereas more general volunteer activities often involve the provision of assistance to people who are not fellow congregants. Second, the discussion of more general volunteer activities in the previous section focused solely on the health-related benefits that accrue to volunteers from helping others, but an emphasis is placed in the discussion that follows on the benefits that formal church-based support may provide for older shut-ins themselves (i.e., the help recipients).

The discussion that follows begins by exploring the ways in which participation in formal church programs for the homebound may be associated with the health and well-being of older service recipients. Following this, methodological and conceptual issues are examined that confront researchers who wish to study the effects of formal church services for the homebound.

Formal Programs for the Homebound and Health in Late Life

Although it is important to focus on the health-related benefits that may arise from participating in programs that are designed to minister to the needs of homebound elders, this issue cannot be evaluated properly without taking a second issue into consideration. More specifically, researchers must reflect carefully on the best way to assess health-related outcomes when conducting this type of research. Both issues are examined closely below.

The Health-Related Benefits of Programs for Homebound Elders. There are at least three ways in which participating in church-related programs for the homebound may provide health-related benefits for older help recipients. First, these formal programs may help older people who are homebound confront problems associated with loneliness. Second, taking part in church programs for the homebound may provide respite for those who care for someone who is ill, which may affect the quality of care that older people receive from their caregivers, thereby further enhancing their health. Third, church-related programs for the homebound may help older people strengthen and maintain their faith. The literature on the health-related effects of church-based programs for the homebound is vastly underdeveloped, and as a result, there do not appear to be any studies that empirically evaluate the mechanisms discussed below.

Research reveals that people who suffer from chronic health problems are more likely to be homebound and, therefore, more likely to feel lonely than individuals who do not have a chronic illness (see Beal 2006, for a review of this research). Similarly, a number of studies indicate that individuals who are primary caregivers are also more likely to feel lonely than people who are not caring for someone who suffers from a physical or mental health problem (Ekwall, Sivberg, & Hallberg 2005). Loneliness is defined as "the generalized lack of satisfying personal, social, or community relationships" (Andersson, 1998, 265). Loneliness is an important issue to consider in late life because it has been linked with a wide range of health-related outcomes. Research indicates that people who are lonely are more likely to experience symptoms of depression (Cacioppo, Hughes, Waite, Hawkley, & Thisted 2006), elevated systolic blood pressure levels (Hawkley, Masi, Berry, & Cacioppo 2006), a decline in food intake, and a loss of motivation to eat (Donini, Savina, & Cannella 2003). Moreover, a number of studies suggest that older people who are lonely are more likely to commit suicide (Waern, Rubenowitz, & Wilhelmson 2003), and they are at greater risk for premature death (Meller, Fichter, & Schroppel 2004). The regular social contact afforded by participation in church-based programs for the homebound and the social relationships that are likely to emerge as a result of this interaction may go a long way toward alleviating feelings of loneliness among older shut-ins.

Although precise estimates are difficult to obtain, research suggests that as many as 52 million individuals provide care to a disabled family member or friend annually (Schulz & Martire 2004). Moreover, this research further reveals that caregivers experience a wide range of physical and mental health problems (Schulz, Newsom, & Mittelmark 1997). Consequently, it is hardly surprising to find that a number of interventions have been devised to help alleviate the deleterious effects associated with caregiving. Although these interventions involve a number of different strategies and techniques, one procedure that has received significant attention is respite care, which involves temporarily relieving the caregiver of his or her duties in order to provide a break from the heavy demands encountered on a daily basis. Although evaluation of respite care is complex, the literature generally suggests that it has beneficial effects for caregivers (Jeon, Brodaty, & Chesterson 2005). As Richards (2003) discusses, regular visits by church members through formal programs for shut-ins may provide time for older women and men to get away from their caregiving duties. In fact, the regular social interaction these visits provide may prove to be a valuable source of respite in its own right.

The third benefit of relationships that arise in formal church programs for the homebound may be found by returning to the data presented earlier. Recall that unpublished data from the RAH Survey reveal that 27.9 percent of people who do not go to church often report that church members come to their home to help them worship. Many times this may take the form of administering Communion, or it may involve the provision of audiotapes or videotapes of church services. Providing religiously focused services to the homebound may help homebound elders maintain their faith. Support for the notion that continued participation in religious rituals helps to maintain one's faith may be found in the work of Whitehouse and McCauley (2005) on the cognitive foundations of religion. These investigators argue that repetition of religious rituals serves to enhance semantic memory for religious principles and teachings, thereby keeping them salient and fresh in the minds of participants. This point is important, because there is an extensive amount of evidence which suggests that participation in religious rituals is associated with better physical and mental health across the life course (Koenig, McCullough, & Larson 2001).

Identifying Health-Related Outcomes in Research on Church Programs for the Homebound. Initially, it might appear as though research on participation in formal programs for homebound elders and health should be conducted by merely correlating involvement in these programs with the presence or absence of some physical or mental health problem among the help recipients. If the theoretical issues discussed in the previous section are valid, this research should show that involvement in formal church programs helps homebound elders avoid becoming ill. But if a number of people are shut-in because they already suffer from physical health problems, then this may not be the best way to proceed. Instead, researchers may more profitably spend their time by seeing whether involvement in programs for the homebound improves the health of older people who are already experiencing physical health problems. Clearly, the two issues are not the same. This discussion points to a broader problem in the literature on religion and health. More specifically, as Levin (1996b) points out, many studies on religion and health are solely concerned with whether involvement in religion helps people avoid becoming ill. However, he goes on to argue that religion may also help those who are already sick recover from their physical health problems. This is not a new issue. Over four decades ago, John Cassel, a prominent social epidemiologist, raised the same concern when he pointed to a significant gap in research on psychosocial risk factors and health: "greater attention must be given to the possibility that those sets of 'causes' which are responsible for the onset of conditions may be very different from those responsible for the lack of recovery from those conditions" (Cassel 1964, 1486). Cassel (1964) went on to argue that the study of factors that inhibit or promote recovery from existing physical health problems "has not yet found general acceptance" (1486). Unfortunately, this is still true today.

In view of these insights, it appears that not one, but two questions need to be addressed when studying the potential health-related benefits of participating in formal church programs for the homebound. First, do these programs improve the health of those who are already suffering from some sort of physical health problem? Second, because some people who are homebound are not ill themselves but are instead caring for someone who has health problems, does participation in formal church programs for the homebound help caregivers avoid developing new physical diseases?

The notion that programs can improve the health of homebound elders who are sick makes a good deal of sense, but another way to think about this issue further extends the scope of inquiry. Many of the illnesses that are experienced by homebound elders are chronic, and as a result, recovery is not a likely option. So it is important to reflect on how the health of these elders might be affected by church-based programs for older shut-ins. Instead of helping these elders recover from an illness, perhaps relationships that are formed with church members who work in programs for the homebound merely slow the downward progression of a chronic disease. The empirical assessment of this issue has implications for the way data are collected and analyzed. More specifically, in order to see whether help for the homebound slows the downward progression of chronic conditions, researchers must obtain multiple assessments of an older person's health over fairly extended periods of time. Three observations are the minimum that is needed, but more would provide greater data analytic flexibility. Then, individual growth curves could be estimated to identify trajectories of change in health over time (Raudenbush & Bryk 2002). Following this, researchers could see whether participation in programs for the homebound is associated with a more gradual decline in a given chronic condition, whereas trajectories of decline are more steep and accelerated for older people who do not participate in this type of church program.

Conceptual and Methodological Challenges

Because so little empirical work has been done in the field, a number of challenges face researchers who wish to study the health-related effects of church-based programs for elderly members who are homebound. Three issues are examined below that may help move research in this area forward.

First, research was discussed in chapter 1 which indicates that attendance at formal worship services is associated with better health. In fact, as pointed out in that chapter, this relationship is perhaps the most well-documented in the literature on religion and health. Although it is difficult to identify the underlying aspects of participating in church services that drive this relationship, one possibility is that the very act of worship itself conveys health-related benefits. For example, perhaps the positive emotions that arise when taking Communion exert a direct beneficial effect on the immune system. To the extent that this is true, researchers who study the effects of help for the homebound are faced with an interesting data analytic and conceptual challenge. Assume that a member of a congregation goes out to the dwelling of a homebound elder in order to help that person celebrate Communion. It will be difficult to tell if health-related benefits of these visits are due to the helping relationship that is formed with the visitor from church or whether the positive health outcomes arise from the opportunity to take Communion. In order to address this issue, two sets of measures must be devised and contrasted data analytically. First, researchers must ask if someone from church visits a homebound elder in order to help them celebrate Communion. Second, questions must be devised that ask about specific aspects of the relationship that is formed with the visiting church member. Then the effects of the two types of measures on health can be compared and contrasted using multivariate data analytic procedures.

Second, a number of secular programs have been developed to help older shut-ins, such as the Friendly Visitor Program (Denney 1988). Researchers need to know if church-based programs for homebound elders are more effective than secular programs or whether the secular programs are just as likely to improve the physical or mental health of homebound older people. Much like the research on secular and church-based informal social support discussed in chapter 2, this type of study can go a long way toward demonstrating whether something is truly unique about social relationships that develop in the church.

Third, in order to estimate correctly the relationship between social ties that arise from church-based programs for shut-ins and health in late life, investigators must be sure they measure and control for other possible sources of assistance that homebound elders may be receiving. For example, research reviewed by Schulz and Martire (2004) suggests that assistance from secular programs (e.g., Alzheimer's disease associations) as well as informal social network members (i.e., family members and close friends who do not reside with the homebound elder) may provide significant benefits to those who care for older people who are shut-in.

Conclusions

As the discussion in this chapter reveals, older people may enter into relationships through formal roles in the church in a number of ways. A number of formal roles were examined, including those that arise around formal pastoral counseling services, social relationships that arise in formal Bible study groups and prayer groups, as well as volunteer groups and programs that are designed to help homebound elders. In each instance, religious and secular constructs were evoked in an effort to show how participation in these formal roles may influence the health and well-being of older adults. The religious constructs examined ranged from developing a close relationship with God to prayer expectancies, whereas the secular constructs that were linked with health and well-being ranged from hope to feelings of generativity. These theoretical formulations were coupled with a host of methodological and conceptual challenges that should be addressed if the research in the field is to move forward.

Three broad methodological and conceptual issues yet to be discussed cut across all the formal relationships discussed in this chapter. First, unlike the previous chapters, nothing has been said about how to measure social relationships that arise in formal church programs and activities. This reflects the current state of the literature. More specifically, no survey items probe the underlying nature and function of social ties that arise in formal church programs. Instead, extant measures merely reflect whether a person participates in activities like church-based volunteer programs or Bible study groups. However, as House and Kahn (1985) observed some time ago, it is necessary to distinguish between the structure and the function of social relationships. Measures that assess the structure of social ties merely capture whether a person participates in a given type of social relationship. Although having the opportunity to participate in a given type of social relationship is important, it says little about the nature, quality, and function of the social ties that may arise. This gap was encountered in the early attempts to study secular social support. Some investigators used a simple measure of marital status to assess social support. Although being married is an important determinant of whether a person will receive social support, it does not necessarily guarantee they always will, because not all marriages are supportive. So in order to move forward the study of formal social relationships in the church, researchers need to devise measures that explicitly assess the nature, quality, and functions of social ties that arise in the various formal contexts discussed in this chapter. Perhaps the best way to proceed is to conduct a detailed series of qualitative studies similar to those used in the RAH Survey (Krause 2002a).

Second, greater insight into the nature of formal church-based social relationships may be obtained by delving into the underlying motives that people have for engaging in them. The informal social relationships discussed in chapters 2 (social support) and 3 (church-based companion friendships) are likely to be driven, at least in part, by interpersonal attraction. Moreover, older people have a fair degree of latitude in selecting the specific church members with whom to form supportive or friendship ties. But these factors are less likely to play a major role in formal relationships that arise in the church. Older people do not play a role in determining who attends Bible study groups and prayer groups, nor do older adults who participate in church-based volunteer programs choose the specific individuals they will help. Moreover, it seems that interpersonal attraction plays a less important role in determining the development of various types of formal relationships in the church. Instead, formal relationships in the church are more likely to arise from a deep sense of religious motivation and commitment. For example, the primary motive to participate in Bible study groups and prayer groups is likely to involve the desire to learn more about and deepen one's faith. In addition, people are likely to participate in formal church volunteer programs because they are committed to religious principles that involve helping others who are in need. Religious motivation and commitment are likely also to influence informal ties in the church, but the role played by religious motivation and commitment is likely to be even more evident in formal church-based social relationships. Researchers have been studying religious motivation and commitment for decades (e.g., Hoge 1972), but relatively little effort has been made to see if religious commitment and motivation are related to health and well-being in late life. Studying religious commitment in the context of formal church-based social relationships provides an important opportunity to address this gap in the literature. It is not difficult to imagine a causal model in which religious motivation and commitment affect participation in formal relationships in the church, and formal church-based social ties, in turn, affect health and well-being through the mechanisms discussed throughout the current chapter. Devising and testing this kind of causal model would provide an exciting opportunity to ground research on religious motivation and commitment in the health arena, thereby demonstrating the applicability and utility of these fundamental aspects of religion.

Third, when viewed from a distance, the wide range of issues and conceptual formulations discussed in this chapter may create the sense that the literature on formal relationships in the church is in a sense of disarray; it may seem that there are too many loose ends and that the formal ties investigated in this chapter are at best loosely integrated. However, a broader issue helps bind into a tighter whole the various types of formal roles in the church. This issue was identified by Wuthnow (1994). He writes, "If there is a single key to spiritual development that takes place in groups, it is not so much the dynamics of the whole group or the information given by the leader, but the one-on-one relationships that develop between individuals in the group. They become special friends" (Wuthnow 1994, 270). Simply put, one of the greatest contributions of engaging in formal roles in the church may involve the close informal relationships they tend to promote, especially the kinds of informal ties discussed in chapters 2 and 3.

A key issue that arises at this juncture involves specifying how close informal ties emerge in the process of occupying formal roles in the church. Although very little is known about this process, some valuable insights may be found in the work of Rook (1991). She argues that close informal relationships evolve slowly and cautiously as individuals carefully feel each other out and gradually reveal more intimate notions about themselves once they feel the shared social environment is safe. This idea is not new. Seneca was a Stoic philosopher born around 4 BCE. He offered the following advice when forming new friendships: "Those people who...judge a man after they have made him their friend instead of the other way around certainly put the cart before the horse. Think for a long time whether or not you should admit a given person to your friendship" (Seneca 2004, 34). Rook (1991) helps show how this may take place in the context of formal roles in an organization. She maintains that non-intimate shared activities, such as volunteer activities, provide an arena in which the cautious and fragile process of developing informal relationships, such as close companion friendships, may unfold. More specifically, she maintains, "Such shared activities...allow participants to make discreet assessments of each other's suitability as potential friends, avoiding awkwardness and self-consciousness that can accompany an explicit focus on the extent of mutual attraction" (105).

As the discussion provided by Wuthnow (1994) and Rook (1991) reveals, the task facing investigators who wish to study social relationships in the church is complicated by the fact that they must not only investigate the various kinds of social ties individually; they must also take into account the ways in which one type of social relationship in the church may give rise to another. This, in turn, presents further challenges for the study of church-based social ties and health because investigators must find ways to tease out the unique contributions of each type of social relationship as well as the potentially important joint benefits they may provide. Social and behavioral scientists often neatly partition the social world into various conceptual domains, such as formal and informal social ties in the church. Yet these distinctions are largely artificial because they are experienced as a seamless whole in the daily lives of older people. As a result, something is likely to be lost when these various types of social relationships are viewed in isolation from each other. It is important to keep this fundamental fact firmly in mind when elaborate categorization schemes are devised that differentiate between various types of formal and informal social ties in the church.

Chapter 5

Negative Interaction in the Church

Exploring the Dark Side of Religion

Up to this point, the discussion has focused primarily on the positive or beneficial aspects of church-based social relationships. This reflects the emphasis in the literature and may be traced, in part, to the belief that church-based social ties are particularly close and especially efficacious (Ellison & Levin 1998). But some studies suggest that social relationships in the church are not always pleasant and that, at times, interaction with fellow congregants may be conflicted, undesirable, and unpleasant (e.g., Becker 1999). However, a good deal of this research does not relate negative interaction in the church with health or psychological well-being. Instead, a number of researchers have been concerned with issues like the effect of church conflicts on organizational change and the development of religious sects (Stark & Bainbridge 1987), or the predictors of conflict in the church, such as liberal versus conservative worldviews (Becker 1999). The goal of the current chapter is to address this gap in the literature by examining the ways in which interpersonal conflict in the church may affect the health and well-being of older churchgoers.

Based on insights that have emerged from studies done in secular settings (Rook 1984), negative interaction in the church is defined as unpleasant social encounters with fellow congregants that are characterized by disagreements, criticism, rejection, and invasion of privacy. Excessive helping as well as ineffective helping are included under the broad rubric of this construct as well.

Studying negative interaction and health in the church is important for two reasons. First, a fairly extensive body of research conducted in secular settings suggests that interpersonal difficulties may have an adverse effect on physical health (Krause 2005b) and psychological well-being in late life (Okun & Keith 1998). One longitudinal study of negative interaction and health in secular settings is especially noteworthy. This research, by Newsom, Mahan, Rook, and Krause (2008), uses sophisticated trait-state error models to examine the effects of stable negative interaction on health in late life over a two-year period. The findings reveal that high levels of stable negative interaction were significantly predictive of unfavorable self-rated health, greater functional disability, and a larger number of chronic and acute health conditions during the follow-up period.

The second reason for focusing on negative interaction in the church has to do with the relative magnitude of positive and negative interpersonal encounters. Some investigators maintain that the effects of negative interaction on health and well-being are greater in magnitude than the effects of positive support. For example, after reviewing research on this issue, Taylor (1991) concluded, "Negative events appear to elicit more physiological, affective, cognitive, and behavioral activity and prompt more cognitive analysis than neutral or positive events" (67; see also Okun & Keith 1998). However, this idea is not new. The essence of this perspective was captured over two hundred years ago by Adam Smith (1759/2002), who observed, "Pain...is in almost all cases, a more pungent sensation than the opposite and corresponding pleasure. The one, almost always, depresses us much more below the ordinary, or what may be called the natural state of happiness, than the other raises us above it" (141). Similar views were expressed by Schopenhauer in 1851: "As a rule, we find pleasure much less pleasurable, pain much more painful than we expected" (1851/2004, 42).

When the key characteristics of negative interaction are examined closely, it becomes evident that interpersonal conflict may be construed as a specific type of stressor. In fact, ever since the early days of survey research on stress, investigators routinely included interpersonal difficulties in checklists assessing stressful life events. For example, as discussed in chapter 1, the widely used checklist devised by Holmes and Rahe (1967) lists trouble with in-laws, trouble with the boss, and marital separation as stressful events. Viewed in this way, it can be seen that negative interaction occupies a somewhat unusual position in the literature because it is considered to be a facet of interpersonal relationships as well as a type of stress. No attempt is made to resolve this issue here, nor is it necessary to do so. Instead, negative interaction in the church is viewed as a key aspect of interpersonal relationships in the church that may have an adverse effect on the health and well-being of older church members.

The discussion that follows is divided into six main sections:

1. Issues in the measurement of informal church-based negative interaction are examined first.
2. Research suggesting that negative interaction in the church may have an adverse effect on health and well-being is presented.
3. A series of theoretical issues are explored that help explain how the pernicious effects of church-based negative interaction on health-related outcomes may arise.
4. Negative interaction with the clergy is evaluated.
5. Age-related effects of church-based negative interaction are explored after this.
6. Methodological and conceptual challenges that arise in the process of studying negative interaction in the church are identified and discussed in detail.

Measuring Negative Interaction in the Church

Two broad approaches are generally taken to assess church-based negative interaction. First, some investigators focus on interpersonal conflict that arises around institutional issues and problems that face the members of a congregation as a whole. For example, Becker (1999) examined conflict involving church finances, the format and content of worship services, as well as disagreements arising over issues involving gender (e.g., the role of women in the church) and sexuality (e.g., whether homosexuals should be welcomed into the church) (see also Krause, Chatters, Meltzer, & Morgan 2000b). Second, other studies have examined negative interaction in the church emerging around issues that are more social-psychological in nature, that are found inside and outside the church, and that primarily involve more informal aspects of social relationships. More specifically, this latter type of church-based negative interaction arises when fellow congregants are critical of each other, make too many demands on each other, are unwelcoming, and fail to provide assistance when a focal person is counting on it (e.g., Krause, Ellison, & Wulff 1998).

The current chapter focuses primarily on informal church-based conflict rather than negative interaction that arises around institutional issues. This strategy was adopted for the following reason: the overall goal of this volume is to see if church-based social relationships are associated with health and well-being. Only very limited attention has been given to the relationship between institutional religious conflict and health. In contrast, research on informal negative interaction in the church, health, and well-being is beginning to appear in the literature, and the findings from this work suggest that further investigation into the linkages involving this particular type of negative interaction is justified (e.g., Krause et al. 1998; Krause & Wulff 2005).

Only four studies appear to provide closed-ended survey items that focus exclusively on informal negative interaction in the church. Other investigators have developed indicators of interpersonal difficulties in the church, but these items have been embedded in more comprehensive scales that assess others types of religious conflicts, such as alienation from God (e.g., Exline, Yali, & Sanderson 2000; Nielsen 1998). Table 5-1 contains the indicators from the studies that focus exclusively on informal negative interaction in the church. The first set of items was developed by Pargament, Zinnbauer, Scott, Butter, Zerowin, and Stanik (1998). As shown in Table 5-1, these questions assess whether an individual had disagreements with family members and friends about religious principles and whether he or she felt that people at church failed to provide support and comfort when needed. These items are important, but they appear to mix negative interaction with people inside church (i.e., fellow church members) with interpersonal conflicts among people who may not be in the same congregation as the study participant or who may not be involved with any religious institution at all (i.e., family members and friends).

The second set of indicators that assess negative interaction in the church was developed by the Fetzer Institute/National Institute on Aging Working Group (1999). Their brief composite consists of three items. The first asks how often fellow church members make too many demands on the respondent, how often they are critical of the study participant, and how often study participants feel fellow congregants have taken advantage of them. The first two indicators were also used recently in a study by Ellison, Zhang, Krause, and Marcum (2007). Although the items in these studies take an important first step toward assessing informal negative interaction in the church, it seems unlikely that the content domain of this complex construct can be captured adequately with two or three items.

A longer, six-item scale of church-based negative interaction was devised by Krause (2002a). Evidence that the reliability of this scale is satisfactory is provided by Krause (2002b). Two of these indicators were

Table 5-1. Measures of Negative Interaction in the Church

1. Negative Interaction Items Devised by Pargament et al. (1998)[a]
   A. Family or friends spoke to me about religion in a way I didn't agree with.
   B. Argued with family or friends about faith, God, and religion.
   C. Felt that the church did not support me in my time of need.
   D. Felt angry that no church members comforted me.

2. Negative Interaction Items Devised by the Fetzer Institute/National Institute on Aging Working Group (1999)[b]
   A. How often do the people in your congregation make too many demands on you?
   B. How often are the people in your congregation critical of you and the things you do?
   C. How often do the people in your congregation try to take advantage of you?

3. Negative Interaction Items from the RAH Survey[b]
   A. How often has someone in your congregation made too many demands on you?
   B. How often are people in your congregation critical of you and the things you do?
   C. How often do people in your congregation gossip about you?
   D. How often are you bothered by cliques in your congregation?
   E. How often are people in your congregation unwelcoming to you?
   F. How often have people in your congregation failed to provide support when you were counting on it?

[a] Neither the entire question stem nor the response options are provided by Pargament et al. (1998).
[b] These items are scored in the following manner (coding in parentheses): never (1); once in a while (2); fairly often (3); very often (4).

taken from the scale devised by the Fetzer Institute/National Institute on Aging Working Group (1999), but the other four items were based on Krause's (2002a) extensive qualitative research with older people. A common theme involving inclusiveness in a congregation appears to cut across these additional items. More specifically, these indicators reflect whether others at church gossip about an older person, form cliques, are unwelcoming toward them (i.e., whether study participants felt they were accepted and wanted by the members of their congregation), and whether older church members fail to provide assistance when they are expecting to get it. As discussed later in this chapter, issues involving inclusiveness may be especially important in late life.

Preliminary unpublished analyses of the negative interaction items devised by Krause (2002a) for the RAH Survey suggest that between 7.2 percent and 17.3 percent of the study subjects indicated they experienced these unpleasant social encounters once in a while or more often. These descriptive data suggest that negative interaction in the church may be relatively rare, but as research reviewed in the next section reveals, it may nevertheless have an adverse effect on the health and well-being of older church members.

Prior Research on Negative Interaction in the Church, Health, and Well-Being

Only four studies in the literature appear to assess the impact of negative interaction in the church on health and well-being. The first study was conducted by Krause, Ellison, and Wulff (1998). These investigators analyzed data from a nationwide survey of clergy, elders, and rank-and-file members of the Presbyterian Church (USA). Negative interaction in the church was assessed with two of the items devised by the Fetzer Institute/National Institute on Aging Working Group (1999). The findings from this study reveal that greater negative interaction with fellow church members is associated with more symptoms of depression and diminished feelings of positive well-being. However, the results further indicate that negative interaction exerts a more noxious effect on clergy and elders than on rank-and-file church members. The authors explain these findings by turning to the basic tenets of identity theory (Stryker 2001; Thoits 1991). According to this theoretical perspective, people occupy multiple roles, such as father, husband, and church member. These roles are arrayed in a hierarchy reflecting the importance of the role to the individual and the amount of effort and time invested in it (Thoits 1991). As a result, identity theory specifies that problems arising in roles that are more highly valued (i.e., roles at the top of the salience hierarchy) will have a more pernicious effect on health and well-being than difficulties emerging in roles that are less important to study participants. Cast within the context of the church, the impact of negative interaction on well-being should be more pronounced among individuals who place a higher premium on religion and are more involved in it. Although there are clearly exceptions, members of the clergy and elders are likely to invest more time and effort in religion, and they are likely to be more deeply committed to religion than most rank-and-file church members. Because church-related roles are a more integral part of the identities of clergy and elders, they are therefore more likely to be troubled when they encounter negative interaction with the members of their congregations.

The second study on negative interaction in the church and health was conducted by Krause and Wulff (2005). The data for this study came from the U.S. Congregational Life Survey, a large survey of rank-and-file members of a diverse array of congregations across all fifty states. Negative interaction in the church was also assessed in this study with two items from the scale devised by the Fetzer Institute/National Institute on Aging Working Group (1999). Krause and Wulff (2005) report that people who encounter more negative interaction at church tend to be less satisfied with their health. Consistent with the observations of Taylor (1991), Smith (1759/2002), and others, Krause and Wulff (2005) found that the effects of negative interaction in the church were larger in magnitude than the corresponding impact of positive interaction (i.e., emotional support from fellow church members).

Pargament et al. (1998) conducted the third study. These investigators found that greater interpersonal religious conflict was associated with higher trait anxiety scores.

Ellison et al. (2007) conducted the fourth study, with the data from the same nationwide survey of Presbyterians that Krause et al. (1998) evaluated. However, the study by Krause et al. (1998) was based on cross-sectional data, whereas Ellison et al. (2007) used longitudinal data gathered at a later point in time. The findings from the Ellison et al. (2007) study suggest that negative interaction tends to increase or exacerbate depressive symptoms over time. In the process, these investigators show that some types of negative interaction (e.g., excessive demands) are more likely to affect depressive symptoms over time than other kinds of unpleasant interaction (e.g., criticisms) with fellow church members.

The findings from the studies that have been done so far underscore the potential importance of unpleasant interaction in the church on the health and well-being of the people who worship there. Nevertheless, this research has at least three limitations. First, the studies by Krause et al. (1998) and Ellison et al. (2007) focused solely on Presbyterians, making it difficult to tell if the findings can be generalized to people in other denominations. The second problem has to do with the age composition of the samples in all four studies. As discussed later in this chapter, negative interaction in the church may be especially troublesome for older people, but evaluating this issue directly is not possible because the samples used in the studies reviewed in this section were

comprised of adults of all ages, and no effort was made to test for age differences in the data. The final problem is that data in three of the four
studies were cross-sectional, which makes it difficult to know, for example, whether negative interaction creates more depressive symptoms, or
whether people who are initially more depressed subsequently tend to
have more interpersonal difficulty with fellow church members because
of their mental health problems.

Negative Interaction in the Church and Health: Examining Conceptual Linkages

Church-based negative interaction may exert a pernicious effect
on health and well-being through several of the mechanisms that have
been discussed in previous chapters. For example, unfavorable feedback
that arises during negative interpersonal exchanges may quite likely
have a deleterious effect on an older person's sense of self-worth. Nevertheless, consistent with the approach taken throughout this volume, an
emphasis is placed in this chapter on identifying the relatively unique
ways in which church-based negative interaction may exert an adverse
effect on the health and well-being of older people.

Researchers have identified a number of reasons why negative interaction may have a pernicious effect on health and well-being. Although
a good deal of this work focuses on negative interaction in secular settings, a number of the points that these investigators discuss apply to
negative interaction in the church as well. Because Rook (1984) is a pio-
neer in the study of negative interaction, it is fitting to begin the discussion with an overview of the explanations she offers for the relationship between unpleasant social encounters with health. Then, based on
the work of other investigators, anger and religious doubt are explored
as potentially important intervening mechanisms as well. After this, a
final mechanism is reviewed that involves the role negative interaction
may play in the decision to leave a congregation.

Rook's Theoretical Explanations

Rook and Pietromonaco (1987) provide three reasons why negative interaction arising in secular settings may have an adverse effect on
health and well-being. First, they point out that most people typically
experience a disproportionately greater amount of positive than negative interaction during the course of daily life. This creates the expectation that social relationships will continue on a desirable course. But
negative interaction tends to violate these expectancies, often stunning

the recipient. This perspective has deep roots in the literature. Writing in 1759, Smith observed, "Relations being usually placed in situations which naturally create their habitual sympathy, it is expected that a suitable degree of affection should take place among them. We generally find that it actually does take place; we therefore naturally expect that it should; and we are, upon that account, more shocked when, upon any occasion, we find that it does not" (Smith 1759/2002, 258). Because the goal of religion is to promote feelings of love, brotherhood, compassion, and forgiveness, negative interaction may be especially shocking and unanticipated when it arises within the church. These unpleasant feelings and emotions may, in turn, be associated with more physical and mental health problems.

The second explanation that Rook and Pietromonaco (1987) offer has to do with the attributions that are typically made about social interaction. When people interact, they try to make inferences about the motives of others. But as Rook and Pietromonaco (1987) maintain, one reason it is sometimes difficult to gauge the underlying motives behind positive supportive behaviors may be that people may help because they genuinely care for the recipient, or because they feel they have a duty or obligation to do so. In contrast, there is little ambiguity when negative interaction arises. The sheer force of the starkly negative and undeniable motives behind an unpleasant social encounter may be difficult to face and hard to comprehend, but they are also impossible to overlook. As a result, the motives for initiating an unpleasant encounter may foster considerable distress, especially, perhaps, with negative interaction in the church. When it arises, church members may feel bewildered, unprepared, and unable to come to grips with spiteful, malicious, and vindictive motives that deviate so blatantly from the fundamental principles of the faith.

Third, because of inherited adaptive mechanisms, Rook and Pietromonaco (1987) argue that people are especially vigilant to threats in the environment. As a result, they are more attuned to and more influenced by negative than positive social encounters. This problem may be exacerbated when negative interaction continues for some time. More specifically, as the research of Krause and Rook (2003) reveals, negative exchanges are quite stable over a six-year period, suggesting that, over time, the victim of negative interaction may experience a protracted state of hyperarousal or hypervigilance that may have an especially adverse effect on his or her health.

Anger and Hostility

Negative interaction may make people feel angry and hostile, especially when they believe it is not justified. Some insight into how this may happen in a religious context may be found by extending insights in the work of Pargament and his colleagues on sanctification theory (Pargament, Magyar, Benore, & Mahoney 2005). They maintain that some people sanctify various facets of their lives by infusing them with spiritual character and significance. Social relationships, such as marriage and other close interpersonal ties, are among the things that people sanctify. Pargament et al. (2005) go on to argue that severe undesirable consequences can arise when sanctified aspects of people's lives are either lost or violated (i.e., desecrated). Although interpersonal relationships may be desecrated in a number of ways, negative interaction may be a potentially influential factor. Pargament et al. (2005) report that the experience of desecration is associated with a range of negative outcomes, including higher levels of state anger. It seems likely that people at church may sanctify some of the relationships they establish with fellow church members, and if they do so, it follows from sanctification theory that they are likely to become angry and hurt if these relationships are desecrated by negative interaction.

The emphasis in the study by Pargament et al. (2005) on anger is noteworthy because a vast literature links anger with a wide range of physical and mental health problems (Everson-Rose & Lewis 2005). A good deal of this work is discussed in a comprehensive review by Williams (2002) that focuses on hostility, a construct that is closely akin to anger. The roots of research on hostility go back at least to the work on the type A personality (Friedman & Rosenman 1974). As studies with this construct evolved, investigators became aware that a good deal of the relationship between the type A personality and health outcomes can be explained by hostility. More specifically, Williams (2002) reports that hostility is associated with a range of physical health problems including coronary heart disease. In addition, Everson-Rose and Lewis (2005) report that anger and hostility are linked with an excess risk of hypertension as well as carotid atherosclerosis.

Williams (2002) provides a number of explanations for how the undesirable cardiovascular effects of anger and hostility arise. To begin with, greater hostility is associated with an increased incidence of health-damaging behavior, including greater intake of caffeine and the use of tobacco. He also reviews research showing that greater hostility is associated with impaired immune functioning.

Although negative interaction may promote anger, the process may be more elaborate and more subtle than it appears initially. As noted above, research by Krause and Rook (2003) suggests that negative interaction that arises in secular settings tends to be fairly stable over time; an older individual may be exposed to conflict that is protracted and ongoing, or he or she may encounter multiple bouts of interpersonal conflict. If the theoretical rationale that is presented in this section is valid, then negative emotions, such as feelings of anger, should either emerge repeatedly or continue unabated. Under these circumstances, these negative emotions may intensify, thereby exacerbating their undesirable effects.

The notion that anger may grow and intensify is not new. In fact, this possibility was of great concern to the ancient Stoic philosophers. For example, Epictetus warned, "If you have given way to anger, be sure that over and above the evil involved therein, you have strengthened the habit, and added fuel to the fire.... Habits and faculties are necessarily affected by the corresponding acts. Those that were not there before, spring up; the rest gain in strength and extent. This is the account which philosophers give of the origin of diseases in the mind" (Plato & Eliot 1909, 144). Perhaps this is one reason why Newsom et al. (2008) found that stable negative interaction exerts an especially noxious effect on the physical health of older people.

Religious Doubt

Additional insight into the relationship between negative interaction and health-related outcomes may be found by extending some of the insights in a recent paper by Park (2005). She proposes an intriguing mechanism: unpleasant interaction at church may cause some individuals to have doubts about their faith. This proposal is important because, as noted in chapter 2, a longitudinal study by Krause (2006e) reveals that greater religious doubt is associated with a diminished sense of life satisfaction, self-esteem, and optimism over time.

Although Park's (2005) hypothesis regarding the relationship between interpersonal difficulty in the church and religious doubt makes a good deal of sense, there is relatively little empirical evidence to support it, especially with respect to studies involving older adults. Fortunately, some evidence may be found in a recent study by Krause and

Ellison (2007) that is based on data from the RAH Survey. A set of analyses were performed to assess the relationship between negative interaction in the church and change in religious doubt over time. The relationship between these constructs was evaluated after controlling for a number of factors that should dispel doubts about religion. Included among these potentially protective factors were the frequency of attendance at church services, Bible study groups, and prayer groups, as well as the frequency of private prayer and spiritual support. The findings from this research reveal that more negative interaction at the baseline survey is associated with greater religious doubt at the follow-up interview. The results further indicate that older adults who encounter interpersonal conflict in the church try to cope with subsequent doubts about their faith by denying them when they arise. Perhaps older people tend to use denial as a coping strategy because the dissonance they experience when negative interaction arises in church raises painful questions about core religious principles involving compassion, helping others, and forgiveness. The emphasis on the denial of doubt in the Krause and Ellison (2007) study is important because their analyses further show that the denial of religious doubt is associated with a decline in physical health status over time.

Negative Interaction and Leaving Communities of Faith

Earlier, in chapter 1, insights from the work of Tillich (1987) were cited to underscore the social foundation of religion. More specifically, he maintained that there is no faith without a community of faith, suggesting that people who are deeply committed to religion draw their spiritual sustenance from association with like-minded religious others. But when negative interaction arises among members of a religious community, the bonds between them are threatened, and social ties that previously provided assistance and acted as a vehicle for personal growth may instead become a source of distress, consternation, and dismay. In effect, negative interaction in the church may drive a wedge between older church members and the congregation that had previously embraced them. This may, in turn, have implications for the continued practice of their faith as well as their health.

Older people may potentially react to negative interaction in the church in several ways. For example, some may sever their connection with the congregation and become apostates (i.e., abandon religion altogether), others may leave the church and join another congregation in the same denomination, whereas others may switch to a different religious denomination altogether. Although little empirical research on the topic is available, it is unlikely that many older adults abandon religion altogether and become apostates when they encounter negative interaction in their place of worship. Instead, it seems more likely that some will leave the church when conflict has arisen. Research by Loveland (2003) suggests that up to one-third of Americans switch congregations at some point in their lifetime. Unfortunately, as Spilka et al. (2003) point out, getting a good sense of why this happens is difficult. Clearly, switching congregations is a complex phenomenon that is driven by a number of factors. For example, as Loveland (2003) reports, people may switch to a different church because they marry outside their faith, because they move, or because of complex childhood socialization issues (i.e., whether their parents instilled a deep sense of faith in them when they were young). But a number of these explanatory factors do not appear to be relevant for older churchgoers. For example, rates of marriage are typically low among older people, and geographic relocation is a relatively rare event as well. Instead, some other factor must come into play during late life.

A basic premise in this chapter is that negative interaction in the church may have something to do with switching congregations or denominations in late life, but this issue has rarely been examined empirically in the literature with data from older adults. At least part of the problem arises from the fact that negative interaction in the church has not been measured directly in research on switching or leaving congregations. Nevertheless, it is not hard to see why interpersonal conflict may drive a person from a congregation, and why leaving a congregation may, in turn, be a significant source of distress. Evidence of this may be found in a qualitative study by Krause et al. (2000b). An older woman who participated in one of their focus groups described her experience with negative interaction in the following way: "It took many years to realize how these dynamics develop and how they're allowed to get out of hand and why there's a lack of tolerance in people's opinions and how certain groups seem to smother other people's opinions. They don't want any input because...it's my way or the highway....I don't think it ever heals. I think it does such emotional and spiritual damage, that while you may resume somewhere else in another church, the damage is done" (Krause et al. 2000b, 521). These observations are important because they suggest that negative interaction in the church may drive some individuals from the congregation and because interpersonal conflict may have an adverse effect on health.

Support for the insights provided by Krause et al. (2000b) may be found in two studies. The first was conducted some time ago by Hartman (1976). He studied people who left five Methodist churches and found that the most frequent reason for leaving was that study participants did not feel accepted or wanted by the people in their congregation. This reason is closely akin to one of the indicators of church-based negative interaction that is provided in Table 5-1 ("How often are the people in your congregation unwelcoming to you?").

The second study that is relevant to research on negative interaction and leaving the church was conducted by Olson (1989). He studied five Baptist churches in the suburban St. Paul–Minneapolis area. All members and regular attendees age fifteen and older participated in the study. Olson (1989) found that the number of friendships formed with fellow congregants had a fairly substantial influence on the decision to remain in the congregation. But perhaps more important for the purposes of the current chapter, Olson (1989) also reports that cliques in the church tended to depress participation, especially among individuals who had relatively few friends in the church. Once again, this issue is captured in the measures of church-based negative interaction provided in Table 5-1 ("How often are you bothered by cliques in your congregation?").

Although neither Hartman (1976) nor Olson (1989) cast their research in terms of church-based negative interaction, the close correspondence between the factors associated with church participation in their work obviously relate to this issue. Unfortunately, two methodological problems are present with the studies by Hartman (1976) and Olson (1989). First, the samples in both studies comprised five churches from the same denominations, which makes it difficult to know if the findings apply to people who are members of other denominations. Second, the samples in both studies comprised individuals of all ages, making it hard to know if the results can be generalized to older adults as well.

Although negative interaction may be associated with leaving a congregation, it is still not clear why leaving a church may, in turn, be associated with health-related outcomes, especially psychological distress. Even though pinpointing the intervening mechanisms precisely is difficult, different sets of factors may come into play for older adults who have been members of a congregation for some time and older people who are relatively new to a congregation. With respect to relatively long-time members, leaving the church may be a source of distress because it signals a loss of comfort and security that arises from knowing that social ties have been severed with people who were once a source of predictable and supportive interaction. Moreover, the feeling of being let down, of expecting support but encountering negative interaction instead, may have an especially deleterious effect on well-being. Evidence of this may be found in research that has been conducted in secular settings by Edwards, Nazroo, and Brown (1998). Their work suggests that being let down by someone who formerly was a trusted other can more than double the odds that a person will subsequently experience clinical depression.

In contrast, older people who are relatively new to a congregation may find the sense that they were never accepted and fully integrated into the group to be especially troubling because research reveals that being excluded or rejected is a significant source of distress (Williams, Forgas, & von Hippel 2005). In addition, the deep sense of disappointment arising from the realization that the underlying social principles of the faith have been violated may come into play as well. Finally, regardless of whether a person has been with a congregation for a long time or not, the sheer process of being uprooted, finding a new congregation, and becoming integrated into it may pose a significant challenge for some older people. Regardless of the factors that may be at work, the relationships among negative interaction in the church, switching congregations, and psychological distress are clearly areas that are ripe for further investigation.

Negative Interaction with the Clergy

As discussed in chapter 4, formal social relationships with members of the clergy can be an important source of health and well-being for older church members, but relationships with members of the clergy can also assume a more informal nature as well. When they do, older people may encounter the same problems that are found in informal relationships with their fellow rank-and-file church members. More specifically, informal relationships with the clergy may become conflicted and unpleasant, as is evidenced in the qualitative study by Krause et al. (2000b). One woman in their focus groups shared how stressful interaction with her pastor had become: "For one thing, he refused to let our daughter have another pastor, that we had earlier, perform her marriage ceremony. He was very strict, and there just was no reasoning with him. He did more harm than good, I think. A lot of people left" (Krause et al. 2000b, 522). Given the trusted, prestigious, and highly respected position occupied by the clergy, it is not difficult to see how conflict and negative interaction with them would be especially distressing for rank-and-file members of the congregation.

Unfortunately, very little empirical research exists on the relationship between negative interaction with the pastor and health-related outcomes in late life. Once again, few investigators have developed survey items to assess conflict with the clergy. Fortunately, Krause (2002a) devised a series of closed-ended survey questions to measure negative interaction with clergy. These indicators are provided in Table 5-2.

Members of the clergy occupy a trusted and respected position in the church for a number of reasons. However, one that was identified by Stark and Bainbridge (1987) may be especially useful for understanding how negative interaction with the clergy can affect the psychological well-being of older church members. These investigators note that almost everyone would like to live forever. Consequently, people reach out to the only source they believe can grant immortality: God. However, Stark and Bainbridge (1987) go on to point out that many individuals feel they either cannot establish direct contact with God or they cannot be certain about life after death. Therefore, they must rely on intermediaries to do this for them, thereby gaining reassurance that the immortality they seek will indeed be forthcoming. These intermediaries, whom Stark and Bainbridge (1987) call religious specialists, are, in essence, members of the clergy.

The importance of having members of the clergy who can help allay fears about death is underscored by research on terror management theory. This perspective, based on the work of Becker (1973), suggests that the motivation to deny death serves as a unifying principle that can explain a good deal of people's thoughts and actions. In fact, Becker maintains that the instinct for self-preservation coupled with the awareness of mortality can result in a paralyzing fear of death. He goes as far as to argue that one of the great rediscoveries of modern thought is "that of all things that move man, one of the principal ones is his terror of death" (Becker 1973, 11). Becker (1973) ends his volume with a discussion of the role that religion may play in the management of fear about death. It follows from this work that if people are inherently terrified of dying and members of the clergy can help them find assurance of life after death, then interpersonal conflict with members of the clergy may interfere with this vitally important function, thereby exacerbating the fear of dying.

Unpublished analysis of the relationship between negative interac-

Table 5-2. RAH Survey Items Assessing Negative Interaction with the Clergy

1. How often is your minister, pastor, or priest critical of you and the things you've done?[a]

2. How often do you disagree with your minister, pastor, or priest face-to-face about how money is spent in your church?

3. How often does your minister, pastor, or priest treat some members of your congregation better than others?

4. How often does your minister, pastor, or priest insist on doing things his or her own way?

5. How often has your minister, pastor, or priest failed to provide support when you were counting on it?

[a] These items are scored in the following manner (coding in parentheses): never (1); once in a while (2); fairly often (3); very often (4).

tion with the clergy and death anxiety were examined with the longitudinal data from the RAH Survey (Krause 2002a). Consistent with the focus in the current chapter, an index of negative interaction with the clergy was created by summing the items in Table 5-2 that deal with unpleasant encounters that arise around more personal or informal issues, including being criticized by a member of the clergy, feeling that a pastor or priest treats other members of the congregation more favorably, and feeling let down by a member of the clergy. The frequency of church attendance and private prayer as well as a number of demographic variables were also included in the analysis. The findings reveal that greater negative interaction with the clergy at the baseline survey is associated with an increase in death anxiety at the follow-up interview (Beta = .109; $p < .01$).

Negative Interaction in the Church during Late Life

There are three reasons why negative interaction in the church may have an especially noxious effect on the health and well-being of older people. The first follows directly from the study of negative interaction with the clergy and death anxiety discussed in the previous section. Because older people are closer to death than younger individuals, terror management theory would suggest that older adults should therefore have a greater fear of dying. Although it is not widely known, Erikson recognized this possibility in his work. His views on aging and death can be found in a volume of his unpublished papers edited by Hoare (2002). In this book, Hoare (2002) reports that Erikson believed that older people "can no longer repress death, they harbor fears of 'spiritual meaninglessness' and the sense of depleted time 'accentuates issues of nonbeing'" (82). Hoare (2002) goes on to point out that Erikson believed this heightened sense of death anxiety instills in older people a "wish to fuse with another, with God, with the cosmos, or with one's 'innermost self'" (82). If older people are especially fearful of dying, then the effects of conflict with the clergy, who are in a critically important position to assuage these fears, should be especially troublesome in late life.

The second reason that older people may be more vulnerable to negative interaction may be found by returning to the developmental theories of aging provided by Carstensen (1992) and Tornstam (2005). Both investigators argue that as people grow older, they tend to prefer social relationships that are especially close emotionally. If people value close emotional relationships more highly as they grow older, but encounter negative interaction instead, it follows that they should be especially disturbed by interpersonal conflict that confronts them. Moreover, this may be particularly true if negative interaction arises in the church because, as discussed in chapter 1, older people are more likely than younger people to report that religion is important in their lives. In addition, older people may be especially vulnerable to interpersonal problems that arise specifically with the clergy because research reveals that members of the current cohort of older adults (i.e., those born between 1922 and 1927) have "respect for authority...in ways previously unheard of" (Meredith & Schewe 2002, 101). Because pastors are the principal symbol of authority in the church, conflict with members of the clergy should be particularly unsettling for older people.

The third reason why negative interaction in the church may have a more pronounced effect on the health of older adults may be found by turning to long-standing issues in social and behavioral gerontology. More specifically, some investigators argue that as people enter late life, they exit a number of roles that had previously formed the cornerstone of their lives and that infused their existence with a sense of direction and purpose. For example, as people grow older they retire from the workforce, and become widowed, and their children grow up and leave the home. As noted in chapter 2, this has led some gerontologists to claim that old age is a "roleless role" (Rosow 1976). Simply put, older people may feel excluded from the flow of the wider social order. This problem is exacerbated by the fact that proper cultural apparatus is not in place to fill this vacuum, and as a result, older people are set adrift in an unpredictable and unsettling world (Baltes & Smith 2003). Fortunately, as discussed in chapter 4, the church has been a place where many elderly people have been able to find meaningful roles (e.g., volunteer activities), thereby providing them with an opportunity to feel integrated and included in society. However, if they encounter negative interaction in the church, then a valuable source of integration into the wider social order is threatened, thereby creating a heightened sense of anxiety and uncertainty.

Conceptual and Methodological Challenges

Because research on negative interaction in the church is so underdeveloped, there are numerous ways in which studies in this area can be improved. Moreover, a number of issues involving negative interaction are yet to be examined. Nine ways to enhance research on church-based negative interaction are reviewed below. Exploring these issues in detail provides further insight into the essential nature and impact of interpersonal conflict in the church.

The Genesis of Negative Interaction in the Church

First, researchers need to know more about how negative interaction arises in the church. Simply put, more studies are needed that treat church-based negative interaction as a dependent variable. The study by Becker (1999) provides an important point of departure, but it does not exhaust all the possible factors that may cause interpersonal difficulty. Tracing the genesis of negative interaction in the church is important because this kind of knowledge is essential for the development of interventions that can help heal conflict in congregations. Undoubtedly, negative interaction can emerge in a church for many reasons. As a result, reviewing them all here is not possible. Two factors that may play an important role in the genesis of negative interaction are reviewed below. In order to highlight the breadth of research that can be conducted on this issue, the first is more cognitive or psychological in nature, whereas the second has to do with the potentially important influence of wider social forces that arise from the broader social milieu of the church.

Pride is one psychological construct that may influence negative interaction in the church and which has attracted a good deal of attention in the work of religious scholars. In his insightful review of work on pride, LaMothe (2005) outlines how it has been a major concern of theologians ever since Christianity first emerged. For example, LaMothe (2005) describes how Cassian, a fourth-century desert monk, saw pride as giving rise to hatred, alienation from God, and, ultimately, spiritual death. LaMothe (2005) goes on to point out how similar negative views of pride were expressed by other well-known luminaries, such as Thomas Aquinas and Augustine.

Negative views of pride also may be found in the work of more contemporary scholars. For example, in *Mere Christianity* (1942/2001), C. S. Lewis considers pride to be the most heinous of the seven deadly sins. The reasons for taking this stance clearly arise from his concerns about the impact of pride on social relationships. More specifically, Lewis (1942/2001) maintains that pride is "*essentially* competitive—is competitive by its very nature.... Pride gets no pleasure out of having something, only out of having more of it than the next man" (122, emphasis in original). Lewis (1942/2001) goes on to point out that "power is what pride really enjoys, there is nothing makes a man feel so superior to others as being about to move them about like toy soldiers" (123). It is not difficult to see how negative interaction could be fueled by the basic characteristics of pride, including the drive to enhance the self by feeling superior to others, as well as the need to exercise power and control over social network members.

But Lewis was by no means the only contemporary scholar concerned with pride. As Cooper (2003) points out, Reinhold Niebuhr was one of the most influential theologians in American history. In his seminal work, *The Nature and Destiny of Man* (1964), Niebuhr maintained that pride is the primary problem of mankind. He went on to identify four distinct types of pride, but regardless of the type, Niebuhr (1964) saw them all leading to the same outcome. As Cooper (2003) summarizes it, "Niebuhr strongly argues that our essence as persons is in our bond with God and others. We are created for relationships. For Niebuhr, this liberates us from a frantic attempt to find satisfaction and fulfillment in ourselves" (56). Niebuhr (1964) went on to discuss how pride undermines the ability of people to develop close relationships with other individuals because it leads them to approach social relationships in a self-centered way, thereby depriving social ties of the warmth, empathy, equity, and trust they need to flourish.

Although a number of theologians have viewed pride as sinful, other, and primarily secular, scholars present a different view. In particular, they maintain that a certain amount of pride is necessary for a "healthy" sense of self-worth (Goffman 1959; Rorty 1990). Moreover, they go on to point out that pride in one's group (e.g., church, race, or nation) is also important because it can promote group solidarity, thereby enhancing the overall functioning and effectiveness of the collective.

Taken as a whole, the discussion provided so far points to a rather ambiguous view of pride in the literature. Some scholars view it as necessary and good, whereas others (especially some theologians) see pride as something that is entirely negative and that should be avoided at all cost. Perhaps, as Becker (1973) and others point out, pride becomes problematic only when it becomes grandiose and narcissistic.

Assuming that excessive pride lies at the root of the problem, it is important to delve more deeply into how it may promote negative interaction in the church. Some insights have already been provided above, but other more illuminating factors are identified by LaMothe (2005). He observes that an over-elevated sense of pride and self-worth may create a sense of "destructive hostility toward those perceived to be of lesser value" (LaMothe 2005, 244). Moreover, as LaMothe (2005) goes on to point out, an excessive sense of pride also tends to foster distrust in others, as well as feelings of irritation and resentment toward them. Unfortunately, researchers have not taken advantage of the debate on pride and conducted studies that are designed to identify whether it leads to negative interaction in the church, and ultimately, undesirable mental and physical health outcomes.

In contrast to the micro-level influence of pride on negative interaction, the wider social climate of a congregation may come into play as well. A long-standing principle in sociology stipulates that the behavior of people in institutions, such as churches, is shaped by the wider social climate in which these organizations are embedded. This view was captured succinctly by Berger and Luckman (1966), who maintain, "Institutions...by the very fact of their existence, control human conduct by setting up predefined patterns of conduct, which channel it in one direction as against many other directions that are theoretically possible" (55). Although important, this proposition is challenging to evaluate empirically because institutions may influence behavior in many ways.

Several researchers have attempted to delineate the different facets of religious institutions that may shape the behavior of the people who worship there. Pargament, Silverman, Johnson, Echemendia, and Snyder (1983) conducted one of the more comprehensive studies. These investigators propose that the social climate of a congregation is determined by a range of factors, including the stability of church leadership, the level of autonomy and openness in church meetings and committees, and the extent to which congregants are involved in church activities. Although this study makes a number of valuable contributions to the literature, the findings are somewhat limited for the purpose of the current chapter for two reasons. First, Pargament et al.'s (1983) study is based on a nonrandom sample of adults from all age groups, which makes it difficult to determine whether the results can be generalized to older people. Second, the goal of their study was to see if the congregational climate is related to self-esteem and life satisfaction. These outcomes are important, but we also need to know if the congregational climate affects social relationships in the church, especially negative interaction.

The study by Krause (2002c) approached the influence of the congregational climate from a more circumscribed point of view and, in the process, evaluated the relationship between the congregational environment and social relationships in the church. More specifically, this study focused on only one facet of the wider church setting: congregational cohesiveness. This construct reflects the extent to which church members believe that their values, beliefs, and outlook on life are shared by the people with whom they worship. It seems as though the common values, beliefs, and shared outlook on life that Krause (2002c) studied underlie many of the facets of the congregational climate that Pargament et al. (1983) identified. For example, one might expect that when people in a congregation share common values and beliefs, their committee meetings tend to be more open and they may become more involved in church activities. But perhaps more important, Krause's (2002c) empirical findings suggest that greater congregational cohesiveness is associated with receiving more emotional and spiritual support from fellow church members.

If a highly cohesive congregational climate contributes to positive social relationships in the church, then perhaps a congregational climate that is not cohesive may have the opposite effect. When church members hold different views, beliefs, and outlooks on life, these differences will likely lead to disagreements about how the church should be run. Earlier, when the measurement of negative interaction in the church was discussed, disagreement over church issues (e.g., the format of worship services and church finances) was identified as one broad way of assessing interpersonal conflict in the church. This approach to assessing negative interaction in the church has not been discussed up until now because researchers have not shown if it affects health and well-being. Recent research by Ellison, Krause, Shepherd, and Chaves (2007), identified an intriguing mechanism. Based on data from a nationwide survey of adults of all ages, these investigators report that conflict over institutional issues may lead to more informal interpersonal conflict that forms the cornerstone of the current chapter. For example, when people in a church finance committee fall into deep disagreement over monetary issues, the unpleasant feelings may carry over into their informal interaction outside the church committee. In fact, people may try to identify and focus on negative attributes of those they are in conflict with as a way of further justifying the legitimacy of their own position on how church funds should be spent. The relationship between the climate of a congregation and negative interaction in the church represents yet another facet of religious life that is ripe for further study.

Creating Topologies of Negative Interaction in the Church

The second problem with research on negative interaction in the church has to do with the way measures of this construct have been developed. Negative interaction in the church may take many forms. For example, everything from gossip to criticism and being let down by previously trusted others are included under the broad rubric of this construct. So far, researchers have combined indicators of diverse types of negative interaction to form a single summary score. However, this measurement strategy is based on the assumption that all types of negative interaction in the church affect health and well-being and that they do so to roughly the same extent. Yet it is not clear that gossip at church has the same effect on health and well-being as open social conflict in the form of criticism and overt rejection. Moreover, as discussed earlier in this chapter, the fact that Ellison et al. (2007) found that excessive demands, but not criticism, are related to change in depression over time provides further evidence that great care should be taken when pooling items that assess church-based negative interaction into a single index.

Two steps can be taken to resolve problems associated with the differential effects of various types of negative interaction in the church. First, researchers must carefully stake out the content domain of church-based negative interaction, being sure that all the diverse ways it is manifest are represented adequately, which is another way of saying that indices of negative interaction in the church must be developed that have good content validity. Then, once items have been developed to measure the various forms of interpersonal conflict in the church, different kinds of negative interaction must be classified and topologies can be created from them. Both exploratory and confirmatory factor analysis would greatly facilitate this process. This type of work has already been done with negative interaction in secular settings (Newsom, Rook, Nishishiba, Sorkin, & Mahan 2005). More specifically, these investigators developed multiple indicators to assess each of four types of negative interaction: unwanted advice, failure to receive help when it is needed, unsympathetic behavior, and rejection and neglect. The same approach could be used in the study of church-based negative interaction. The importance of developing such topologies is illustrated in a recent study by Krause, Newsom, and Rook (2008) that was conducted in a secular setting. The work of these investigators suggests that one form of negative interaction (not getting help when it is expected—that is, being let down) is more likely to intensify the unwanted effects of financial strain on health than three other types of negative interaction identified in the work of Newsom et al. (2005).

Methodological Challenges in Studies on Leaving the Church

The third difficulty facing researchers who wish to investigate negative interaction in the church was introduced earlier in this chapter. If interpersonal conflict in the church becomes especially acute, older people may simply decide to leave the congregation and find another place to worship. This creates clear data analytic challenges, especially for studies based on cross-sectional designs. An example can help clarify the nature of the problem. It is highly unlikely that physical health problems will emerge as soon as negative interaction is encountered in the church. Instead, a certain amount of time must transpire before the pernicious health-related fallout from interpersonal conflict becomes manifest. Evidence of this delay may be found in a study Krause (2005b) did in secular settings. This research reveals a lag of approximately two years between exposure to negative interaction and the subsequent development of heart disease. During a two-year period, an older person could encounter significant interpersonal difficulty in his or her church and leave the congregation for a new one where no conflict is encountered. If older individuals are interviewed two years after they move to the new congregation, they would report experiencing low levels of negative interaction in the new congregation even though they are suffering from health problems that can be traced to the social environment in their previous place of worship. Without information on experiences in the prior congregation, it would not be possible to estimate properly the relationship between negative interaction in the church and health. This problem clearly illustrates why researchers must collect data at more than one point in time. But it points to a second important methodological issue as well. More specifically, this example shows that knowledge about the lag between exposure to negative interaction in the church and health is important because this information is critical for determining when follow-up interviews should be conducted in studies that have a longitudinal design. For example, if follow-up surveys are conducted too soon (e.g., six months after exposure to interpersonal conflict), then researchers may miss the opportunity to observe the health-related effects of negative interaction in the church. Viewed more broadly, these problems point to the need to develop congregational histories so that transitions in church membership may be taken into account when researchers explore the interface between negative interaction in the church and health.

Moving beyond Negative Interaction in Dyads

The fourth problem with research on negative interaction in the church is more subtle. Most studies of negative interaction in the church do not specify the number of people who are involved in a given social conflict. Yet the number of people who take part in negative interaction may make a difference. Although no research on this issue is available, there is reason to believe that negative interaction involving more than two people may have more pernicious effects on health and well-being than interpersonal conflict arising in a dyad, especially when a number of church members direct negative interaction toward a single congregant. Under these circumstances, the greater the chorus of accusations and criticism, the greater the effects of unpleasant interaction. Arguments in favor of this view may be found in two sources. Adam Smith (1759/2002) spoke directly to this issue two centuries ago: "The violence and loudness, with which blame is sometimes poured upon us, seems to stupify and benumb our natural sense of praise-worthiness and blame-worthiness.... We scarce dare to absolve ourselves when all our brethren appear loudly to condemn us" (151). A similar notion was expressed by Edward Alsworth Ross. Writing in 1907, Ross observed that, "In praising and blaming each of us exerts a power over his fellows. When the praises and blames of many men run together, they become a torrent no one can withstand" (vii). These observations bring to the foreground subtle issues about the way people cope with negative interaction. More specifically, it seems only natural that a person's initial reaction to criticism would be to dismiss it as being unfounded. In this way, he or she may protect his or her sense of self. However, it should be easier to engage in this type of coping response when criticism comes from one person rather than from a larger number of individuals. When a number of other church members are involved in negative interaction, empirical research is needed to see if there is a tipping point—precisely how many critics are needed to overwhelm the defensiveness of a focal older person, and where does the maximum undesirable effect on health emerge?

Unjustified Negative Interaction

The fifth problem with research on church-based negative interaction has to do with the fact that researchers rarely gather sufficient information about the context in which interpersonal conflict arose. For example, when older people encounter negative interaction in the church, they are likely to ask themselves whether it is justified. Sometimes, targets of negative interaction may believe they are indeed at fault and therefore deserve the unpleasant feedback they receive. Other times, people may feel that negative interaction is not justified and they are being treated unfairly. Researchers need to know which scenario has the greatest impact on health. On the one hand, one might argue that the sense of guilt or shame that arises from knowing that one is at fault will bring about the most pernicious effects on health. But in contrast, the anger and hurt associated with being unjustly attacked may cause even more damage. Once again, Adam Smith provides some insight into this issue. He maintained, "Unmerited reproach, however, is frequently capable of mortifying very severely even men of more than ordinary constancy....There is no greater tormentor of the human breast than violent resentment which cannot be gratified" (1759/2002, 138–139).

Studying Perpetrators of Negative Interaction

The sixth problem with research on negative interaction in the church arises from the fact that researchers tend to view interpersonal conflict solely from the perspective of the victim, while ignoring the effects it may have on the perpetrator. A host of issues arise at this juncture. For example, researchers need to know if initiating interpersonal conflict exerts a deleterious effect on the health and well-being of the perpetrator. Although this issue has not been examined empirically, doing so should be given a high priority because being critical of and rejecting others runs directly counter to the teachings of the church. Researchers need to see if initiating behavior that is explicitly forbidden by the church has an adverse effect on health and well-being. The well-known philosopher Spinoza (1677/2005) seemed to believe that initiating negative interaction has adverse effects on the perpetrator. Spinoza is credited with writing one of the first scientific treatises on psychology: *Ethics and on the Improvement of Understanding* (1677/2005). In this work, he derived a series of explicit propositions about basic human nature. One proposition (Proposition XXX) speaks directly to the effects of negative interaction on the perpetrator: "If anyone has done something which he conceives as affecting other men pleasurably, he will be affected by pleasure, accompanied by the idea of himself as a cause; in other words, he will regard himself with pleasure. On the other hand, if he has done anything which he conceives as affecting others painfully, he will regard himself with pain" (Spinoza 1677/2005, 148). In the subsequent justification of this proposition, Spinoza (1677/2005) explicitly invokes the notion of shame, which is noteworthy because a number of studies indicate that a deep sense of shame is associated with greater psychological distress (e.g., Pineles, Street, & Koenen 2006).

Researchers also need to understand the motives for initiating an unpleasant encounter and how different motives may influence health and well-being. Negative interaction is sometimes a cry for justice from an individual who believes that he or she has been treated unfairly. But other times, darker motives are involved. More specifically, negative interaction may arise from an unhealthy and misguided effort to shore up one's own sense of self-worth, which is especially evident with gossip. One of the founders of social psychology, George Herbert Mead (1934/1962), discussed this issue some time ago. He pointed out, "There is a certain enjoyableness about the misfortunes of other people, especially those gathered about their personality. It finds its expression in what we term gossip" (Mead 1934/1962, 206). It seems likely that negative interaction arising from darker, self-serving motives is likely to have a more noxious effect on health and well-being than negative interaction that arises from a sense of injustice. In fact, the latter may actually be a healthy response to unfair treatment by others.

Exploring the Role of Third Parties

The seventh unexamined issue in the study of church-based negative interaction has to do with the reaction of significant others who are not directly involved in the negative social encounter. Their reaction and input may have a major influence on the way the victim responds to what has transpired. For example, upon being told of an infraction, significant others may fan the flames of righteous indignation by underscoring the unfounded nature of the injustice that has been perpetrated, which may, in turn, lead to acts of retaliation and revenge that serve to further and deepen the conflict. In contrast, significant others may contribute to the healing process by helping the victim of negative interaction work toward a resolution of the problem, thereby setting the stage for forgiveness and reconciliation. This is important, because a number of studies suggest that forgiveness is associated with a greater sense of health and well-being across the life cycle (Krause & Ellison 2003; McCullough, Pargament, & Thoresen 2000). Viewed more generally, this raises the unexplored possibility that third parties who are not directly involved in negative interaction may help broker a solution. Being an intermediary, moreover, may provide the third party with an opportunity to implement fundamental teachings of the church, thereby strengthening his or her own faith. Support for this notion may be found in the vast secular literature on attitude change. As research reviewed by Chaiken, Wood, and Eagly (1996) reveals, persuading others to adopt an attitude or behavior reinforces and strengthens the persuader's own feelings about the attitude or behavior. Perhaps strengthening his or her own faith in this way may ultimately improve the health and well-being of the third party as well.

The Beneficial Effects of Negative Interaction in the Church

The eighth way in which research on negative interaction in the church can be improved may be found by returning to an issue first raised in chapter 3: close companion friends at church may invoke negative sanctions in order to get an older person to adopt a beneficial health behavior or avoid health behaviors that are undesirable. Thus, negative interaction in the church may not always have undesirable consequences, and may in fact perform functions that ultimately have positive outcomes. Researchers need to know more about this. More specifically, it is especially important to determine when negative interaction in the church creates health-related problems and when it is likely to have potentially beneficial effects. One factor may involve the closeness of the relationship between two individuals. On the one hand, negative interaction is likely to be especially troublesome when it arises in relationships that are particularly close; being let down by a previously trusted other may be particularly unsettling. However, there may be more to it than this. Because close relationships involve high levels of interaction, intimacy, and influence, problems are likely to arise within them. As a result, the members of a close dyad need to vent, let off steam, and say potentially negative things in order to clear the air. Doing so makes it possible to get problematic aspects of close relationships out in the open, thereby paving the way for smoother interpersonal functioning in the long run. Moreover, the process of airing grievances, coupled with the subsequent reconciliation of these differences, may lead to renewed commitment to the relationship, thereby making it stronger than it was before the negative interaction arose.

The fact that a certain amount of negative interaction is likely to arise in especially close social relationships points to a different way of estimating the relationship between interpersonal conflict and health. More specifically, researchers need to see if there is a nonlinear relationship between the two constructs. Relatively low levels of conflict may be associated with better physical and mental health, but beyond a certain threshold, further increases in negative interaction may have an adverse impact.

Further benefits of negative interaction may be found by returning to the notion of forgiveness. Learning to forgive others for the things they have done may be construed as a towering personal achievement and a marker of significant personal and spiritual maturity in the Christian community. Yet without an initial transgression, without the initial spark created by some form of negative interaction, there would be no need for forgiveness. Without forgiveness, there would therefore be no opportunity for growth.

Beyond these specific examples, the general notion that negative interaction may have beneficial as well as harmful effects is hardly new. Support for this assertion comes from two well-known sources. The first is Cooley's (1902/2003) classic work, *Human Nature and the Social Order.* In this volume, he devoted an entire chapter to the discussion of hostility. In his view, a certain amount and type of hostility is necessary for social life: "The mass of mankind are sluggish and need some resentment as a stimulant.... Surround a man with soothing flattering circumstances, and in nine cases out of ten he will fail to do anything worthy, but will lapse into some form of sensualism or dilettantism.... Common sense and careful observation will, I believe, confirm the opinion that few people who amount to much are without a good capacity for hostile feeling, upon which they draw freely when they need it" (Cooley 1902/2003, 273).

The second source that highlights the potential benefits of negative interaction comes from Walt Whitman's classic collection of poems, *Leaves of Grass* (1892/2001). A short poem in this volume, titled "Stronger Lessons," goes directly to the heart of the matter:

> Have you learn'd lessons only of those who admired you, and were tender with you, and stood aside for you?
> Have you not learn'd great lessons from those who reject you, and brace themselves against you? or who treat you with contempt, or dispute the passage with you? (649)

The general principle that is provided by both of these historical figures is an important one; negative interaction may be a source of significant growth. Viewed more generally, these observations suggest that in order to understand fully the impact of negative interaction in the church, researchers must strive to identify the benefits as well as costs of what may initially appear to be a wholly undesirable facet of congregational life. There is far too little research on this issue to date.

Taking Relationship Histories into Account

The impact of negative interaction on the health and well-being of an older person may depend, in part, upon the history of the relationship he or she has with the perpetrator. For example, it seems that older adults will be more likely to brush off or downplay an unpleasant encounter with a fellow church member they have known for some time and with whom they have previously had a close supportive relationship. In this instance, they may, for example, simply dismiss a sharp word or criticism as evidence that the fellow congregant was merely having a bad day. But the same type of negative encounter may not be taken so lightly if the perpetrator is a casual acquaintance. Simply put, church members with whom an older adult has had a good long-standing relationship are likely to have built up a store of positive social credits that can be used to offset the relatively rare instances of negative interaction they have instigated. In contrast, fellow church members who have not had this kind of relationship history with an older person lack this kind of social capital, and as a result, they are more likely to be taken to task for their unacceptable behavior.

Relationship histories may come into play in the study of negative interaction in the church in another way. Although an occasional incident of negative interaction is likely to be overlooked when the perpetrator is a relatively close other, repeated offenses are likely ultimately to overtax the store of social credits they have managed to accumulate so that, at some point, the older victim may handle repeated offenses in a more serious way. Researchers need to know where this tipping point occurs.

The study of relationship histories will not be easy because it requires the collection of much more fine-grained data than has appeared in the literature so far. Instead of asking global questions, such as those in Table 5-1, that assess negative interactions with fellow church members taken as a whole, researchers will have to ask about unpleasant social interaction on a relationship-by-relationship basis. This approach will obviously take a good deal of space in a questionnaire, forcing investigators to make difficult choices about what to cover in a given wave of interviews. Nevertheless, it is possible to implement this strategy, as the work of Newsom et al. (2005) reveals.

Conclusions

Research on the relationship between negative interaction in the church and health is in its infancy. Even so, finding so little work in this field is surprising for three reasons. First, members of the clergy have speculated for centuries that the powerful negative emotions generated by interpersonal conflict may have an adverse effect on health. For example, Jonathan Edwards was a leading theologian of his day. In 1746 he wrote a book, *The Religious Affections*, that dealt with a range of positive and negative emotions that arise in the church. In fact, for Edwards (1746/2004), emotions were the primary way in which the basic tenets of religion are acquired and maintained. Some emotions identified by Edwards (1746/2004) were positive, like love and gratitude, but others were negative, such as hatred and anger. As Edwards (1746/2004) proposed, "All affections whatsoever have in some respect and degree an effect on the body....The greater those affections be, and the more vigorous their exercise...the greater will be their effect on the body" (59). The second reason it is surprising to find so little research on negative interaction in the church and health may be found in studies that were conducted in secular settings. As noted earlier, this research reveals that negative interaction may be more consequential for health and well-being than the positive aspects of social relationships (Okun & Keith 1998). To the extent this is true, researchers need to pay more attention to it when it arises in the church. Third, the wider social world is replete with interpersonal conflict, and because people live in both secular and religious settings, there is little reason to believe that interpersonal difficulties do not carry over into the church as well. In fact, a study by

Krause and Rook (2003) conducted in a secular setting shows that inter-personal conflict in one sphere of life (i.e., with a spouse) tends to spill over into relationships with other individuals (i.e., children, other rela-tives, and friends). This raises the possibility that interpersonal difficul-ties in the secular world may spill over into the church, and vice versa. After all, the secular and religious social worlds form a seamless whole, and whatever boundaries exist between them are highly porous.

These issues aside, the study of negative interaction in the church is essential because it provides a much needed sense of balance in a literature that is overwhelmingly concerned with the potential bene-ficial effects of religion on health. Religious institutions are built and maintained by human beings, and because human beings are inherently flawed, so are the institutions they create. Focusing only on the bene-fits of church-based social relationships ignores this fundamental aspect of human nature and in the process unwittingly discourages efforts to improve interpersonal relationships in congregations. This approach is unfortunate because members of the clergy have, for decades, played an important role in providing counseling that is designed to overcome interpersonal difficulties in congregations (e.g., Clark 2000). Learning more about how negative interaction arises, persists over time, and in-fluences health and well-being may provide valuable insight for pastors who perform these vitally important counseling functions.

Studying the negative facets of religion serves two other important purposes as well. First, as noted in chapter 1, research on religion and health is not without its critics (e.g., Sloan & Bagiella 2002). Explicitly acknowledging and studying the darker underside of religion should go a long way toward taking some of the sting out of the criticisms that have been hurled at research in this field. The second reason for study-ing negative aspects of religion is even more important. If the purpose of a study is to see if religion affects health, and researchers focus only on the benefits of religion while ignoring the detrimental aspects of religion, then the models they evaluate will be misspecified, and estimates of the total effects of religion on health that are derived from these conceptual schemes will be overestimated. This is especially true if negative interac-tion and positive interaction in the church are inversely related. Studying the downside of religion is not an option. Instead, researchers are bound by scientific integrity to bring it to the foreground of the work they do.

Chapter 6

Exploring the Pervasive Influence
of Social Structural Factors

Religious institutions and the people who worship in them do not exist in isolation from the wider society in which they are embedded. Consequently, it is difficult to assess adequately the influence of church-based social relationships on health without taking this wider social context into account. One of the most important influences in this respect is social structure. Social structure is typically viewed as consisting of four basic elements or dimensions, including race, gender, socioeconomic status (SES), and age. Because issues involving age have been infused throughout the current volume, the discussion in this chapter focuses on the three remaining components of social structure.

There are two reasons why it is important to single out social structural factors for inclusion in the study of social relationships in the church and health in late life. First, extensive evidence links each social structural component with health, especially with respect to physical health status. Based on their extensive review of the literature on race differences in health during late life, Hummer, Benjamins, and Rogers (2004) conclude, "We have documented continuing racial/ethnic disparities in health, activity limitations, and active life among U.S. elders. Non-Hispanic black, Native American, and, to a lesser degree, Mexican Americans and other Hispanic elders were shown to have overall worse health across a number of indicators compared to Non-Hispanic whites" (88–89). A large body of research suggests that there are also gender differences in physical health status, but the picture provided by these data is complex. More specifically, the literature suggests that older women tend to report higher levels of hypertension, asthma, chronic bronchitis, and arthritic symptoms than older men. In contrast, older men report higher levels of heart disease, cancer, diabetes, and emphysema. More-over, research consistently shows that women tend to live longer than men (Federal Interagency Forum on Aging Related Statistics 2004). In contrast to research on gender, there is little doubt about the relation-ship between SES and physical health status. A recent volume by Mar-mot and Wilkinson (2006) contains reviews of a vast literature show-ing that a wide range of physical health problems are more prevalent in lower than in upper SES groups throughout the life course. In addition, as these investigators show, rates of mortality are inversely associated with SES as well.

The findings regarding the influence of social structural factors on mental health problems are less consistent than the results involving physical health status. Part of the problem has to do with whether men-tal health is measured in terms of symptoms of psychological disorder, such as depressive symptoms, or whether mental health is assessed with scales that are designed to detect clinical cases of psychiatric disorder. As George (2004) points out, there is some evidence that older whites tend to experience more symptoms of depression than older blacks. More-over, she reports that the few studies available in the literature indicate that older Hispanics report higher levels of depressive symptoms than either older whites or older African Americans. However, George (2004) goes on to point out that several studies suggest that race differences in mental health problems tend to disappear once the effects of SES are taken into account. The evidence regarding gender differences in men-tal health outcomes during late life is also mixed (George 2004). Some studies suggest that older women experience more symptoms of depres-sion than older men, but this pattern of findings fails to emerge when clinical major depression is under consideration. In contrast, research reviewed by Gurland (2004) indicates that rates of alcoholism and sui-cide tend to be higher among older men than among older women. Per-haps the most prevalent mental health problem in late life is dementia. The influence of social structural factors is more evident in this instance. More specifically, as Gurland (2004) reports, rates of dementia are higher among older people with lower levels of educational attainment (i.e., a key indicator of SES). There also appear to be race differences in demen-tia during late life, but as Gurland (2004) indicates, they also tend to dis-appear once the effects of SES (i.e., education) are taken into account.

The second reason for taking social structural factors into account when studying social relationships in the church may be found in research suggesting social structural variations in the relationships that people form at church as well. However, the interface between social structural factors and church-based social ties has not been explored extensively. Even so, research consistently shows that older African Americans receive more church-based social support than older whites (Krause 2002b; Taylor, Chatters, & Levin 2004). Similarly, data provided by adults of all ages suggest that men tend to receive less emotional support from fellow church members than women (Krause, Ellison, & Marcum 2002). Unfortunately, much less is known about socioeconomic variations in church-based social relationships during late life. This is part of a larger gap in the literature on SES and religion in general that Wuthnow (2003) discusses. He observes, "Social class, perhaps curiously, has received less attention in studies of religion than one might have imagined, given the continuing importance of social class as a reality and as a topic of sociological inquiry" (Wuthnow 2003, 24). The potentially important interface between SES and church-based social relationships is addressed later in this chapter with unpublished analyses from the RAH Study (Krause 2002a).

Taken together, the research reviewed up to this point begins to lay the groundwork for exploring an important series of issues. Specifically, this work raises the possibility that the long-standing and frequently observed relationship between social structural factors and health may be explained, at least in part, by church-based social relationships. The goal of the current chapter is to take a preliminary step toward addressing this issue. This discussion will be accomplished in four sections. An overall conceptual strategy for studying social structural factors, church-based social relationships, and health is presented first. Following this, separate sections are devoted to applying this framework to the study of race, gender, and SES on social ties in the church and health in late life.

A Strategy for Studying Social Structural Variations in Church-Based Social Ties and Health

At first, it may appear as though research on the relationships among social structural factors, church-based social ties, and health is relatively straightforward. However, as Krause, Ellison, and Marcum (2002) point out, this issue is not as simple as it seems. Focusing on an example provides the best way to explain the nature of the challenge that confronts investigators who are interested in working in this field. Assume the purpose of a study is to examine the relationship between church-based companion friends and health among older blacks and older whites. Assume further that an investigator hypothesizes that having close companion friends at church is more likely to benefit the health of older African Americans than older whites. There are two potential ways in which the hypothesized race difference in the effect of church-based companion friends on health may be manifest. The first is referred to by Krause et al. (2002) as the differential involvement perspective, whereas the second is called the differential impact perspective. The intellectual roots of this conceptual framework go back at least to the work of Kessler (1979).

Differential Involvement in Church-Based Social Ties

The differential involvement approach specifies that older blacks are more likely than older whites to benefit from having close companion friends at church simply because they are more likely than older whites to form close friendships with fellow congregants in the first place. The health-related effects of the differential involvement perspective can be evaluated with the following two-step process. First, church-based companion friendship is regressed on race. If the study hypothesis is correct, the data should reveal that older African Americans are more deeply involved with companion friends at church than older whites. In the second step, health is regressed on church-based companion friends. If the differential involvement perspective is valid, the findings should show that older people with greater levels of involvement with church-based companion friends, in turn, have better health than older adults who are not as deeply involved with companion friends in their congregations. A fundamental assumption lies at the core of the differential involvement perspective. The slope representing the relationship between church-based companion friends and health should be the same for older blacks and older whites. This would signify that at comparable levels of involvement with church-based companion friends, older blacks and older whites receive the same health-related benefits. However, the hypothesized race differences arise in this instance because older blacks are likely to be more deeply involved with church-based companion friends than older whites in the first place (i.e., race differences emerge in the first, but not the second step, outlined above).

Differential Impact of Church-Based Social Relationships on Health

In contrast, the differential impact perspective states that something is qualitatively different about the nature of close companion friendships that older blacks and older whites form at church. Some unmeasured historical, cultural, or religious factor serves to enhance the nature and functioning of church-based companion friendships in the Black Church, and as a result, older African Americans derive more health-related benefits from this kind of relationship than older whites. In this instance, the impact of church-based companion friendships on health would not be the same for older blacks and older whites, even when members of both racial groups are equally involved in the close friendships they have formed with fellow congregants. Instead, the regression slope representing the relationship between church-based companion friendships and health would be larger for older blacks than for older whites. The differential impact perspective is evaluated by testing for a statistical interaction effect between involvement with church-based companion friends and race on health. The reasons for the differences in these slopes that emerge from these analyses may not be known or measured explicitly, but the presence of a statistically significant interaction effect should alert researchers to their presence, thereby setting the stage for further work on the ways in which church-based companion friendships differ in black and white congregations.

It should be emphasized that the differential involvement and differential impact perspectives are not mutually exclusive and that both may operate at the same time. To continue with the current example, older blacks may derive greater benefits from the companion friends at church because they are more deeply involved with them than older whites and because the nature and functioning of close companion friends is more efficacious than the nature and functioning of companion friendships that older whites form with their fellow church members.

It should be evident at this point that the differential involvement and differential impact perspectives are important tools for deriving greater conceptual insight into the finer points of the relationships among social structural factors, church-based social relationships, and health. At the most basic level, the distinction between the two views comes down to tracing differences in the health-related benefits of social ties in the church for people in different social structural groups to either the *quantity* of the social relationships that are available to them (i.e., differential involvement) or the unique *quality* of these social ties (i.e., differential impact). For this reason the differential involvement and differential impact perspectives form the bedrock of the discussion provided throughout this chapter.

Variations by Race: Studying Older African Americans

The discussion that follows focuses entirely on the relationship between church-based social relationships and health among older African Americans and older whites. This analysis will be accomplished by exploring the historical and cultural reasons why church-based social ties may differ between older blacks and older whites. Then data on the differential involvement and differential impact of church-based social ties on health is presented. It would have been desirable to focus on members of other racial and ethnic groups as well, especially Mexican Americans because they represent the fastest-growing minority group of older people in America (Federal Interagency Forum on Aging Related Statistics 2004). However, empirical research focusing specifically on church-based social relationships, health, and well-being among older Mexican Americans simply does not exist. Instead, the handful of studies that have been done with older Mexican Americans focus solely on the relationship between things like the frequency of church attendance and the importance of religion on health-related outcomes (e.g., Hill, Angel, Ellison, & Angel 2005).

The wide majority of studies that have been done on race differences in church-related social relationships focus primarily on social support. And, as noted earlier, this research suggests that older African Americans are more likely than older whites to get more social support from the people they worship with (Taylor, Chatters, & Levin 2004). But before turning to this literature, we should reflect on why race differences in church-based social relationships may arise. Historical and cultural reasons exist for expecting older blacks to be more deeply involved in social relationships in the church than older whites. This discussion is the first time in this volume that the influence of historical factors on church-based social ties has been mentioned, which is unfortunate, because as C. Wright Mills (1959), a classic social theorist, put it, "Neither the life of an individual nor the history of a society can be understood without understanding both" (3). The fact that the influence of history has been overlooked in the current volume reflects the state of the literature. As the discussion provided below reveals, researchers must delve more deeply into historical factors so they can arrive at a better understanding of the reason that differences in church-based social relationships between older blacks and older whites arise.

Historical and Cultural Influences

Historical influences on the development and nature of the church in the black community were discussed some time ago by Nelsen and Nelsen (1975). As these investigators argue, the church has been the center of the African American community since its inception. Due to centuries of prejudice and discrimination, black people have turned to the church for spiritual, social, and material sustenance primarily because it was the only institution in their community that was built, funded, and wholly owned by black people. As a result, the church became a conduit for the delivery of social services, and the first schools for black children were located in churches. In fact, many of the great leaders in the black community have strong ties to the church, and many have been members of the clergy (e.g., Martin Luther King Jr.).

Perhaps no one wrote more on the early history of the church in the black community than W. E. B. Du Bois (2000). Strong themes involving social relationships emerged in his work. Writing in 1887, he concluded, "The Negro church ... provides social intercourse, it provides amusement of various kinds, it serves as a newspaper and intelligence bureau, it supplants the theater, it directs the picnic and excursion, it furnishes the music, it introduces the stranger to the community, it serves as a lyceum, library, and lecture bureau—it is, in fine, the central organ of organized life of the American Negro" (21). Later, in 1899, Du Bois (2000) went on to argue that social ties in black churches were even stronger than those found in churches in the white community: "Without wholly conscious effort the Negro church has become a centre of social intercourse to a degree unknown in white churches even in the country" (34).

Although the observations of Du Bois (2000) were made over a century ago, the strong social ties that exist in black churches are evident in the work of contemporary investigators as well. For example, Mattis and Jagers (2001) conclude, "African American religiosity and worship traditions emphasize both a profound sense of intimacy with the divine, and a horizontal extension of that intimacy into the human community" (523). But the importance of church-based social relationships in the black community is perhaps nowhere more evident than in the work of the noted black theologian J. Deotis Roberts (2003). Specifically, he states, "The black church, as a social and religious body, has served as a kind of 'extended family' for blacks. In a real sense then, thousands of blacks who have never known real family life have discovered the meaning in real kinship in the black church" (Roberts 2003, 78).

In addition to reflecting historical forces, the strong social ties that are thought to flourish in black churches are based on wider cultural factors as well. Baldwin and Hopkins (1990) went to great lengths to identify the key elements of the African American worldview or culture. They persuasively argue that African American culture is characterized by an emphasis on harmony, cooperation, collective responsibility, "groupness," and "sameness." Similar themes emerge in the work of Maynard-Reid (2000), who maintains, "The communal worldview is most evident in the extended family. African cultural tradition sees every woman, for example, as mother, aunt, grandmother, sister, and daughter. All are family. Africans and African-Americans view life as one-in-community.... This cultural worldview of necessity is carried over into worship. Worship therefore is a community happening in which kinship and mutual interdependence are affirmed" (61). Because institutions reflect the elements of the wider culture in which they are embedded, it follows that these key cultural characteristics should permeate the Black Church as well. And because the key elements of black culture that are identified by Maynard-Reid (2000), as well as Baldwin and Hopkins (1990), deal directly with interpersonal issues, one would expect them to be especially evident in the social relationships that are formed in black congregations.

The literature reviewed in this section strongly suggests that social ties in the Black Church may be especially well-developed, and because a vast literature links strong social relationships with better physical and mental health (Krause 2006a), one would therefore expect to find that church-based social relationships have an especially visible influence on the health of older African Americans. There are, however, two reasons why the discussions provided by Du Bois (2000), Roberts (2003), Baldwin and Hopkins (1990), and others make it difficult to determine precisely how these health-related benefits may arise. First, these investigators rarely differentiate between specific types of church-based social relationships, such as spiritual support and church-based companion friendships. As a result, it is difficult to know precisely where race differences in church-based social relationships are likely to emerge. Second, none of these scholars make a distinction between differential involvement in church-based social ties and the differential impact of social relationships in the church on health. However, as the data presented in the next section reveal, doing so provides additional insight into the nature and functioning of church-based social ties among older blacks and older whites.

Differential Involvement in Church-Based Social Relationships

Recall that the differential involvement perspective is evaluated with a two-step process. First, church-based social relationships are regressed on race. Then, in step two, health is regressed on church-based social ties. The second step in this estimation process was completed when data was presented on the influence of informal and formal relationships in the church on health-related outcomes in chapters 2 through 5. This research provides evidence that older people with strong church-based social relationships tend to have better physical and mental health than older adults who are not as deeply involved with their fellow congregants. So in order to complete the preliminary assessment of the differential involvement perspective, differences in church-based social ties between older blacks and older whites must be assessed. Fortunately, fairly extensive research on this issue is provided in three studies by Krause (2002b; 2003e; 2006g). The findings in all three papers are based on data from Wave 1 of the RAH Survey.

Church-Based Social Support. In the first study, Krause (2002b) tested for mean differences between older blacks and older whites in the following dimensions of informal church-based social support using the Wave 1 data from the RAH Survey: emotional support received, tangible support received, satisfaction with emotional support received, satisfaction with tangible support received, spiritual support received, emotional support provided, tangible support provided, and anticipated support. Then, using multivariate analysis of covariance procedures, the mean values of these social support measures were adjusted for the influence of age, sex, education, and marital status. The findings reveal that statistically significant race differences emerged in six of the eight measures of church-based social relationships. More specifically, older African Americans reported higher levels of giving and receiving emotional and tangible assistance with fellow church members than their older white counterparts. Older blacks also reported receiving more spiritual support and more anticipated support from their fellow congregants than older whites. In contrast, significant race differences failed to emerge with respect to satisfaction with emotional support received and satisfaction with tangible support received from fellow church members. Put another way, older whites did not score higher than older blacks on any of the church-based social support measures that were examined in this study.

Church-Based Companion Friendships. Recall that two ways of measuring close companion friendships at church were introduced in chapter 3. The first involves simply assessing whether older study participants have an individual in their congregation whom they consider to be an especially close friend. Data from the third wave of the RAH Survey were examined to see if older blacks are more likely than older whites to have a close companion friend in the place where they worship. This was accomplished by estimating a logistic regression model in which a binary measure denoting respondents who did and did not have a close companion friend at church was regressed on age, sex, education, race, and marital status. The findings reveal that older whites were significantly less likely than older African Americans to report having a close companion friend at church ($b = -.785$; $p < .001$; odds ratio = .456). The second measure of close companion friendships at church was designed to capture the nature and function of this type of social relationship. Race differences in the composite measure of this construct were evaluated with a univariate analysis of covariance model. This model tested for mean differences between older blacks and older whites in the nature and function of close companion friendships. The demographic measures used in the previous set of analyses were included in this model as covariates. The data suggest that adjusted mean value of the measure assessing the nature and functioning of close companion friendships at church for older whites ($\bar{x} = 32.839$) was not significantly larger than the corresponding mean for older African Americans ($\bar{x} = 31.773$).

Formal Social Relationships in the Church. As discussed in chapter 4, social relationships arise in the church around a number of formal activities, including attendance at Bible study groups and prayer groups, as well as volunteering to help people who are in need and helping older church members who are homebound. The second study by Krause (2006g) involved testing for race differences in participation in each of these formal activities. The findings revealed that, compared to older whites, older blacks were more likely to attend Bible study groups and prayer groups. In addition, older African Americans were also more likely to be involved in church programs that are designed to help people in need. Finally, the data suggest that older blacks were significantly more likely than older whites to worship at home with fellow church members.

Research on pastoral counseling was reviewed in chapter 4 when formal social relationships in the church were examined. The respondents in the RAH Survey were not asked if they received counseling from the pastor in the church they attend. Fortunately, this issue has been evaluated in other studies. This research reveals that churches in the black community are more likely to provide mental health services to rankand-file members than churches in the white community (Blank, Mahmood, Fox, & Guterbock 2002).

Negative Interaction in the Church. Research involving negative interaction was discussed in chapter 5. Two ways of assessing negative interaction in the church were examined. The first involved negative exchanges with fellow rank-and-file church members. Data in the study by Krause (2002b) reveal that there were no differences in the amount of negative interaction that was encountered by older whites and older blacks with fellow church members. The second way of assessing negative interaction in the church involved negative interaction with the clergy. Findings from a third study by Krause (2003e) suggest that compared to older whites, older blacks encounter significantly *more* negative interaction with members of the clergy.

When coupled with the data presented in chapters 1 through 5, the findings presented above provide strong support for the differential involvement perspective. A total of sixteen tests with the RAH Survey data are reported above: eleven favor older blacks, four are not statistically significant, and only one favors older whites. In addition, research conducted by other investigators suggests that blacks are more likely to get pastoral counseling services in their church than whites (Blank et al. 2002). Viewed in more general terms, these results reveal that older African Americans are more likely to enjoy the health-related benefits of church-based social relationships than older whites because older blacks are likely to be more deeply involved in these various types of social ties in the first place.

One set of findings reported above merits a closer look because it points to some intriguing possibilities that are not discussed often in studies on race differences in church-based social relationships between older whites and older blacks. Recall that the data show that older blacks report giving and receiving more emotional and tangible support with their fellow church members than do older whites. Given the high level of positive informal social exchanges in the Black Church, one might expect to see lower levels of negative interaction among older blacks as well. Yet the data indicate that there are no race differences in negative interaction with rank-and-file church members. In addition, the findings reveal that older blacks may encounter *more* negative interaction with members of the clergy. Although additional data were not available in the RAH Survey to pursue this issue further, speculating briefly on what these findings may mean provides new avenues for investigators to explore.

Researchers have known for some time that giving and receiving social support in secular settings is typically a positive experience. However, a small cluster of studies suggest there may also be limits associated with becoming more deeply involved with others. More specifically, there is some evidence that very high levels of social support do not always exert a beneficial effect on health-related outcomes (Krause, 1987). Stated in more technical terms, there may be a nonlinear relationship between social support and well-being: initially, increments in social support may bolster health and well-being, but beyond a certain threshold point, further increases in support may have the opposite effect because older people may begin to feel smothered, enmeshed, and put upon by significant others. Two key issues arise at this point that need to be investigated in the future. First, research on these nonlinear effects is based on data that were gathered in secular settings. Researchers need to find out if the same situation emerges in the church. Second, if there are limits to the beneficial effects of church-based social support, then researchers need to learn more about how these limits are manifest specifically.

Research by Ellison and Sherkat (1995) provides an intriguing way to address the second issue. These investigators maintain that the Black Church is so deeply entrenched in the community that it has become a "semi-involuntary institution" (1415), especially in the rural South. Specifically, these investigators argue that social norms and expectations involving church participation are so strong in these geographical areas that individuals experience significant social pressure to become involved in church activities. Although greater involvement in the church may provide access to greater social support, the social pressure and control associated with being in a semi-involuntary institution may also create unpleasant feelings (e.g., resentment) that give rise to levels of negative interaction that one might not expect to see in an otherwise highly supportive environment. Moreover, the tension that is created under these circumstances may spill over into the relationships that older blacks have with the clergy as well as the informal ties they maintain with rank-and-file members. As Wheaton (1985) pointed out some time ago in his discussion of secular coping resources, there can be too much of a good thing. The research discussed here suggests that it is time to see if this conclusion is true with respect to church-based social relationships as well. Doing so will help provide more balance in a literature that presents what may be construed as an overly positive view of an inherently complex social process.

Differential Impact of Church-Based Social Relationships on Health

A comprehensive assessment of the differential impact of church-based social relationships on the health of older whites and older African Americans has not appeared in the literature. Consequently, a preliminary first step is taken here by presenting findings from tests of this perspective based on unpublished analyses of the RAH Survey data. These analyses are all conducted with OLS multiple regression and use the covariates identified in the previous section. In addition, with the exception of worshiping at home with fellow church members, all the analyses are based on data from Wave 2 and Wave 3 of the RAH Study. In contrast, data from Wave 1 are used to assess race differences in the effect of worshiping with others at home because this was the only time this question was asked in the study. Data from Wave 2 and Wave 3 are used to assess the differential impact perspective for the remaining types of church-based social relationships for three reasons. First, a full complement of health-related outcomes were not administered until Wave 2. These health variables include a single item assessing global self-rated health ("How would you rate your overall health at the present time?"), the number of acute and chronic health problems, and an index of functional disability. In addition to these physical health measures, a brief four-item index of depressive symptoms taken from the Center for Epidemiologic Studies Depression Scale (CESD, Radloff 1977) was also used as an outcome so that findings involving the differential impact perspective could be evaluated with a mental health outcome as well. The second reason for turning to the Wave 2 data to conduct tests of the differential impact perspective arises from the fact that church-based social support is used primarily to help people deal with the effects of stress, and measures of stressful life events were not administered in the study until this time. This forty-nine-item stressful life event checklist was developed by Krause (1994) for use specifically with older people. Third, using data from Wave 2 and Wave 3 makes it possible to look at the relationship between church-based social relationships and change in health-related outcomes over time.

Church-Based Social Support. Unlike tests of the differential involvement perspective, assessing the differential impact perspective is more complex, especially with respect to church-based social support. The nature of this problem can be seen by returning to the essential function of church-based social support. As discussed in chapter 2, the social support from fellow church members helps offset the deleterious effects of stressful life events on health and well-being in late life. Stated in more technical terms, this function is evaluated by testing for a statistical interaction effect between stress and church-based social support on health. However, if the differential impact perspective is valid, older blacks should be more likely than older whites to enjoy the stress-buffering properties of church-based social support. Consequently, a more complex data analytic model is needed that tests for a three-way interaction effect between race, stress, and church-based social support on health.

As shown in Table 2-1, measures of eight different dimensions of church-based social support were assessed in the RAH Survey. Tests were performed for the three-way interaction between race, each type of social support, and stress on change in each of the four health-related outcomes identified above. Rather than review each set of findings, better insight may be obtained by focusing on the overall pattern of results that emerge across them. Altogether, thirty-two tests were performed. Statistically significant three-way interactions involving race, stress, and church-based social support failed to emerge in any of the analyses. Taken as a whole, these data therefore provide no support for the differential impact perspective.

Church-Based Companion Friendship. Unlike social support that is provided by fellow church members, church-based companion friendships do not perform a stress-buffering function. Consequently, tests of the differential impact of companion friends on health for older blacks and older whites can be evaluated with a simpler two-way interaction between race and companion friends on the four health-related outcomes identified above. As discussed in chapter 3, two measures of companion friendships at church were available in the study: the presence of a close companion friend and the nature and functioning of this important social tie. Taken as a whole, then, eight tests of the differential impact perspective can be performed with close companion friendships at church. The measures of church-based companion friendships appeared for the first time in the Wave 3 survey. As a result the eight tests were based on this wave of interviews only. The findings suggest that not one of the eight tests produced statistically significant results. Once again, these results provide little support for the differential impact perspective.

Formal Social Relationships in the Church. As noted in the previous section, measures of four different types of formal social relationships in the church were included in the RAH Survey: participation in Bible study groups, prayer groups and formal volunteer activities, and elders who worship at home with fellow church members. Once again, tests of the differential impact perspective involved models that contain a two-way interaction between race and each of the formal social relationships on change in the four health-related outcomes over time. Altogether, sixteen tests were conducted. None were statistically significant, suggesting that formal social relationships in the church do not exert a more advantageous effect on the health of either older African Americans or older whites.

Negative Interaction in the Church. Measures of interpersonal conflict in the church were available for two sources in the RAH Survey: negative interaction with fellow church members and negative exchanges with a member of the clergy. Tests were conducted to see if a significant two-way interaction was present between race and these two measures of church-based negative interaction on change in the four health outcomes over time. Altogether, eight tests were performed. Three were statistically significant. First, the data suggest that negative interaction with fellow church members is more likely to be associated with a decline in self-rated health over time for older whites than older blacks ($b = -.089$; $p < .05$). In addition, the results reveal that negative interaction with the pastor was associated with an increase in the number of acute and chronic conditions over time ($b = .276$; $p < .05$) as well as greater difficulty with physical functioning ($b = .770$; $p < .01$). In both instances, negative interaction with the clergy had a more adverse effect on older whites than older African Americans.

The findings involving negative interaction are intriguing. When coupled with the results involving differential exposure to negative interaction, the data suggest that even though older blacks encounter as much unpleasant interaction with fellow church members as older whites, and even more negative interaction with the clergy than older whites, older whites seem to be more vulnerable to the effects of interpersonal conflict in the church than older blacks. Although it is not possible to pursue this issue further with the data on hand, research by Krause and Ellison (2003) may provide some insight. Their work sug-

gests that older blacks are more likely than older whites to forgive transgressors for the things they have done. Perhaps forgiving, in turn, allows
older blacks to set aside unpleasant encounters with others and move
on with their lives, thereby avoiding the deleterious health-related consequences of negative interaction in the church. Even so, the findings
involving negative interaction must be viewed with considerable caution. Taken as a whole, results from sixty-two tests of the differential
impact perspective were performed with all the social relationship measures in the RAH Survey. Only three were statistically significant. Given
the large number of tests, some are quite likely to have arisen by chance
alone.

Summary

Researchers have argued for some time that the social ties maintained by older blacks in the places where they worship are more tightly
knit than the social relationships that older whites establish at church
(Du Bois 2000). Even so, translating these general observations into specific research hypotheses is difficult because there are many different
kinds of social relationships in the church, and these ties may affect
health and well-being in at least two different ways, as reflected by the
differential involvement and differential impact perspectives. The data
presented in the current chapter strongly favor the differential involvement perspective. More specifically, any health-related advantages that
older blacks may accrue from social relationships in the church appear
to arise because they are more likely than older whites to form social ties
in the first place, and they are more likely to be more deeply involved in
them. In contrast, little evidence appeared that social relationships in the
church confer any special or unique health-related advantages to older
blacks. Simply put, the data from the RAH Survey support the differential involvement, but not the differential impact perspective. It should
be emphasized, however, that this conclusion is tentative because health
and psychological well-being were evaluated with only four measures.
There are obviously many other ways to conceptualize and assess these
outcomes, and as a result, evidence supporting the differential impact
perspective may emerge when other health-related dependent variables
are examined.

Gender, Church-Based Social Ties, and Health in Late Life

Gender roles are a master status that tends to influence virtually every area of life. For example, as discussed earlier in this chapter, important gender differences in health arise in late life (Federal Interagency Forum on Aging Related Statistics 2004). Significant gender differences also emerge in secular social relationships (Antonucci 2001). More specifically, this research suggests that older women have larger, more well-developed secular social networks than older men, and elderly women tend to be more deeply involved in the lives of their social network members than their male counterparts. Finally, research reveals that older women tend to be more deeply involved in religion than older men (Levin, Taylor, & Chatters 1994). Even though fairly extensive gender differences emerge in a number of life domains, the literature is still underdeveloped. As Sinnott and Shifren (2001) concluded in their review of the secular literature on gender and aging "... much research shows little to no theoretical reasoning behind the examination of gender similarities and differences as we age" (460). This is especially true with respect to gender differences in the church-based social relationships.

The discussion that follows is divided into three main sections. Literature on gender, social relationships, and health is reviewed first. Second, in an effort to infuse research in this field with a gerontological perspective, a series of theoretical perspectives are examined that suggest different ways in which gender roles may change with advancing age. If gender roles change as people grow older, then relationships that have been found with younger people in studies of gender, religion, and health may not accurately depict what happens in late life. Third, consistent with the overall data analytical focus taken in the current chapter, empirical findings from a preliminary analysis of the differential involvement and differential impact perspective are presented and discussed within the context of gender.

Current Research on Gender, Social Ties, and Health

There do not appear to be any studies in the literature that systematically examine gender differences in the relationship between multiple dimensions of church-based social relationships and health in late life. Instead, researchers provide either theoretical discussions of gender variations in religion in general (e.g., Payne 1994; Payne-Stencil 1997), or empirical studies of gender differences in religion are conducted without considering the impact these gender differences may have on health (e.g., Levin et al. 1994).

Krause, Ellison, and Marcum (2002) conducted one of the few studies in the literature that examined the relationships among gender, church-based social support, and health. Only one dimension of social support was evaluated in this study: emotional support received by fellow rank-and-file church members. The findings from this longitudinal study reveal that women receive more emotional support at church than men, thereby providing support for the differential involvement perspective. However, the data provided a somewhat surprising manifestation of the differential impact perspective. Specifically, the results suggest that emotional support at church is more likely to enhance the health of men than women.

Although the study by Krause et al. (2002) provides some useful insights, several limitations are apparent in the work they have done. First, the study included adults of all ages, and as a result, knowing if the findings can be generalized to older people is difficult. Second, only one type of social relationship in the church was examined: emotional support received from fellow church members. As the discussion in previous chapters of this volume reveals, older people are involved in many other kinds of church-based social relationships. Third, only one health outcome was examined (i.e., global self-rated health), leaving open the possibility that different findings may emerge when other health-related dependent variables are evaluated. Fourth, as the theoretical rationale provided in chapter 2 suggests, it is best to examine the effects of emotional support at church in conjunction with stress. But the data set used in this study did not contain stress measures. Fifth, the data in the study by Krause et al. (2002) came from a nationwide survey of Presbyterians, and as a result, it is difficult to tell if the findings from this work apply to people who are members of different denominations.

Although Krause et al. (2002) did not have additional data to help evaluate why church-based emotional support may bolster the health of men, but not women, they offer several explanations that are worth pursuing in future studies. In particular, they argue that women face two relatively unique challenges in the church that may diminish or offset the potential benefits of receiving emotional support from their fellow church members. First, a number of studies indicate that women often occupy subordinate roles in the church. More specifically, research reviewed by Heyer-Grey (2000) indicates that women are less likely than men to lead or say prayers during worship services, and they are less likely to assist in serving Communion or reading to the congregation from the Bible. In contrast, Heyer-Grey (2000) further notes that women are more likely than men to clean the church, staff the nursery, and cook, serve, and clean up after church meals. Being relegated to subordinate positions may be a source of distress for women that may negate the potential benefits of having strong social ties in the church.

Studies conducted in secular settings provide a second reason why women may fail to reap health-protective benefits from the social support they receive at church. Research consistently shows that women receive more social support than men (Umberson, Chen, House, Hopkins, & Slaten 1996). Initially, this would appear to suggest that women should therefore have better physical and mental health than their male counterparts. But maintaining extensive social networks may extract a price, evidence for which may be found in Kessler's insightful research on the costs of caring (Kessler, McLeod, & Wethington 1985). Their work suggests that women tend to become more deeply involved in a wider circle of relationships than men. Although women may consequently receive more assistance from others, they must also provide more assistance when their social network members are in need. Moreover, in the process of making these exchanges, women may become more deeply involved in the lives of significant others and grow more concerned about the problems that loved ones face. As a result, being more deeply immersed in the lives of others tends to be emotionally demanding, and may even lead to higher levels of psychological distress among women, which may be especially true for women who maintain extensive social networks inside as well as outside the church.

The situation of men may be quite different from that of women. Because they receive less support in the secular world than women, men may, therefore, be in need of and benefit more from support that arises in religious settings. But the support men receive in church may convey benefits that would otherwise not be available in secular settings. The social support process is complex, and as noted in chapter 2, it is likely to be effective only if it is provided in a way that makes the potential support recipient feel comfortable (Eckenrode & Wethington 1990). Krause et al. (2002) maintain that the church may provide the opportunity for men to receive assistance in a way that is more palatable to them. The literature on gender roles helps explain why this may be so. This research suggests that the social skills possessed by men are not as well developed as those possessed by women (Hobfoll & Stokes 1988).

As a result, men may not know the best way to seek out assistance from others nor may they feel comfortable when asking for it. The church may help men overcome these obstacles in at least two ways. First, as discussed in chapter 4, many religious institutions encourage church members to participate in Bible study and prayer groups. As Wuthnow (1994) reports, these groups provide a forum for members to share personal problems and help each other. So instead of having to initiate a request for help entirely on their own, the norms and protocols that guide formal groups in the church provide a structured way of getting support that may help men surmount the problems arising from the lack of adequate help-seeking skills. In fact, research on the Promise Keepers movement provides compelling evidence on how religious organizations may be geared specifically toward meeting the social support needs of men (Bartkowski 2000). In addition to these more overt functions, religious institutions may promote the formation of socially supportive ties through less structured social gatherings (e.g., coffee hours after worship services) that can be fertile ground for the development of helping relationships as well.

But there is another, more subtle way in which the church may facilitate the helping process for men. In particular, structured worship services may make it easier for men to bond with others in the congregation. Most religions require the faithful to engage in certain rituals, such as the singing of hymns during worship services, taking Communion, and tithing. As Sosis (2000) points out, engaging in these religious rituals conveys important information to the members of a congregation. In particular, these rituals tell church members that fellow congregants share the same beliefs, are committed to the same faith, and, therefore, have much in common with them. Under these circumstances, members of a congregation may be more attractive to each other and they may be more likely to trust each other (McPherson, Smith-Lovin, & Cook 2001). These subjective perceptions are important because social psychological research suggests that direct requests for assistance are likely to arise more freely when potential support providers and potential support recipients are sure about each other's commitments (Cutrona, Suhr, & MacFarlane 1990). Regardless of the social and psychological forces that are at work, the fact that women receive more support than men, but the impact of church-based social support is greater for men than women, underscores the importance of distinguishing between differential involvement in church-based social ties and the differential impact of church-based social ties on health.

Age-Related Change in Gender Roles

The findings from the study by Krause et al. (2002) may be thought-provoking, but they are limited because they do not speak directly to the situation of older people. As the following discussion reveals, a number of researchers argue that gender roles may change over the life course. To the extent that this is true, then the relationships among gender, church-based social ties, and health may also change as people grow older. A thorough review of the literature makes it possible to derive at least four different views on how gender differences may either emerge over the life course or vary across different cohorts. Speculating on how gender-related changes may affect social relationships in the church provides an important way to encourage further research in the field.

The first perspective specifies that women are more involved in religion than men and that these gender differences are evident across the life course. According to this view women have less access than men to secular sources of power, prestige, and other resources in American society (Saltzman-Chafetz 2001). This is especially true for the current cohort of older women. Consequently, older women are more likely than older men to compensate for these social structural constrains by turning to religion (Pargament 1997). There is some indirect empirical support for this view. More specifically, Levin et al. (1994) report that compared to older men, older women are more likely to attend church, pray, and report that religion is more important to them. However, this study does not empirically link greater involvement in religion specifically with power differentials. Moreover, like other studies in the field, gender differences in church-based social relationships are not evaluated empirically. Nevertheless, the study by Levin et al. (1994) is important because people who go to church more often, pray more frequently, and believe religion is more important to them are also more likely to have well-developed social ties in the church.

The second perspective also states that women are more involved in church-based social relationships than men and that these gender differences are visible across the life course. However, proponents of this view turn to the sex role socialization literature to explain these gender differences. In their comprehensive review of the literature, Beit-Hallahmi and Argyle (1997) note that boys are socialized to be competitive, aggressive, and independent, whereas girls are taught to be obedient, sociable, helpful, and nurturing of others. Beit-Hallahmi and Argyle (1997) argue that because of these socialization practices, women are more likely than men to be attracted to religion because obedience to God is the cornerstone of many faiths, and nurturing others is a core religious value. Because the current cohort of older women are more likely than younger women to have been raised in an environment where these sex role socialization practices were more strictly endorsed, one would expect to find that older women are more immersed in church-based social relationships than older men, and older women may be more skillful in extracting the benefits these church-based social ties have to offer.

In contrast to the first two perspectives, the third point of view specifies that there may be no gender differences in church-based social relationships by the time people reach late life. Based on Erikson's (1959) developmental framework (see chapter 2), Sinnott and Shifren (2001) maintain that as people enter old age, they grapple with the crisis of integrity versus despair. These investigators argue that this final stage of adult development involves a shift away from stereotyped roles for men and women (especially child-rearing roles) to an emphasis on finding wholeness and meaning in life. As a result, Sinnott and Shifren (2001) speculate that, "In older age, gender is psychologically transcended" (459). Although these investigators did not focus specifically on church-based social ties, their discussion, nonetheless, provides an important strategic context for evaluating the interface between gender, church-based social relationships, and health in late life. If the struggle to attain a sense of integrity helps older people transcend gender roles, then gender differences in church-based social relationships should be less pronounced as people reach and go through late life.

A fourth perspective may be found by extending the widely cited research of Gutmann (1987). He marshals an impressive body of evidence which suggests a gradual reversal of gender roles as people grow older. In young adulthood, men are aggressive and competitive, whereas women are nurturing and focus primarily on tending to the needs of others. But by late life, Gutmann (1987) maintains that men assume roles that are similar to those of younger women. More specifically, older men become more nurturing and more concerned about caring for others. In contrast, older women tend to become more competitive and more aggressive. Because religion often emphasizes taking care of people who are in need, men who are more involved in religion should therefore become more attuned to tending to the needs of others as they grow older. And if they do, then the social networks they develop in church should rival, or even exceed, those of older women in terms of size and depth of involvement.

The discussion that has been provided up to this point treats church-based social relationships in a rather general or generic way. We need more focused and specific theoretical orientations that specify how gender differences may arise in particular types of church-based social ties. For example, virtually nothing is known about the influence of gender on church-based companion friendships. On the one hand, women may benefit more than older men from church-based companion friendships because they possess greater social skills than their male counterparts. However, a case may be made for why church-based companion friendships may be especially important for older men. Older men are more likely than older women to have been employed outside the home during young adulthood and midlife (Henretta 2001). During this time, men are therefore more likely than women to have developed companion friendships with co-workers. However, the wider majority of men retire by age sixty-five or so, and as a result, they may no longer be able to maintain companion friendships that were in place for decades. In contrast to older men, older women are less likely to be confronted by the prospects of losing close ties with work-based companion friends because the current cohort of older women were less likely to be employed outside the home. Because older men are more likely than older women to have lost companion friends in the secular world, the opportunity to develop and maintain companion friends at church may take on added significance and meaning for men as they reach late life. Under these circumstances, church-based companion friendships may play an especially important compensatory role in the maintenance of the health and well-being of older men.

Researchers also need to know if there are gender differences in the level of negative interaction in a congregation, and they need to know if the impact of negative interaction in the church is greater for older women than older men. If older women are more attuned than older men to social relationships as Beit-Hallahmi and Argyle (1997) maintain, then older women might be more troubled by the interpersonal conflict they encounter with fellow church members. But if the developmental process described by Gutmann (1987) is valid, then older men may be more vulnerable than older women to the effects of negative interaction in the church.

As discussed in chapter 4, having a formal relationship with the pastor, minister, or priest is also an important part of social life in the church, but once again, virtually nothing is known about whether gender differences arise in the extent to which these formal ties are cultivated and maintained, and there do not appear to be any studies that assess the differential impact of formal social ties with the clergy on the physical and mental health of older men and women.

As this brief review of unanswered research questions reveals, the field that encompasses the interface of gender, social relationships in the church, and health is wide open. In fact, pursuing these and other related issues may well constitute a research agenda that could envelop an entire career. Even though it is not possible to provide a comprehensive empirical analysis of gender differences in church-based social relationships in the current volume with the RAH Survey data, a preliminary assessment of the differential involvement and differential impact of relationships formed in the church may help show why further research on these issues is needed.

Differential Involvement in Church-Based Social Relationships

Consistent with the analyses provided in the section on race, the differential involvement perspective is evaluated below by seeing whether older women are more likely than older men to be involved in church-based social support, church-based companion friendships, formal social relationships in church, and negative interaction in church. However, the bulk of the analyses on these issues that are presented below have not appeared before in print. In an effort to make the analyses on social structural variations in church-based social relationships as consistent as possible, the empirical tests of variations by gender were conducted with the same measures, the same data analytic procedures, and the same waves of interviews that were used to explore variations by race.

Church-Based Social Support. A series of analysis of covariance models were estimated to see if there are mean differences between older men and older women in the following dimensions of informal church-based social support: emotional support received, tangible support received, satisfaction with emotional support received, satisfaction with tangible support received, spiritual support received, emotional support provided, tangible support provided, and anticipated support. These means were adjusted for the influence of age, race, education, and marital status. Consistent with the analyses on race, the data come from Wave 1 of the RAH Survey only. Five of the eight tests that were conducted to see if gender differences emerged in the data were statistically significant. More specifically, the findings suggest that compared to older men, older women receive more emotional support from fellow church members (older women $\bar{x}$ = 8.634; older men $\bar{x}$ = 7.810; $p < .001$) and more tangible help from the people with whom they worship (older women $\bar{x}$ = 6.619; older men $\bar{x}$ = 5.851; $p < .001$). Older women also report receiving more spiritual support from fellow church members than older men (older women $\bar{x}$ = 7.636; older men $\bar{x}$ = 7.242; $p < .05$), and older women have higher levels of anticipated support than their male counterparts (older women $\bar{x}$ = 10.403; older men $\bar{x}$ = 10.096; $p < .05$). The findings further reveal that older women report providing more emotional support to fellow congregants than older men (older women $\bar{x}$ = 8.869; older men $\bar{x}$ = 8.068; $p < .001$). However, statistically significant gender differences failed to emerge with respect to giving informal tangible help to people in church (older women $\bar{x}$ = 6.317; older men $\bar{x}$ = 6.187; ns). Similarly, significant gender differences were not found with either satisfaction with emotional support received (older women $\bar{x}$ = 3.643; older men $\bar{x}$ = 3.639; ns) or satisfaction with tangible help received from others at church (older women $\bar{x}$ = 3.596; older men $\bar{x}$ = 3.599; ns).

Taken as a whole, the data suggest that older women report receiving and providing more informal church-based social support on five of the eight measures in the RAH Survey. On the remaining three measures, older women were neither higher nor lower than older men. Viewed the other way around, the data suggest that older men did not score higher on any of the informal church-based social support measures than older women.

Church-Based Companion Friendships. Gender differences in the probability of having a close companion friend at church were assessed with a logistic regression analysis in which a binary measure denoting whether a study participant had a close companion friend at church (scored 1) or not (scored 0) was regressed on age, sex, education, marital status, and race. Recall that measures of church-based companion friendships were available only in the Wave 3 RAH Survey data. The findings reveal that older men were less likely than older women to have developed a close friendship with a fellow church member (b = −.404; $p < .05$; odds ratio = .668). Gender differences in the composite index that was designed to capture the nature and functions of close companion friends at church were evaluated with a univariate analysis of covariance model. The demographic control variables that were used in the previous set of analyses were included in this model as covariates. The data failed to show that there are significant gender differences in the nature and functioning of close companion friends at church (older women $\bar{x}$ = 32.633; older men $\bar{x}$ = 31.415; ns). Taken together, the two sets of findings suggest that even though older women are more likely than older men to have a companion friend at church, once a close companion friendship has been forged, the nature and function of these close ties do not differ significantly by gender.

Formal Social Relationships in the Church. Unlike the data that have been presented so far, analyses of gender differences in formal social relationships at church have been published with data from the RAH Survey (Krause 2006g). The findings reported in this study reveal that compared to older men, older women are more likely to attend Bible study groups and prayer groups. But in contrast, the data further indicate that older men and women were equally involved in church programs that are designed to help people who are in need and older women who were no more likely than older men to worship at home with fellow church members.

Negative Interaction in the Church. Unpublished findings based on the first wave of the RAH Survey were used to evaluate whether gender differences emerge in negative interaction with fellow church members as well as negative interaction with a member of the clergy. These analyses were performed by two univariate analyses of covariance models. The demographic variables that have been used throughout the analyses reported in this chapter were used as covariates. The data suggest that older women are no more likely than older men to report encountering negative interaction with fellow rank-and-file church members (older women $\bar{x}$ = 3.382; older men $\bar{x}$ = 3.479; ns). Similarly, the data suggest that older women do not report experiencing more interpersonal conflict with a member of the clergy than older men (older women $\bar{x}$ = 3.382; older men $\bar{x}$ = 3.479; ns).

An intriguing pattern of findings begins to emerge when the results involving gender differences in church-based social relationships are viewed in conjunction with the data on race differences in church-based social ties. Older blacks and older women report being more deeply involved in positive exchanges than either older whites or older men. Yet neither older blacks nor older women encounter less negative interaction with fellow church members than older whites or older men.

Viewed in a more general way, these data reveal that being more deeply immersed in beneficial social ties does not have a protective effect for older blacks or older women when it comes to unpleasant encounters with people at church. For older blacks, this pattern of findings was explained by turning to social constraints, such as the semi-involuntary nature of church attendance that was discussed by Ellison and Sherkat (1995). But a different set of constraints may operate for women. Recall that Kessler et al. (1985) argue that costs are associated with the relatively larger social networks that women maintain, and these costs are manifest in terms of greater demands for reciprocity and higher levels of emotional concern when social network members are in need. When the findings on race and gender are viewed in a more general way, they point to the possibility that greater social involvement at church is a mixed blessing, and that having more extensive and more intimate ties does not necessarily protect older people from encountering certain costs as well. This, in turn, raises a whole host of issues about the gross or overall impact that these seemingly offsetting effects may produce. Although pursuing this issue is not possible here, examining the joint influence of positive and negative exchanges at church on the health and well-being of older men and women, as well as older blacks and older whites, should be a high priority in the future.

Differential Impact of Church-Based Social Relationships on Health

There do not appear to be any studies in the literature that provide a comprehensive assessment of the differential impact of social relationships in the church on the health of older men and older women. Such an analysis would involve a wide range of health-related outcomes assessed in conjunction with the sixteen measures of church-based social relationships in this volume. As a result, only a preliminary set of analyses is presented below that is based on unpublished data from the RAH Survey. These analyses use the same health-related outcomes that were used in the analyses involving race (i.e., self-rated health, acute and chronic conditions, physical functioning, and depressive symptoms) and the same waves of data that were utilized when evaluating the differential impact perspective among older whites and older African Americans.

Church-Based Social Support. Recall that tests of the differential impact perspective call for a three-way interaction effect between gender, church-based social support, and stress on the health-related outcomes. Measures of eight different types of church-based social support are available in the RAH Survey. Altogether, thirty-two tests were performed. Statistically significant three-way interaction effects emerged in only three of these tests with the longitudinal data from Waves 2 and 3 of the RAH Survey. First, the findings reveal that the deleterious effects of stressful life events on change in self-rated health are offset or buffered when older people receive more spiritual support from their fellow church members. However, these benefits were more likely to be enjoyed by older men than older women ($b = .016$; $p < .05$). Second, the data suggest that receiving more tangible assistance also helps to reduce the noxious effects of stressful life events on change in self-rated health over time. But once again, these benefits were more evident among older men than older women ($b = .033$; $p < .01$). Third, the results indicate that receiving tangible help from fellow church members when stressful life events arise appears to increase depressive symptoms over time for older women, but not older men ($b = -.078$; $p < .05$).

Church-Based Companion Friends. Two sets of cross-sectional analyses were performed with the Wave 3 RAH Survey data to see if having a companion friend exerts a differential impact on the health of older men and older women. The data suggest that older women who report having a close companion friend at church tend to have fewer physical functioning problems, but the same health-related benefits are not enjoyed by older men ($b = 1.253$; $p < .05$). For older men, having a close companion friend at church did not have a statistically significant effect on physical functioning. The second set of analyses focused on gender differences in the relationship between the composite measure of the nature and functioning of companion friendships on the health-related outcomes. No statistically significant gender differences emerged from these analyses.

Formal Social Relationships in the Church. Sixteen different tests were conducted to see if gender differences emerged between the four measures of formal social relationships in the church and the four health outcomes. All of these tests were performed with longitudinal data. The findings reveal that only one test was statistically significant. More specifically, the results indicate that older men who worship at home with members of their congregation tend to have more favorable ratings of their health. But in contrast, the same effect was not evident among older women ($b = .713$; $p < .01$).

Negative Interaction in the Church. A series of eight tests was performed to see if gender differences emerged in the relationship between negative interaction with fellow church members and negative interaction with members of the clergy and health. No statistically significant interaction effects emerged from the data.

Summary

The data reviewed in this section suggest that older women tend to be more deeply involved in church-based social relationships than older men. Cast within the context of the analytic framework that was developed for this chapter, support was found for the differential involvement perspective, but only mixed support was found for the differential impact perspective. Specifically, only five of sixty-two tests of the differential impact perspective produced statistically significant results, and when significant findings emerged from the data, four of the five tests suggest that older men may reap greater benefits from social ties at church than older women. These findings are largely consistent with the results reported by Krause et al. (2002) in their study of Presbyterians of all ages. However, it is important to once again emphasize that these results should be viewed cautiously because of the large number of tests that were conducted. Nevertheless, when all the results involving gender are taken as a whole, more consistent gender differences appear to emerge with the differential involvement perspective than with the differential impact perspective.

The findings from the empirical tests of the differential involvement and differential impact perspectives did not fit neatly into any of the four theoretical perspectives on gender and aging that were discussed at the beginning of this section. Despite the speculation of Sinnott and Shifren (2001), there was little evidence that gender is transcended in late life. Instead, it appears that gender still matters. The fact that women are more deeply involved in church-based social relationships (as assessed by testing for the differential involvement perspective) is consistent with the observations of Beit-Hallahmi and Argyle (1997) on the influence of traditional sex role socialization practices. However, the sparse evidence that emerged from tests of the differential impact perspective suggests that older men may reap greater health-related benefits than older women, which is not consistent with what one would expect from the sex role socialization literature. Viewed more generally, the empirical findings involving gender point to significant gaps in the theory on gender, church-based social relationships, and health. If researchers hope to move the field forward, then creating more well-developed theories that are capable of explaining the complex web of empirical findings that are just now beginning to emerge should be a top priority in the future.

Church-Based Social Ties and Health: Variations by Socioeconomic Status

Ever since the founding of the discipline, sociologists have maintained that social class exerts a profound influence on a wide range of social behaviors. For example, Cooley (1902/2003) argued, "There is nothing more important to understand, or less understood, than the class atmosphere in which nearly all of us live" (72). Sociologists of religion are certainly aware of the influence of social class on religious behaviors and beliefs (e.g., Davidson & Pyle 2005; Smith & Faris 2005), but as noted at the beginning of the current chapter, very little attention has been paid specifically to the relationship between socioeconomic status and church-based social relationships in late life. The purpose of the discussion provided below is to address this issue. This discussion is accomplished in three sections. The first focuses on issues in the measurement of socioeconomic status (SES) in late life. The second section is concerned with identifying the ways in which SES may influence the social relationships that older people form and maintain at church. Because so little research has been done in this area, the discussion in this section deals primarily with studies that have examined SES differences in social relationships that arise in secular settings. The purpose of the third section is to provide a preliminary empirical assessment of SES differences in church-based social relationships using the data from the RAH Survey. Consistent with the approach taken to assess race and gender, these analyses focus on differential involvement in church-based social ties as well as the potential differential impact of social relationships in the church on health and well-being among older people in different SES groups.

Measuring SES in Late Life

Before turning to an examination of substantive issues involving SES and church-based social relationships, it is important to take a close look at the measurement and meaning of SES among older people. SES is typically assessed with indicators of either income, occupational status, education, or some combination of them. More recently, some investigators have turned to more comprehensive measures of wealth to assess SES. Unfortunately, a number of challenges arise in using income, occupation, and wealth that are especially vexing when studying older adults.

Income is typically assessed by presenting study participants with a single item that asks them to report their total yearly family income before taxes from all sources for the year prior to the survey. Two major problems arise when this type of measure is used to assess SES among older people. First, although there do not appear to be any comprehensive studies in the literature, questions on total yearly family income tend to contain more nonresponse than other survey items (see, for example, Kahn & Fazio 2005). For example, total annual family income was assessed in the first wave of the RAH Survey. A total of 27.7 percent of the older people who participated in the study either refused to provide their income or said they were not sure what it was. This is substantially more missing data than was encountered with any other variable in the data set.

Second, and far more serious, are findings from studies which suggest that self-reports of total yearly family income contain a substantial amount of measurement error. Moreover, this problem appears to be especially true when the data are provided by older people. In a revealing study, Crystal (1986) compared self-reports of annual income with income contained in Social Security Administration payment records. He found that, on average, the income of older people is underestimated by a startling 46 percent. Problems like this are a concern to the U.S. Bureau of the Census, and as a result, they conducted a series of studies to determine the potential amount of measurement error in the data they collect on income and a range of other demographic variables (U.S. Bureau of the Census 1975). In order to determine the extent of the problem, they created a measure they call the Index of Inconsistency, which is closely akin to a test-retest reliability coefficient. The highest score on this index (i.e., a value of 100) reflects total inconsistency in reports of income over time, whereas the lowest score (i.e., a score of 0) denotes perfect consistency. The U.S. Bureau of the Census (1975) reports that the index of inconsistency for income among men of all ages is 50 while the corresponding estimate for women of all ages is 43. Once again, the findings suggest that self-reports of income contain a significant amount of measurement error, and as researchers have shown for decades (e.g., Bohrnstedt 1983), measurement error of this magnitude is likely to bias study findings.

Although measurement error creates problems when researchers focus on the additive and linear relationships among variables like SES and church-based social relationships, the problems associated with measurement error are compounded when evaluating the differential impact perspective. Recall that in order to assess the differential impact perspective, a researcher must test for a statistical interaction effect between things like SES and church-based companion friendships on health. As Bohrnstedt and Marwell (1978) forcefully demonstrated some time ago, the reliability of the multiplicative term that is formed to assess this interaction effect is always lower than the reliability of either of the components that are used to create it (e.g., SES and church-based companionship). So if income is measured with significant error, then reliability of a cross-product term containing income is likely to be quite low. And if the reliability of the cross-product term is low, the substantive study findings that are generated with it are likely to be biased significantly.

In contrast to income, a different set of problems arise when occupational status is used as a measure of SES. More specifically, as Mirowsky and Ross (2003) point out, compared to younger women, older women are more likely to have never been employed outside the home, which makes it difficult to classify their occupational status. In addition, many older adults are no longer in the labor force, and as a result, it is often hard to give them an occupational status score. Problems arise when attempting to do so because a number of older people were in one occupation for the majority of their working years, but subsequently shifted to a different occupation shortly before retirement (Henretta 2001). This raises questions about whether these bridge jobs or one's lifelong occupation should be used to assess SES in late life.

More recently, a number of investigators have turned to the assessment of wealth as an indicator of SES among older people (e.g., Kahn & Fazio 2005). In addition to encountering the problems with item nonresponse that are discussed above, measures of wealth are problematic because a fairly long battery of items is typically needed to assess this construct. For example, Kahn and Fazio (2005) determined the overall wealth of older people by asking a number of questions on the value of their homes and automobiles, total debt arising from credit card balances and car loans, as well as a number of items on financial assets. The problem arises because a fairly large number of items are also needed to assess other domains in a survey, such as church-based social relationships and health, thereby creating significant competition for scarce questionnaire space. But perhaps more importantly, it is not clear whether older people can accurately recall and report data like the value of their home or the value of their automobile.

In contrast to the indicators of SES that have been discussed up to this point, there are two reasons why education may be the measure of choice in studies on church-based social relationships and health in late life. First, income and occupation are determined by education. In fact, as Mirowsky and Ross (2003) conclude, "Education is the key to one's place in the stratification system" (30). As a result, models may be misspecified if they do not contain measures of education. This problem arises because a relationship between either income or occupation and health may be confounded because of the joint dependence of these SES measures on education. Second, extensive research by Mirowsky and Ross (2003) clearly indicates that education is the "root cause" of good health in late life. More specifically, the findings from their extensive study of SES and health reveal that the effects exerted by education tend to be more pronounced than those of income or occupation. As these investigators conclude in the last paragraph of their book: "Why does health increase with social status? Not because of the money, much less the authority, but because learned effectiveness creates the ability to achieve something everyone wants: health. Education develops the skills, habits, and attitudes that help individuals take control of their own lives" (Mirowsky & Ross 2003, 206).

Some investigators argue that it is best to use an aggregate index of SES that is created by combining income, occupation, or education to form some sort of composite measure. However, as Mirowsky and Ross (2003) point out, the various indicators of SES capture different underlying constructs that may affect outcomes, such as health, in different ways. More specifically, education reflects accumulated knowledge and skills, whereas income is obviously focused solely on economic resources, and occupation reflects job-specific skills and prestige. Each may influence health, but for different reasons. Consequently, combining the different SES measures into a single index serves to obfuscate these potentially important differential influences. This may be especially problematic if some, but not all, of the underlying mechanisms affect health.

Taken as a whole, this somewhat cursory review of how to measure SES suggests that education may be the best marker for studying the relationship between church-based social relationships and health in late life. For this reason education is used in tests that are provided in this chapter of the differential involvement and differential impact perspectives.

Current Research on SES and Social Relationships

As noted above, there is virtually no research on SES differences in church-based social relationships, especially with respect to studies that focus specifically on older people. Consequently, a reasonable strategy for setting up the empirical analyses that are reported in the next section involves turning to research on SES and social relationships in secular settings and speculating on how the findings from this work may be adapted to the study of social ties in the church.

A good deal of the secular literature on SES and social relationships focuses on social ties in lower SES neighborhoods. In fact, researchers have been exploring this relationship for over fifty years. During this time a number of qualitative and quantitative studies have appeared that suggest that the social networks of people who live in lower SES neighborhoods are not as well developed as the social networks maintained by people in upper SES areas. For example, the Stirling County Study was one of the first to examine the mental health of people living in the community (Hughes, Tremblay, Rapoport, & Leighton 1960). Based on a series of ethnographic studies that were embedded in this comprehensive research program, Hughes et al. (1960) report that people who live in dilapidated neighborhoods frequently take advantage of each other, are suspicious of outsiders, and provide little assistance to their co-residents. More specifically, these investigators describe people who live in run-down areas of town in the following way: "They find difficulties in family and community relationships, and expect inconsistency of affection and support from their fellows. Meeting hostility from their nearest human contacts, they react to many situations with avoidance and apathy" (Hughes et al. 1960, 250). Similar observations were made by Stephens (1976), who conducted a qualitative study of older people living in a single-room-occupancy hotel. She observes, "In this society of the alone, suspicion is institutionalized" (Stephens 1976, 33). The findings reported by Hughes et al. (1960) and Stephens (1976) are corroborated in yet another qualitative study by Rubin (1976). The title of her book succinctly captures social life in lower SES families: *Worlds of Pain* (Rubin 1976).

The insights from these qualitative studies are supported by findings from a number of quantitative studies. For example, research by Krause (1993) reveals that older people who tend to live in run-down neighborhoods tend to be more distrustful of others, and older people who are more distrustful of others are, in turn, more socially isolated. Similar findings are reported by Woldoff (2002). Her data indicate that physical disorder in the neighborhood (e.g., abandoned and run-down buildings) tends to foster more social disorder (i.e., greater mistrust of others), and greater mistrust of others is, in turn, associated with less social contact. More recently, Feldman and Steptoe (2004) report that greater neighborhood deterioration is associated with lower levels of social interaction.

A study by Belle (1982) paints a bleak picture of social life in economically deprived areas of the city and, in the process, helps to identify some of the underlying mechanisms that may be at work. She reports that women living in run-down neighborhoods are afraid of accepting social support from others because they feel they will not be able to reciprocate when former support providers need assistance. A somewhat different set of intervening mechanisms may be found in a qualitative study by Black and Rubinstein (2000). These investigators report that the social relationships of older women living in poverty are hampered by a number of factors: "Physical distance, dissimilar values and the need to be considered independent and not be a burden to family were named as reasons why our respondents did not ask for emotional or physical assistance" (Black & Rubinstein 2000, 118).

Perhaps the clearest statement of why individuals in lower SES groups may have underdeveloped social relationships is found in Hobfoll's (1998) notion of the pressure-cooker effect. He begins by arguing that social networks tend to be homogeneous with respect to SES. Therefore, if a focal person is suffering from economic deprivation, there is a good chance that the members of his or her social network are confronted by the same problems as well. The resulting stress contagion that arises in lower SES social networks serves to undermine the social support process. More specifically, Hobfoll (1998) maintains, "Since no one in the system is free of threat, individuals who themselves have great need to depend on others must serve as supporters and lose precious resources they themselves need at this time" (208).

A slightly different mechanism is identified and empirically evaluated in a study by Krause and Shaw (2000). They argue that a lower SES elder may try to help a social network member who is experiencing financial difficulty. However, because both parties in this exchange lack adequate resources, the situation of the support recipient is not likely to change over time. As a result, the benefits that normally accrue to a person for helping someone else fail to materialize, so they may become frustrated with the lack of progress and ultimately cease to engage in the helping process altogether. Recall from chapter 2 that research suggests that helping others tends to bolster the self-esteem of older support providers. The longitudinal study by Krause and Shaw (2000) reveals that initially, helping others tends to bolster the self-esteem of lower as well as upper SES elders. However, consistent with the conceptual framework that was developed by these investigators, these benefits began to taper off over the course of their longitudinal study. By the time the third wave of interviews was conducted, the salutary effects of helping others were evident only among older adults in upper SES groups.

Although there appears to be considerable evidence that the social relationships maintained by people in lower SES groups do not function as well as the social ties maintained by upper SES individuals, other investigators fail to reach the same conclusion. For example, a number of studies highlight the important role played by extended kin and close friends in enhancing the quality of life of poor, inner-city African Americans (Liebow 1967; Stack 1974). Similar views are reached in another of the classic psychiatric epidemiologic studies: the Midtown Manhattan Study (Langner and Michael, 1963). Specifically, Langner and Michael (1963) report that people in lower SES areas of Manhattan have more extensive family network structures than are typically found in upper SES areas of the city. In addition, these investigators find that when well-to-do areas of the city are contrasted with economically depressed areas, there are no differences in the number of neighbors with whom a respondent is friendly. Similarly, research by Sokolovsky and Cohen (1981) failed to find that the social ties maintained by elders living in disadvantaged areas of the city are deficient in any way. In fact, these researchers argue that the notion that inner-city elders who live in single-room-occupancy hotels are isolates and loners is a myth. These views are supported by a recent review of the literature on SES, social relationships, and health by Young (2004). He argues that the claim that social ties explain the relationship between SES and health is unfounded empirically and that the personal or psychological resources of lower SES individuals are more likely to come into play.

Although the lack of consensus in the literature on SES and secular social relationships is puzzling, there are at least two ways to reconcile these contradictory findings. First, as reflected throughout the current volume, the content domain of social relationships is vast and subsumes a wide array of specific kinds of social ties. If this is true, then a better

view of SES differences in social relationships may be found by probing for SES differences in a comprehensive battery of social relationship
measures. One of the few studies to begin to address this issue was conducted by Krause and Borawski-Clark (1995). Using data from a nationwide survey of older adults, these investigators assessed the relationship
between education and six different types of social ties: contact with
family, contact with friends, support provided (as assessed by a composite measure in which emotional, tangible, and informational support were combined), support received, negative interaction, and satisfaction with support. Significant SES differences emerged, but in only
three of the six dimensions. More specifically, the findings suggest that
compared to older people with higher levels of educational attainment,
older adults with fewer years of schooling tend to have less contact with
friends, provide less support to their social network members, and are
less satisfied with the assistance they received from significant others.
In contrast, significant SES differences failed to emerge with respect to
contact with family, support received from others, and negative interaction. These findings suggest that merely asking whether there are SES
differences in social relationships is too simple. Instead, a more focused
research agenda is called for in which an effort is made to assess the relationship between SES and different types of social relationships.

The second reason why findings from studies of SES differences in
secular social relationships are inconsistent may be found by returning
to the work of Black and Rubinstein (2000), who found that the social
ties maintained by older women living in poverty are constrained by a
number of factors. But they go on to argue that the women in their study
do not respond to these social challenges in a passive way. Instead, Black
and Rubinstein (2000) report, "Women's faith was their primary coping
mechanism, as well as their main route to seeking emotional, spiritual,
and financial support. To ignore older women's experience of God is to
diminish an all-encompassing reality in their lives" (234; see also Barusch 1999).

If religion helps lower SES individuals compensate for problems that
arise in their secular social relationships, then a key issue involves pinpointing the precise aspects of religion that may be responsible for these
beneficial effects. Although a number of different facets of religion are
likely to come into play, perhaps social ties in the church have something to do with it. But if Hobfoll (1998) is correct, then it is not clear
why social ties in the church would be immune to the same kind of pres-

sure-cooker effect that is thought to plague lower SES interpersonal ties in secular settings. There are three reasons why church-based social ties may be more effective than secular social relationships in this respect.

First, as noted throughout the current volume, basic tenets of the faith encourage church members to love one another and to take care of those who are in need in a nonjudgmental way. Moreover, basic teachings of the faith help instill a sense of trust and belief in the basic goodness of others. The element of trust may be especially important because, as research reviewed earlier in this section reveals, older people who live in run-down neighborhoods may be especially distrustful of others (Krause 1993).

Second, as discussed in chapter 2, one function of religion is to help older people adopt a set of specific coping skills and responses, such as trusting in God for guidance and advice as well as forgiving other people for the things they have done. Because these coping responses arise from, and are maintained through, social relationships with religious others, the mutually endorsed responses to SES challenges may serve to bolster and maintain ties with fellow church members that might otherwise have been eroded by the kind of interpersonal strain discussed by Hobfoll (1998).

The third reason why social ties in the church may be able to withstand SES-related pressure may be found by returning to the work of Belle (1982) that was reviewed briefly above. She argued that lower SES women may withdraw from social relationships because they feel they will be unable to reciprocate when former support providers are faced with the need for assistance. Perhaps the church provides a way to help lower SES elders reciprocate. More specifically, the pooling of resources may provide the raw grist necessary for reciprocity that would otherwise have been unavailable to the isolated individual. Moreover, the opportunity to become involved in formal volunteer programs that provide assistance to people in need may help older church members feel they have found a way to pay others back for the help they have received.

The notion that church-based social ties may be immune to social forces that typically corrupt secular social relationships is provocative and thought provoking, but this key issue has never been evaluated empirically. If social ties in the church convey benefits that are truly unique, and if access to these relationships is open to all, then lower SES elders should be as likely as upper SES elders to be deeply involved with other people in the place where they worship. Moreover, if church-based social ties provide coping skills and other benefits to people who

have few secular resources, then the relationship between social relationships in the church and health-related outcomes should be especially evident among older adults in lower SES groups. These issues are
evaluated empirically in the sections that follow by using data from
the RAH Survey to assess the differential involvement and differential
impact perspectives.

Differential Involvement in Church-Based Social Relationships

Consistent with the rationale provided earlier in this chapter,
education is used as the key indicator of SES in late life. A series of ordinary least squares (OLS) multiple regression analyses were performed
in which each of the church-based social relationship measures were
regressed on education as well as age, sex, martial status, and race. The
same waves of observations from the RAH Survey that were used in the
previous sections were used in the analyses presented below.

Church-Based Social Support. Altogether eight tests were conducted
to see if the frequency of receiving and providing various types of
church-based social support varies by SES. Statistically significant findings emerged in two sets of analyses. First, the data indicate that older
adults with higher levels of educational attainment report receiving less
spiritual support from their fellow church members than older people
with fewer years of schooling (Beta = $-.222$; $p < .001$). But in contrast,
the findings further reveal that more highly educated elders are more
likely than less educated elders to believe that fellow church members
would be willing to provide help in the future if it is needed (i.e., anticipated support; Beta = .108; $p < .001$). Statistically significant differences
failed to emerge with respect to received emotional support (Beta = .107;
ns), received tangible support (Beta = $-.055$; *ns*), emotional support provided to others (Beta = .026; *ns*), tangible help given to coreligionists
(Beta = .058; *ns*), satisfaction with emotional support received (Beta =
$-.006$; *ns*), and satisfaction with tangible help received from fellow rank-
and-file church members (Beta = .023; *ns*).

Church-Based Companion Friendships. Recall that two measures of
church-based companion friendships were administered in Wave 3 of
the RAH Survey. The first was designed to determine whether older study
participants had a close companion friend in the congregation where
they worship. Variations by SES in this binary outcome were assessed
with logistic regression. The data indicate that upper SES elders are not
more likely than their lower SES counterparts to report having a close

companion friend at church ($b = -.019$; ns; odds ratio $= 1.019$). However, different results emerged with respect to the second companion friendship measure. The findings reveal that older people with fewer years of schooling were more likely than older adults with higher levels of educational attainment to feel that their close companion friendships at church are more intimate, more open, and contribute more to their self-development (Beta $= -.151$; $p < .01$).

Formal Relationships in the Church. Four measures were administered in the RAH Survey to determine the extent to which older study participants were involved in formal social relationships in the place where they worship. Significant SES differences emerged in only one. In particular, the data suggest that higher levels of educational attainment are associated with more frequent attendance at Bible study groups (Beta $= .080$; $p < .01$), but the magnitude of this relationship is rather modest. In contrast, statistically significant variations by SES failed to emerge with respect to prayer groups (Beta $= .031$; *ns*), participation in volunteer activities (Beta $= .031$; *ns*), and the frequency of worshiping with church members at home among homebound elders (Beta $= .010$; *ns*).

Negative Interaction in the Church. Based on the data from Wave 1 of the RAH Survey, the findings reveal that older adults with lower levels of educational attainment do not encounter more negative interaction with their fellow rank-and-file church members than older people with more years of formal schooling (Beta $= .029$; *ns*). Moreover, statistically significant variations by SES also failed to emerge with respect to negative interaction with a member of the clergy (Beta $= .066$; *ns*).

Summary. Viewed in general terms, substantial variations by SES did not emerge in the analysis of differential involvement in church-based social relationships. Only four of sixteen tests were statistically significant, and of these, two favored more highly educated elders (i.e., anticipated support and participation in Bible study groups), whereas two favored older people with fewer years of schooling (i.e., spiritual support and the nature and functioning of close companion friendships at church). Although care must be taken in interpreting these findings, the results hint at some potentially important underlying mechanisms. Greater anticipated support among more highly educated churchgoers suggests that these individuals may have a greater sense of stability, security, and permanence in the overall relationships they form with fellow church members. Perhaps this greater sense of anticipated support arises from the awareness that the church-based social network members of upper SES elders possess greater resources and are therefore in a better position to provide assistance in the future if it is needed. Moreover, higher levels of participation in Bible study groups among older people with more years of formal schooling may reflect the fact that these groups provide the kind of forum that challenges and taxes the more well-developed intellectual and reasoning skills possessed by older people with higher levels of educational attainment.

The fact that older people with fewer years of schooling report receiving more spiritual support from fellow church members may reflect the influence of denominational differences. More specifically, a number of studies reveal that people with less education are more likely to attend fundamentalist churches (Spilka et al. 2003). Perhaps the informal sharing of religious experiences and religious teaching among rank-and-file church members is more prevalent in fundamentalist than in more liberal congregations. The findings involving companionship friends at church are especially thought provoking because they point to a potentially important source of resilience among lower SES elders, especially when these findings are viewed in conjunction with the results that emerged with anticipated support. The items that were developed to assess anticipated support were designed to measure assistance that participants feel would be provided in the future by members of their congregations taken as a whole. Since congregations tend to be homogeneous with respect to SES, older people with more education may correctly realize that the members of their congregation have the resources at their disposal to help out if need be, whereas lower SES elders do not have the same luxury. Even so, lower SES elders may be more likely to compensate for the lack of overall church network responsiveness by forming a close alliance and cultivating deeper ties with a specific individual in their congregation. This understudied source of potential resilience in lower SES churches deserves careful consideration in future studies.

Differential Impact of Church-Based Social Relationships on Health. SES variations in the relationship between social relationships in the church and health were evaluated with the same data analytic procedures, the same waves of data, and the same demographic control measures that have been used throughout the current chapter. The findings from these analyses are easy to summarize for the following reason. A total of sixty-two tests of the differential impact perspective were conducted. Not one was statistically significant. Consequently, little would be gained by presenting the coefficients associated with each type of church-based social relationship and health. Instead, it makes more sense to reflect on the broader conclusions that may be drawn from these findings. Taken together, the fact that there are no statistically significant differences in the data suggests that if lower SES elders are able to attain the same level of involvement as upper SES elders in the social relationships at church, then lower SES elders are just as likely as upper SES elders to enjoy the health-related benefits associated with them.

Summary. Although researchers have argued for decades that the social relationships of lower SES groups are likely to be compromised, the research reviewed in the two previous sections provides little evidence that this is true with respect to social ties in the church. Specifically, data from the RAH Survey failed to uncover substantial SES differences with respect to differential involvement in church-based social ties, and no evidence whatsoever of a differential impact of church-based social relationships on health-related outcomes emerged from the data. Stated another way, these findings provide little support for the pressure-cooker effect discussed by Hobfoll (1998). However, these results are only preliminary. At least two steps must be taken to evaluate the pressure-cooker effect more fully. First, as discussed above, it is entirely possible that even though social networks in the secular world are subject to the kinds of stresses and strains described by Hobfoll (1998), religious teachings and principles help ensure that the same is not true with respect to church-based social ties. This issue needs to be examined empirically with data on social relationships in both secular and church settings. In the process, researchers need to measure church teaching and religious beliefs regarding social relationships directly and evaluate them empirically. Doing so is necessary because the extent to which religious teachings and precepts are endorsed in a congregation is likely to vary. Second, the analyses presented throughout this section were based solely on one marker of SES: education. As Mirowsky and Ross (2003) correctly point out, the various indicators of SES have different functions. Developing a well-articulated theory of how the functions that are associated specifically with education affect social ties in the church should be a high priority for investigators wishing to move research on SES differences in church-based social ties forward. A sense of how to begin developing this kind of theory may be found in the discussion of the functions of education that Mirowsky and Ross (2003) provide. They argue that education "develops the ability to write, communicate, solve problems, analyze data, and develop ideas, and implement plans...Education also develops broadly effective habits and attitudes, such as dependability, good judgment, motivation, effort, trust, and confidence....Because education develops competence on many levels it gives people the ability and motivation to shape and control their lives" (51–52). Factors like communication skills, trust, and control have emerged as important intervening constructs throughout this volume. Evaluating them in conjunction with education and social relationships in the church may provide valuable insights.

Conclusions

The research reviewed in this chapter suggests that social structural factors may exert an important influence on the social relationships that older people form at church. However, the various facets of social structure did not appear to exert comparable effects. Instead, the greatest differences emerged with respect to race, followed by gender, and then SES. These findings need to be replicated by other investigators. If these results are verified by others, then we need to know more about why the influence of race overshadows the impact of either gender or SES. Perhaps the influence of the larger cultural influences identified by Baldwin and Hopkins (1990) come into play here.

The data presented in this chapter also provide fairly consistent support for the differential involvement perspective whereas less support was garnered for the differential impact perspective. Thus, social structural variations in the health of older people are likely to arise primarily because older blacks and older women tend to be more deeply involved in developing social ties with fellow church members than either older whites or older men. But it cannot be reiterated often enough that the tests of the differential impact perspective were very preliminary because only a limited range of health outcomes were examined. In addition, only one type of stressor was used to assess the differential impact of church-based social support on health (i.e., stressful life events). However, as discussed in chapter 2, it is crucial to explore the potentially important influence of other types of stress in this context. Chief among these alternative stressors are chronic strains and lifetime traumas.

A host of other issues need to be examined in addition to providing more complete tests of the differential impact perspective. For example, the discussion and data on race differences in church-based social ties focused exclusively on older African Americans. As discussed earlier in this chapter, research is needed on older members of other racial and ethnic groups, especially older Mexican Americans. Fortunately, the National Institute of Aging has provided funds to expand the scope of the RAH Survey to include older Mexican Americans. However, it will be some time before the data on older Mexican Americans will be collected and analyzed.

Research on social structural differences in church-based social relationships and health would also benefit from the valuable insights provided by Schieman and his colleagues (Schieman, Pudrovska, & Milkie 2005). The research presented throughout the current chapter focused solely on the unique influences of race, gender, and SES (i.e., the effects when each social structural component was examined separately). However, as Schieman et al. (2005) demonstrate, greater insights may be obtained by looking at the joint effects of these social structural factors. More specifically, these researchers report finding important variations in the effects of divine control on self-esteem whereby the greatest benefits were enjoyed by older black women, followed by older black men, older white women, and older white men, respectively. This pattern of results was interpreted, in part, by turning to the deprivation-compensation hypothesis, which states that individuals who experience social and economic disadvantage are more likely to turn to, and benefit from, involvement in religion. And because both women and blacks are disadvantaged in American society, it is not surprising to find that the joint influence of race and gender is an especially important factor.

Unfortunately, researchers are likely to encounter significant data analytic challenges when attempting to implement the approach used by Schieman et al. (2005) to study the health-related effects of social relationships in the church. This problem is especially evident with respect to the study of church-based social support on health. Tests of the differential impact of race, for example, were evaluated in the current chapter by testing for a three-way statistical interaction effect on health between race, church-based social support, and stress. Expanding these analyses to include the effects of gender would require that tests be performed for a four-way interaction. At least three problems arise when four-way interaction effects are proposed in a study. First, scientists have argued for decades that parsimony is an important prerequisite for the development of viable theories in virtually any field. For example, Albert Einstein argued, "A theory is the more impressive the greater the simplicity of its premises, the more different kinds of things it relates, and the more extended is its area of applicability" (as quoted in Jammer 1999, 136–137; see also discussions of Occam's razor, Bolles 1957). The theoretical rationale needed to justify tests for four-way interactions appears to violate this long-standing principle of parsimony. Second, the cell sizes in a four-way interaction are likely to be quite small even in surveys that have relatively large overall sample sizes. This is especially true when the variables of interest are skewed, as measures of church-based social support often are (i.e., few older people fail to get any support from the people with whom they worship). To the extent this is true, tests of complex interaction terms may suffer from the well-known problems associated with data sparseness (see Cohen, Cohen, West, & Aiken 2003, for a discussion of how this problem affects substantive study findings). Second, tests for four-way interactions require that all lower-order interaction terms be added to the model, including the two-way and three-way interaction effects. As Aneshensel (2002) warns, the multiple correlation among multiple interaction terms can become quite high, creating data estimation problems associated with multicollinearity. It is important to emphasize that the multiple correlation among cross-product terms remains high even when the individual variables that are used to create them are centered on their means.

Although clear challenges face those who wish to examine social structural variations in research on church-based social relationships and health, continued work in this area is essential because it sketches out the wider social context in which church-based social ties operate, and it brings the porous boundaries between social life in the church and social life in wider society to the foreground. In the process, it helps merge research that is more psychological in nature with research that is decidedly sociological. This underscores yet another benefit of studying social relationships in the church: it provides a forum for merging and integrating research from diverse disciplines, thereby enhancing the quality of the work that is done.

Chapter 7

Conclusions

Taking a Broader Perspective
and Identifying Next Steps

There are two straightforward ways to document the important role that religion plays in social life. The first has to do with historical issues, whereas the second is more anthropological in nature. According to Eliade (1978), the first historical evidence that people were involved in religion may be found in the burial practices of prehistoric man. More specifically, he maintains that relics containing rich religious themes have been unearthed at ancient burial sites that date as far back as 300,000 to 400,000 BC. In addition, research by other investigators reveals that some form of religion may be found in virtually every culture in the world today (Smith 1991). If religion has persisted for so long and it may be found in so many different cultural settings, then it must be performing some basic function; that is, religion must be satisfying some fundamental human needs. Spilka and his colleagues identify three human needs that religion satisfies (Spilka et al. 2003): the need for meaning, the need for control, and the need for sociality (i.e., the need for interpersonal interaction). The current volume has been devoted to the third function, but in a more circumscribed way. Rather than assessing how religion helps people meet the need for sociality per se, the intent has been to trace the health-related implications of church-based social relationships once they are already in place. Drawing on evidence from a host of different disciplines, an effort was made to show the ways in which involvement in church-based social ties may affect the physical and mental health of older people. Although it is too early to make definitive or conclusive statements about these findings, a prudent conclusion is that enough evidence has accumulated to justify further research in this area.

But instead of merely reviewing what is already available in the literature, the goal of writing this book has been to provide a blueprint or road map to guide investigators who are interested in conducting research on the interface between church-based social relationships and health in late life. This blueprint was based on two fundamental principles. First, it was argued that further advances in the field will not take place unless researchers pay careful attention to the interface between measurement and theory. Without good measures, sound theory is of little value, and without sound theory, researchers will not know how to craft good measures of key study constructs. However, recognizing and discussing this widely known dictum does not go far enough. Instead, it must be carried over into practice by presenting measures of key types of church-based social ties and providing a clear theoretical rationale for their development. This is precisely what has been done throughout the current volume.

The second fundamental principle that formed the cornerstone of this book has to do with the type of theory that investigators should endeavor to devise in order to explain how church-based social relationships may affect the physical and mental health of older people. At the present time, it is unlikely that meaningful theoretical advances will be achieved by devising a single overarching conceptual framework that attempts to explain how all the different kinds of social relationships in the church affect health. Instead, based on the insights of Robert Merton (1949), it was proposed that researchers begin more modestly by deriving a series of mid-range theories that illuminate the linkages between each specific type of social relationship in the church and health. The reasons for doing so are straightforward. In order to devise complex models that contain a wide range of constructs correctly, researchers must first understand all the characteristics and finer nuances of each element, which is best achieved by developing a series of models that test more limited mid-range theories. Once the key aspects of each component are fully illuminated, seeing how to best combine them will be easier.

Consistent with this goal, a series of potentially important mid-range theories were identified. Whenever possible, preliminary empirical tests of these linkages were performed with data from the RAH Survey. Some of the intervening constructs in these models were explicitly religious in nature. For example, it was proposed in chapter 2 that one way in which church-based social support affects health is through religious coping responses that fellow church members encourage older people to adapt. Focusing on intervening constructs that are religious in nature is important because it provides one way of creating a sense of order in a literature that has developed in a rather disjointed and unsystematic way. Moreover, searching for theoretically meaningful connections between different facets of religion takes the first step toward devising more comprehensive, higher-order theories of church-based social relationships and health. Other intervening constructs are examined in this volume that are more secular in nature. For example, it was proposed in chapter 5 that negative interaction may affect health by fostering a range of negative emotions, including anger. As noted in chapter 1, linking religious and secular constructs is important because it helps ground research on church-based social ties in the wider secular literature on health in late life.

In addition to adhering to fundamental principles involving measure and the development of mid-range theory, an effort was made to guide further work by highlighting a range of specific conceptual and methodological issues that emerge when studying each specific type of social relationship in the church. For example, when church-based companion friendships were evaluated in chapter 3, a series of conceptual challenges were identified that arise from the potential overlap between social support provided by fellow church members and the functions of companion friendships in church. It was pointed out that the same individual is likely to provide social support and be a close companion friend. To the extent this is true, it may be difficult to differentiate between the health-related consequences of these two types of church-based social relationships.

Taken as a whole, the underlying themes that form the infrastructure of this volume result in a product that is relatively unique and that departs from the way most books on religion and health are written. So far, most of the volumes on religion and health in late life focus primarily on theoretical or conceptual issues (e.g., Koenig 1999; Levin 2001). These works have made invaluable contributions to the field. But the underlying premise in the current book is that even greater insight is likely to emerge when investigators focus on the interface between theory, measurement, and methodological issues. Hopefully, this more pragmatic approach will provide researchers with a concise understanding of the issues they face and give them a concrete set of tools for resolving them.

With the exception of chapter 6, the chapters in this volume provide an in-depth examination of specific social ties in the church. Each type of church-based social relationship was examined individually. But it is important also to discuss wider issues that affect all church-based social relationships regardless of the specific form they take. These issues form the focal point of the current chapter. Three are highlighted in the following discussion. The first has to do with core religious beliefs that bolster and maintain all types of social ties in the church, whereas the second involves conceptual and methodological issues that must be taken into account regardless of the particular type of church-based social relationship under consideration. After examining these factors, this chapter ends with a broader, more philosophical view of the role that is played by subjectivity in research on social ties in church.

Core Religious Beliefs and Church-Based Social Relationships

An emphasis has been placed throughout this book on showing how various types of social ties that arise in the church may enhance the physical and mental health of the older people who worship there. In the process, evidence was presented which suggests that social relationships in the church may be more well developed and more efficacious than social ties that are found in the wider secular world. However, insufficient attention was given to why this may be so. Instead, only passing reference was made to the influence of church teachings regarding issues like compassion, helping people who are in need, and forgiving individuals who have done something wrong. If researchers are to arrive at a deeper understanding of the interpersonal relationships that older people form in the church, then they must delve more deeply into the underlying belief structures that bolster and maintain them. The purpose of the discussion that is provided in this section is to explore the interface between religious beliefs and social relationships in the church. Consistent with the approach that has been taken throughout this volume, this exploration focuses on issues involving the conceptualization, measurement, and empirical assessment of key constructs.

Stark and Glock (1968) identified five key dimensions of religion. Perhaps it is no coincidence that the first dimension they discussed was the belief dimension. The belief dimension involves the expectations and theological outlook that forms the core of all world religions. In fact, Stark and Glock (1968) go as far as to argue, "For all religions it can be said that theology, or religious belief, is at the heart of faith" (16). If beliefs lie at the core of religion, then perhaps greater insight into the religious foundation of church-based social relationships may be found by identifying the belief structures that bolster and maintain the social ties that older adults form with fellow congregants. Even though the potential influence of religious teachings and beliefs on social relationships in the church has been discussed widely in the literature, far less effort has been spent on evaluating this issue empirically.

Davidson (1972) conducted one of the first studies on the interface between religious beliefs and social relationships. In this work, he made a distinction between the vertical and horizontal dimensions of religion. The vertical dimension refers to the relationship that a person establishes with God, whereas the horizontal dimension has to do with the relationships that an individual develops with other people. Davidson (1972) devised a brief measure of the horizontal dimension that consists of two indicators. The first deals with the need to love one's neighbors, and the second involves the importance of helping one's fellow man. Although loving and helping others clearly affects the quality of the social relationships that a person may develop, a deeper and more fundamental set of beliefs may lie behind them. More specifically, it may not be enough to believe that people should love and help each other; instead, these beliefs are likely to have a greater effect on the development of social ties if people have a clear sense of why loving and helping others is important. Recently, Krause and Bastida (2007) attempted to address this issue by arguing that beliefs about loving and helping others arise from a deeper and more fundamental sense of spiritual connectedness. Spiritual connectedness is defined as the belief that a close bond exists among all people, regardless of whether they are religious or not. This sense of oneness arises from the individual's awareness of his or her unity with the wider social whole. When people realize that their fate is tied to the fate of all others, their attitude shifts from one of hostility, competition, or indifference to one of empathy, compassion, and concern. Out of this wider and more enduring sense of oneness and connectedness, the unique aspects of religiously-based social ties are likely to arise.

The notion that human relationships are based on a deep underlying sense of connectedness is hardly new. Evidence of this notion may be found by turning to the work of three classic social theorists who were introduced in chapter 1: Edward Alsworth Ross, Charles Horton Cooley, and Josiah Royce. In his insightful paper on religion, Ross (1896) captured the essence and importance of spiritual connectedness when he wrote, "It is one thing to recognize the manifold interactions of men in social life and to act accordingly; it is quite another thing to believe that apart from, and prior to, the bonds of interdependence, trust, or affection that grow up in the social mechanism, there is a unity of essence that calls for justice and sympathy between men. *The mere perception of likeness fosters sympathy, but the conviction of underlying oneness does more.* It destroys the egocentric world which each unreflecting creature builds for itself.... It fosters respect for others.... It lessens our willingness to use them as means to our own ends" (Ross 1896, 441, emphasis added).

Similar views were espoused by Cooley (1927), who emphasized the importance of seeing the fundamental connectedness and interdependence among all people: "The actual interdependence of human life, of persons, classes, nations, far surpasses our awareness of it, and still more our arrangements for cooperation. Wisdom is largely the perception of this interdependence, and the endeavor to give it organs" (241). Cooley (1927) then went on to ground this sense of connectedness and interdependence specifically within the context of religion: "The best religious education would be one that accustomed us from childhood to cooperation...in service of human wholes. Through family, the play-group, the school, the community, the nation, humanity, we might acquire an enlarging sense of God" (265).

Like Ross (1896) and Cooley (1927), Royce (1912/2001) strongly believed that the road to greater human progress and that attainment of deeper religious insight lay in recognizing the common bond that exists among all people. Specifically, he wrote, "Man is, indeed, a being who cannot be saved alone, however much solitude may help him, at times, toward insight. For he is bound to his brethren by spiritual links that cannot be broken.... Their plight is common; their very need for salvation chains them together" (Royce 1912/2001, 65).

Krause and Bastida (2007) developed a brief three-item index to assess spiritual connectedness that was discussed by these grand theorists. Study participants were asked how strongly they agree or disagree with the following indicators: (1) "My faith helps me see the common bond among all people"; (2) "My faith helps me appreciate how much we need each other"; and (3) "My faith helps me recognize the tremendous strength that can come from other people." These items are grounded specifically in a religious context (i.e., "My faith..."), which is important for this study because a sense of connectedness with others may arise from a number of sources outside religion. In fact, some evidence exists that a sense of connectedness with others may arise from explicitly antireligious sentiments. Evidence of this may be found by turning to the work of two well-known philosophers.

The first is Bertrand Russell. In 1957 he wrote a famous essay titled *Why I Am Not a Christian* (1957/2000). In it, Russell argued that God is little more than a figment of man's superstitious nature and that life is essentially a time of endless pain and suffering. Even so, he saw a deep sense of connectedness among all people: "Let us remember that they are fellow sufferers in the same darkness, actors in the same tragedy as ourselves" (Russell 1957/2000, 76–77). Because of this status, Russell argued, "Be it ours to shed sunshine on their path, to lighten their sorrows by the balm of our sympathy, to give them pure joy of a never-tiring affection" (76).

The same views were expressed in even stronger terms by Schopenhauer. Writing in the nineteenth century, he stated that there is no God and that "the world is Hell and men on the one hand the tormented souls and on the other the devils in it" (Schopenhauer 1851/2004, 48). But just like Russell (1957/2000), Schopenhauer (1851/2004) believed that this shared suffering "makes us see other men in a true light and reminds us of what are the most necessary among all things: tolerance, patience, forbearance, and charity, which each of us needs and which each of us therefore owes" (50). Simply put, for both of these noted philosophers, pain in the world and the absence of God bind people together.

Krause and Bastida's (2007) empirical analyses involve seeing whether their newly devised index of spiritual connectedness was associated with three outcomes: providing emotional support to fellow church members, giving tangible assistance to other people at church, and praying for others. Two points should be emphasized about these outcomes. To begin with, the first two outcomes involve giving assistance rather than receiving it. These particular types of social support were selected for the following reason: if church-based social relationships arise from feeling connected with other people, then the link between these constructs is more likely to be found by focusing on measures of giving support, because the decision to help others is more likely to reflect the influence of these core religious beliefs. In contrast, an older person may accept help from others simply because he or she needs it and not because of feeling a particularly strong sense of spiritual connectedness with the individual who is giving assistance. The measure of praying for others was included in this study because it may be construed as a uniquely religious form of helping others. When people pray for someone else, they are actively doing something to help someone who is in need (i.e., they are interceding with God on behalf of another individual).

Krause and Bastida (2007) used the data from the first two waves of the RAH Survey to examine the relationship between spiritual connect-edness and the three study outcomes. The Wave 1 and Wave 2 measures of spiritual connectedness were included in the latent variable mod-els they evaluated in order to see if change in spiritual connectedness is associated with change in the helping behaviors identified above. The findings suggest that an increase over time in feelings of spiritual con-nectedness is associated with an increase in giving emotional and tangi-ble support to others as well as an increase in praying for other people. Simply put, the data are consistent with the notion that core religious beliefs embedded in the measures of spiritual connectedness may form the basis of social relationships that arise in the church.

Although additional work is needed to see if spiritual connected-ness is associated with other types of church-based social ties, bringing these core religious beliefs to the foreground helps to ground research on church-based social relationships in a deeper and more fundamen-tal context. In the process, this work helps address one of the more challenging aspects of conducting research on religion. As noted above, Stark and Glock (1968) maintain that beliefs lie at the very heart of reli-gion. Even so, researchers often encounter difficulty when studying this facet of religion because there are so many different kinds of beliefs. One way to overcome this problem is to begin by focusing on specific types of religious behaviors, such as providing support to others, and then subse-quently identifying the specific religious beliefs that promote and rein-force them.

General Conceptual and Methodological Challenges

In the process of assessing core religious values that underlie all types of social ties in the church, it is also important to address a series of general methodological and conceptual challenges. Nine are identi-fied and examined in the discussion that follows. These more generic issues include:

1. Exploring denominational differences and investigating other faiths.
2. Identifying and assessing other types of social relationships in the church.
3. Addressing issues involving the direction of causality in studies of church-based social ties and health.
4. Properly interpreting findings from longitudinal studies of social relationships in the church and health.

5. Understanding the limits of social relationships in the church and how their potential benefits are likely to be manifest.
6. Exploring a full range of physical and mental health outcomes that are especially relevant for people in late life.
7. Differentiating between the manifest and latent functions of social ties in the church.
8. Confronting potential problems arising from response bias.
9. Interpreting effect sizes that emerge from empirical studies of church-based social ties and health.

Before turning to these general conceptual and methodological issues, it is important to touch briefly on two points. First, whole volumes have been written on a number of these issues. As a result, reviewing all that is known about them here is not possible. Instead, the discussion provided below is designed to make researchers aware that these issues exist, provide guidance on how to address them in studies on religion and health, and encourage investigators to read more deeply about them. Second, when the general issues discussed below are coupled with the specific conceptual and methodological issues that have been presented throughout this volume, researchers may get the impression that designing sound studies of the relationship between church-based social ties and health is a daunting, if not virtually impossible, task. But there is another way to look at it. Each time effort is exerted to identify and grapple with these issues, researchers obtain a little more insight into the scope and complexity of the task that awaits them. Not only does this incremental learning strategy lead to higher-quality research, it also instills a greater appreciation for the intricate nature of the processes under investigation and the deep sense of mystery from which they emerge.

Exploring Different Denominations and Other Faiths

As noted in chapter 1, this volume focuses on social ties in the Christian Church. However, the Christian Church is not one single entity with a unified doctrine and a set of religious practices that are performed consistently by all of the faithful. Instead, the Christian Church is fractured into a bewildering array of denominations that vary widely in the way fundamental precepts of the faith are taught and implemented in daily life. If religious teachings and practices vary significantly across denominations, then researchers need to know if there are denominational differences in the level and impact of the church-based social relationships that are based upon them. The fact that this issue has not been discussed until now reflects the current state of the literature. Simply put, there do not appear to be any studies that examine denominational differences in the level and impact of church-based social relationships on health and well-being in late life. It is time to correct this glaring oversight.

Evidence that denominational variation may exist in church-based social support may be found by extending the insights in historian Robert Orsi's (2005) thoughtful book on the teachings and practices of the Catholic faith from the 1930s through the 1960s. This time frame is important because it represents the period in which many of the currently older Catholics came of age. Although Orsi (2005) discusses a number of specific practices and beliefs, the way Catholics were taught to deal with adversity during this era is especially relevant for the study of church-based social support: "There was only one officially sanctioned way to suffer even the most excruciating distress: with bright, upbeat, and uncomplaining submissive endurance....No matter how severe your suffering...Jesus' and Mary's were worse, and they never complained" (26–27; emphasis in original).

If Orsi's (2005) observations are accurate, then the notion that it is important to suffer in silence has clear implications for research on denominational differences in the mobilization of social support from fellow church members. For example, the insights provided by Orsi (2005) suggest that older Catholics may be less likely to seek out church-based emotional support than older Protestants because older Catholics believe they should suffer in silence. Some preliminary insight into this issue can be obtained by turning to the data in the first wave of interviews in the RAH Survey. A binary variable was created in these unpublished analyses to compare Catholics (scored 1) with members of all other Christian denominations (scored 0). Then, the simple bivariate correlation was estimated between this binary variable and the frequency of emotional support provided by fellow rank-and-file church members. Consistent with the observations of Orsi (2005), the findings suggest that older Catholics are less likely than older Christians who affiliate with other denominations to turn to fellow church members for emotional support ($r = -.258$; $p < .01$). However, great care must be taken in interpreting this finding. The data should not be viewed as suggesting that all older Catholics therefore lack adequate coping resources. Instead, they may rely on different, more psychological coping mechanisms, such as praying to the saints or saying the rosary. Viewed in a more general way, the data may simply reflect differences in religious cultures.

Denominational differences may also emerge in the relationship between church-based social ties and well-being. For example, recall from chapter 2 that McFadden, Knepple, and Armstrong (2003) studied social support provided by friends at church. In the process, they question whether spiritual support will always be welcomed when it is offered by fellow church members: "We do not yet know...whether some people might be offended if they were offered spiritual support from people they did not consider to be friends" (McFadden et al. 2003, 43). It follows from this observation that spiritual support is not likely to be effective if older people are offended when someone attempts to provide it, but this is likely to happen only under certain circumstances. Perhaps exchanges of spiritual support are more likely to be encouraged in evangelic and fundamentalist churches than in liberal churches (Poloma & Hoelter 1998). If this is true, then fundamentalists should derive greater benefits from receiving spiritual support than either moderates or liberals. Some preliminary insight into these issues may be found by turning to the Wave 1 data in the RAH Survey. An ordinal variable was created that contrasts members of fundamentalist (scored 1), moderate (scored 2), and liberal (scored 3) congregations. The bivariate correlation that emerges from these unpublished analyses suggests that liberals and moderates get less spiritual support from fellow church members than do fundamentalists ($r = -.295$; $p < .001$).

However, the correlation between denominational preference and spiritual support does not reveal if moderates and liberals are more likely than fundamentalists to be offended when spiritual support is offered. Unfortunately, measures of whether people were offended when they were offered spiritual support are not available in the RAH Survey data. It is possible, however, to gain some preliminary insight into this issue by testing the following rationale: if older people are offended when spiritual support is offered, then they should be less likely to enjoy the benefits that arise from receiving this type of assistance. Deriving a greater sense of life satisfaction is among the benefits that are likely to emerge from receiving spiritual support. Therefore, if spiritual support is more likely to be welcomed in fundamentalist congregations, the impact of spiritual support on life satisfaction should be greater among fundamentalists than among moderates or liberals. This reasoning can be evaluated by testing for a statistical interaction effect between the ordinal religious affiliation measure discussed above and spiritual support on life satisfaction. This test was performed with the Wave 1 data from the RAH Survey. Age, sex, education, race, and frequency of church attendance and private prayer were included as control variables. The data suggest that a statistically significant interaction was present in the data ($b = -.057$; $p < .05$). Further analyses reveal that the impact of spiritual support on life satisfaction is greater among fundamentalists than among moderates or liberals.

The analyses presented here are very preliminary. A much more thorough investigation is needed to see whether there are denominational variations in the full range of church-based social relationship measures that have been discussed throughout this volume. Nevertheless, it is hoped that the analyses presented here convince investigators that further work on denominational variations in church-based social ties is warranted.

But studying denominational differences does not go far enough. America is a diverse nation that contains people who practice a number of faiths other than Christianity. Research is needed on social relationships in places where people practice other faiths, such as synagogues and mosques. The importance of this type of work can be highlighted by focusing on forgiveness. As discussed in chapter 2, forgiveness is an important resource for coping with interpersonal problems that arise inside and outside the church. In the process, a study by Krause and Ellison (2003) was discussed which revealed that older people who tend to forgive transgressors right away tend to experience fewer symptoms of depression and death anxiety and are more satisfied with their lives than older adults who require transgressors to perform acts of contrition. However, the data for this study came from the RAH Survey, which consists solely of Christians. This point is important because unconditional forgiveness is a basic tenet that is not necessarily endorsed by all faiths. More specifically, as an insightful paper by Frankel (1998) reveals, people of the Jewish faith receive different guidance on how to go about forgiving others. For Jews, requiring others to perform acts of contrition is important when it is done appropriately (see also Schimmel 2002). So if the study conducted by Krause and Ellison (2003) were to be conducted with older Jewish participants, the results may change dramatically. For this reason, investigators wishing to explore the relationship between social ties and the church should branch out into the study of older people with different faith traditions.

Identifying Other Types of Social Relationships in the Church

A fairly wide range of formal and informal social relationships in the church have been examined throughout this volume. However, as noted in chapter 1, no effort was made to develop a comprehensive taxonomy of all the different types of social relationships that may be found in a congregation. Instead, the goal of the current volume was to identify and discuss at least some of the major types of social relationships that are found in church settings. This modest approach is justified given the current state of the literature. Simply put, this appears to be the first time an effort has been made to explore the nature and effects of a range of different social relationships in the church on the health and well-being of older people. Although this effort may have contributed to the literature, a significant amount of work remains to be done. More specifically, it is important for researchers to identify and evaluate other kinds of social relationships that may arise in the church that have not been discussed here. So, for example, an older person may become an elder, deacon, or lay minister in his or her congregation. These formal roles in the church, and the relationships that arise from occupying them, differ from the formal roles discussed in chapter 4 in at least three ways. First, unlike the other roles that have been examined in the current volume, one of the major functions of these roles is to help preserve the life of the church (i.e., perpetuate the institution). Second, roles such as lay minister, deacon, and elder carry a certain amount of prestige and authority, which may influence the way people who occupy them interact with rank-and-file church members. Third, roles such as lay minister, deacon, or elder may affect health and well-being in ways that have yet to be explored. Some indication of the unique effects of these roles on health and well-being was discussed in chapter 5. Recall the study by Krause et al. (1998) which showed that negative interaction in the church has a greater adverse effect on the well-being of pastors and church elders than on rank-and-file church members.

The pastoral role represents another instance where further research on social relationships in the church is needed. Several ways in which church members interact with the clergy have been examined throughout this volume. For example, the therapeutic relationship that arises between a pastor and a rank-and-file church member was discussed in some detail in chapter 4. But no effort has been made to conduct a full exposition of all the ways in which members of the clergy interact with others at church. It could easily take a separate volume to address this issue properly. However, given the key role that clergy play in the social life of the church, it is important for researchers to conduct a more systematic and comprehensive study of the social ties that members of the clergy forge in religious institutions.

Probing the Direction of Causality

It should be emphasized at the outset that causality can never be determined conclusively with survey data. This problem arises because an investigator will never know if the relationship that is observed between two constructs, such as church-based companionship and health, can be explained by a third variable that has not been included in the analyses (e.g., neuroticism). Nevertheless, an investigator can feel more comfortable with the causal assumptions he or she has made by addressing another of the classic criteria for determining causality (see Bradley & Schaefer 1998, for a detailed discussion of the criteria for establishing causality). More specifically, if longitudinal data are available, then it is possible to see if the cause (e.g., church-based companionship) precedes the effect (e.g., health) in time. Unfortunately, there do not appear to be any studies in the literature that systematically assess whether a full range of church-based social relationship measures precede health-related outcomes in time. Exploring a set of hypothetical analyses highlights the challenges that arise in conducting this kind of work and the payoff from doing it properly.

Assume that the purpose of a study is to see if church-based negative interaction is associated with depression in late life. There are two reasons that these constructs may be related. First, as discussed in chapter 5, something about negative interaction in the church may increase the odds that an older person will subsequently become depressed. However, there is a second way to interpret the relationship between these constructs. A positive correlation between them could simply mean that people who are depressed tend to have more conflicted relationships with people at church because their mental health problems interfere with their ability to interact with others in a positive and constructive manner. A common strategy for addressing this issue involves assessing the relationship between negative interaction at Wave 1 and depression at Wave 2, controlling for depression at Wave 1. The findings from this model would help an investigator see if church-based negative interaction is associated with change in depression. But this model examines only the first of the two possibilities identified above. It says nothing about the potential effect of Wave 1 depression on change in negative interaction. And because this latter issue is not evaluated explicitly, it cannot be ruled out. In order to assess this alternative specification, researchers must estimate a model that contains four constructs: negative interaction and depression assessed at Wave 1 as well as negative interaction and depression assessed at Wave 2. Then structural equation modeling can be used to assess the effects of negative interaction on change in depression at the same time the effects of baseline depression on change in negative interaction are evaluated. Estimating each possibility separately is not good enough, because more precise estimates are derived by evaluating them simultaneously.

Unfortunately, this simple two-wave, four-construct model overlooks another important set of questions. This model looks at lagged relationships only (e.g., the effect of baseline negative interaction on change in depression over Wave 1 and Wave 2). However, it is possible that instead of being lagged, there are contemporaneous relationships among these constructs. This means, for example, that an older person may experience symptoms of depression soon after he or she encounters negative interaction with a fellow church member. In fact, further reflection suggests that this scenario may even be more plausible, especially when a significant amount of time has elapsed between the Wave 1 and Wave 2 interviews. It is not unusual for this between-round interval to be two years or longer. Under these circumstances, it is not clear why two years would have to transpire before the effects of negative interaction on depression would become manifest. The same situation arises with the alternative specification discussed above. If an older person is depressed, then it is likely that the interpersonal tensions created by their mental health problems are likely to arise right away. To the extent this is true, researchers must test for contemporaneous as well as lagged effects. However, data estimation problems arise when both tests are performed with simple two-wave, four-construct models. The problem arises because these models are not identified (i.e., more estimates are requested from the model than it is capable of providing because sufficient information is not available to derive all of them). As Kessler and Greenberg (1981) pointed out some time ago, adding a third wave of observations provides the information that is necessary to estimate both lagged and contemporaneous effects.

The issues discussed in this section are complex, but it is vitally important to recognize them because researchers must be aware of these issues when a study is being planned. Otherwise, sufficient funds will not be requested to collect the data that are needed to address them (i.e., a third wave of interviews). For this reason, problems arising from tests of the classic criteria for determining causality have been reviewed here.

Interpreting Findings from Longitudinal Studies

A subtle issue that is not discussed often in the literature emerges when researchers attempt to interpret findings that surface from longitudinal studies of social ties in the church. This issue is best introduced by focusing on the findings from a recent study by Krause (2007b). Consistent with the theoretical rationale provided in chapter 2, this longitudinal study examined the interface between church-based social support (especially spiritual support from fellow church members) and feelings of God-mediated control over time. The findings revealed that there was a positive, statistically significant relationship between spiritual support at Wave 1 and God-mediated control at Wave 2 controlling for the effects of God-mediated control at Wave 1. The key issue involves how to interpret this result. Most investigators would argue that this positive relationship indicates that spiritual support *increases* feelings of God-mediated control over time. However, as Kessler and Greenberg (1981) argued some time ago, a positive relationship between factors like spiritual support and God-mediated control may reflect not one, but two potentially important influences. In addition to increasing feelings of God-mediated control over time, the positive relationship between these constructs may also mean that spiritual support from fellow church members helps *sustain* feelings of God-mediated control over time. The two are not the same.

Krause (2007b) argued that, if anything, spiritual support may be more likely to sustain rather than increase feelings of God-mediated control in studies involving older people. This hypothesis was based on the following rationale: findings from an earlier study by Krause and Wulff (2005) reveal that older people have typically attended the place where they worship for a longer period of time than younger adults. Consequently, the social relationships that older people have formed with fellow church members are likely to have been in place for a fairly long time. Although social relationships in the church may initially increase an older person's sense of God-mediated control when they are first formed, it is unlikely that close social ties will continue to increase God-mediated control indefinitely. In fact, further reflection suggests this is a logical impossibility. Instead, once social relationships become stable and ongoing, significant others are more likely to help older people sustain and maintain a sense of God-mediated control.

Krause (2007b) provided a preliminary test of this issue by implementing the following strategy: First, God-mediated control values at Wave 1 were subtracted from God-mediated control values at Wave 2. Then, an outcome variable was created that consisted of three ordinal categories that designate three potential patterns of change and stability in God-mediated control scores over time: older people who experienced an increase in God-mediated control, older adults whose feelings of God-mediated control remained the same, and older study participants whose sense of God-mediated control declined over the course of the study. Then, using multinomial logistic regression, the ordinal outcome was regressed on Wave 1 measures of age, sex, education, race, organizational religiousness (i.e., attendance at worship services, Bible study groups, and prayer groups), and spiritual support. The findings reveal that compared to older people who experienced a decline in God-mediated control over time, older people who experienced an increase in God-mediated control do not report receiving more spiritual support from coreligionists. But, in contrast, the data further suggest that, compared to older people who experienced a decline in feelings of God-mediated control, more spiritual support was significantly associated with having the same God-mediated control scores over time. Viewed in a more general way, these analyses provide preliminary support for the notion that spiritual support from fellow church members is more likely to *sustain,* rather than *increase,* feelings of God-mediated control over time (see Kessler & Greenberg 1981, for a more sophisticated way of addressing this issue within a latent variable modeling framework).

The findings from the study by Krause (2007b) are important for two reasons. First, they illustrate how awareness of subtle issues that arise when working with longitudinal data can greatly increase understanding of the precise ways in which the social ties at church influence the lives of older people. Second, it should be evident that the broader issue investigated in this study is generic and applies whenever the relationship between many other facets of religion and health are evaluated over time.

Understanding the Limits of Church-Based Social Ties

Everyone obviously dies at some point. Moreover, research clearly shows that most older people get sick before they die (Federal Interagency Forum on Aging Related Statistics 2004). Given these findings, it is clear that social ties in the church cannot indefinitely prevent illness and death from occurring; at best, social relationships in the church may only postpone these things from happening. Because this is true, the nature of the research question that is under consideration in studies of religion and health changes and becomes more focused. What researchers are really trying to determine is how long church-based social relationships put off or postpone illness onset. Demographers have been aware of this general issue for some time. Writing in 1980, Fries argued that the human life span is relatively fixed, and as a result, all that medical advances and healthy lifestyles can do is reduce or compress the length of time that is spent suffering from various physical health problems. Fries (1980) called this phenomenon the compression of morbidity. This issue has important implications for the way that data in studies on church-based social ties and health are collected and analyzed.

First, thinking in terms of the compression of morbidity affects the way data on health are collected. Instead of merely knowing if an older person has hypertension or diabetes, it is important to know the date of onset for these medical conditions. Second, once these kinds of data have been obtained, special statistical procedures are needed to exploit them properly. For example, hazard rate models can be used to predict the effect of baseline measures of church-based social relationships on the timing of illness onset. In addition, the findings derived with these hazard rate models can provide important insights into issues that arise in the estimation of the latent variable models that were discussed in the section on issues in determining the direction of causality. Two types of effects were examined: lagged and contemporaneous. But if lagged effects arise in the relationship between church-based social ties and health, then it is important to address yet another issue. Specifically, once the baseline data have been gathered, researchers need to know how long to wait before follow-up data are collected at Wave 2. Determining this between-round interval is important, because if data are gathered too soon, investigators will underestimate the true impact of church-based social relationships on health. By focusing on the timing of illness onset, the findings gleaned from the hazard rate models and survival curves can help researchers make a more informed decision about the length of the causal lag, thereby helping to select a more appropriate between-round interval.

Unfortunately, reading the literature on religion and health almost leaves one with the impression that if people become involved in religion they will never get sick and they will never die. But, as noted above, the plain truth of the matter is that everyone dies, and the wider majority of people become seriously ill before they do; this happens to individuals who are deeply religious as well as people who are not. Failing to come explicitly to grips with this issue has opened the door to bitter criticism of research on religion and health (Sloan & Bagiella 2002). One way to counteract these scathing critiques is to describe carefully what religion is and is not capable of doing. Integrating perspectives like the compression of morbidity into research on church-based social ties and health takes an important first step in this direction.

Selecting Physical and Mental Health Outcome Measures

An emphasis has been placed throughout the current volume on the careful and thoughtful measurement of social relationships in the church, but designing and executing a sound study requires more. In particular, study findings are compromised unless equal care and diligence are given to the measurement of physical and mental health outcomes as well. Whole volumes have been written about how to measure physical and mental health status (McDowell & Newell 1996), so adequately covering these vast conceptual domains in only one segment of a single chapter is not possible. Still, the discussion provided below is developed in the hope that touching on a few key issues will help move research forward on church-based social relationships and health. Three issues are especially important. The first has to do with the need to assess biomarkers of physical health status, the second involves selecting mental health outcomes that are best suited for research with older people, while the third focuses on using mental health outcomes that are sensitive to variations in gender and race.

Biomarkers of Physical Health Status. Many studies on religion and physical health status in late life have relied on self-reports of physical health status. For example, study participants are asked whether they have hypertension or whether they have diabetes. In addition, respondents are often asked to rate their overall health status as being excellent, good, fair, or poor. Studies that rely on these measures have produced many valuable findings. However, researchers are becoming increasingly aware that it is important to obtain biomarkers of physical health as well (Seplaki, Goldman, Weinstein, & Lin 2004). Included among these biomarkers are measures of psychoneuroimmunology, blood pressure readings, and various tests that are performed on blood and urine samples. Integrating these types of measures into surveys of church-based social relationships and health are important for at least two reasons. First, there is considerable debate in the literature about the validity of self-reports of various health problems, such as hypertension (Vargas, Burt, Gillum, & Pamuk 1997). Obtaining biomarkers, such as blood pressure readings, will help allay these concerns. Second, including biomakers in research on church-based social ties and health will help integrate this work more tightly into mainstream secular research on health in late life. Fortunately, some preliminary steps have been taken in this direction. For example, Koenig and Cohen (2002b) recently published an edited volume on psychoneuroimmunology and religiousness. In this book, Koenig and Cohen (2002a) provide a conceptual overview of the potentially important role that social support may play in the link between religion and health. However, as these investigators point out, "No research has yet to examine the relationships among religious activity, social support, and immune functioning all in one study" (2002a, 129). It is time to do so.

Unfortunately, integrating biomarkers into studies of church-based social relationships and health poses a number of unique challenges, especially in large-scale nationwide surveys. More specifically, obtaining a range of biomarkers is expensive, and it is difficult to coordinate the collection and analyses of them when study participants are spread across the coterminous United States. One way to address this problem is to supplement nationwide surveys with studies that obtain biomarkers of health from a subsample of older people who reside in more geographically circumscribed areas.

Special Issues When Studying the Mental Health of Older Adults. When a special population, such as older people, is studied, it is important to include outcome measures that are most likely to reflect the mental health problems that older adults are likely to experience. It is easy to see why study findings would be compromised if specific types of mental health problems are overlooked entirely or measured inadequately. Both issues are discussed here.

Cognitive impairment is a mental health problem that is fairly widespread in late life. More specifically, findings from the widely cited Epidemiologic Catchment Area (ECA) surveys suggest that less than 5 percent of the people under age fifty-five suffer from mild cognitive impairment. However, by age seventy-five, over 22 percent of the population suffers from mild cognitive impairment (George, Landerman, Blazer, & Anthony 1991). Yet there do not appear to be any studies that assess the relationship between church-based social relationships and cognitive functioning, even though there is good reason to do so. More specifically, findings from a longitudinal study by Seeman, Lusignolo, Albert, and Berkman (2001) that was conducted in a secular setting suggest that greater baseline emotional support was significantly associated with better cognitive functioning at the follow-up, controlling for baseline cognitive functioning and a range of potential confounding measures. These investigators speculate that the mental stimulation that arises from social interaction serves to maintain and enhance the cognitive abilities of older people. If social relationships in the church are more efficacious than secular social ties as Ellison and Levin (1998) maintain, then church-based social ties may be an especially important determinant of cognitive functioning in late life. Unfortunately, there do not appear to be any studies in the literature that examine the effects of social ties in the church on cognitive functioning. The failure to do so may underestimate the potentially important role played by social relationships in the church in late life.

Even when appropriate mental health outcomes are selected for studies of older people, care must be taken to select measures that capture the way symptoms of these disorders are expressed specifically in late life. Blazer (2002) discusses this issue at length. He points out how depression may be confounded with physical health problems, medication use, and normal age-related changes in sleeping patterns. This requires that special steps be taken to identify these potential confounders when assessing either clinical depression (e.g., major depression) or depressive symptoms. For example, years ago Wells and Strictland (1982) provided a set of special probe questions that can be administered in conjunction with depressive symptom items to screen for these potential sources of contamination. The use of an example helps illustrate the nature of their strategy. The Center for Epidemiologic Studies Depression Scale (CES-D) is perhaps the most widely used measure of depressive symptoms in the literature (Radloff 1977). This scale contains an item that asks study participants if they are experiencing appetite problems, but in addition to being caused by mental health problems, appetite problems can result from physical health problems as well as the use of certain medications. Unless additional probe questions are administered to rule out these confounders, CES-D scores may be inflated unduly. Researchers who study religion and health have yet to include probe questions like those recommended by Wells and Strictland (1982) in their interview schedules. Although doing so will increase the length of the inter-

view, ignoring the issue may lead to study findings that are more difficult to interpret.

Variations in Mental Health by Gender and Race. A detailed discussion
of how the relationship between church-based social ties and health may
vary by gender and race was presented in chapter 6. When exploring
these issues, care must be taken to include outcome measures that best
capture the mental health problems that older men and older women are
likely to experience, as well as the unique mental health problems that
older adults in different racial and ethnic groups encounter.

Researchers have known for some time that men and women do not
express symptoms of psychological distress in the same way. The findings from several studies reveal that when women are exposed to stressful life events, they are more likely to become depressed, whereas men
who have experienced a stressor are more likely to develop problems
with substance abuse (Aneshensel, Rutter, & Lachenbruch 1991; Colbert & Krause 2007). These studies suggest that failure to include gen-
der-appropriate measures of distress can lead to inaccurate findings. For
example, the study by Colbert and Krause (2007) reveals that exposure
to violence is associated with more symptoms of depression, but only
among older women. In contrast, the findings from this research further indicate that exposure to violence is associated with greater alcohol
intake, but only among older men. Had alcohol use not been included
in this study, these investigators would have erroneously concluded that
exposure to violence exerts an adverse effect on older women, but not
older men. The same problem may arise, for example, in studies on gender differences in the relationship between spiritual support, stressful
events, and mental health. Assume that an investigator includes a measure of depressive symptoms in his or her study, but fails to measure
problems with alcohol. Under these circumstances, the study findings
may appear to suggest that spiritual support buffers the effects of stress
on depressive symptoms, but only for older women. As a result, this
investigator may incorrectly conclude that spiritual support therefore
benefits older women, but not older men. However, an entirely different conclusion might have been reached had a measure of alcohol use
been included in the study as well.

A similar problem may arise in studies of racial or ethnic differences
in the relationship between church-based social ties and mental health.
More specifically, an investigator may fail to include measures that capture the way mental health problems are manifest in certain racial or eth-

nic groups. For example, the Diagnostic and Statistical Manual of Mental Disorders–IV (DSM-IV) reports that Latinos may experience a psychological problem called *ataque de nervios* that includes uncontrollable shouting, attacks of crying, and trembling (American Psychiatric Association 1994). The DSM-IV explicitly notes that *ataque de nervios* is likely to arise in response to stressful events, especially those involving family members. If culturally unique ways of expressing psychological distress are not explicitly measured in a study, researchers run the risk of underestimating the relationship between things like stress, church-based social support, and mental health among minority group members.

The Manifest and Latent Functions of Church-Based Social Ties

A number of different types of social relationships in the church were explored in this volume, ranging from social support to companionship to social ties that arise in formal church groups, such as prayer groups. But Robert Merton (1949) posed an intriguing question that cuts across all these relationships. He maintains that when investigators study social processes it is important to focus on the distinction between manifest and latent functions. Manifest functions are outcomes of social behavior that are intended and recognized by the people who engage in the behavior, whereas latent functions are those outcomes that are neither intended nor recognized. Cast within the context of the current volume, it is important to reflect on whether older people at church build and maintain social relationships with fellow church members in order explicitly to improve or maintain their own physical and mental health. Studying the underlying motives for engaging in church-based social ties is important because it highlights an important factor that must be taken into consideration when mid-range theoretical models of social relationships in the church and health are devised. For example, knowing that an older person has deliberately turned to fellow church members in order to reduce the psychological distress they experienced after being exposed to a stressful life event hints at a different social process than if the mental health–related effects of church-based social ties emerge unintentionally during the support-seeking process.

Although no one has studied the underlying motives for establishing and maintaining social relationships in the church, some indirect evidence suggests that at least some people use religion for the explicit goal of improving their health. This evidence may be found, for example, in the recent volume edited by Barnes and Sered, *Religion and Heal-*

ing in America (2005). One chapter in this volume contains findings from a study of ninety-six congregations in the United Church of Christ. The authors, McKay and Musil (2005), report that many congregations set up lay intercessory prayer groups that are explicitly designed to pray for the health of group members and their loved ones. As discussed in chapter 3, participation in these formal prayer groups constitutes a specific type of formal church-based social relationship. But more important than this, participation in a group that explicitly prays for health may bypass many of the intervening psychosocial mechanisms that have been discussed throughout the current volume. Instead, if the controversial research on intercessory prayer is valid (e.g., Harris et al. 1999), then participation in these groups may affect health directly by successfully petitioning God to intervene in a health crisis.

Although there is at least some basis for arguing that the maintenance and improvement of health is a manifest function of church-based social relationships, this conclusion may not apply to all people. In the process of conducting the detailed series of in-depth interviews for the RAH Survey (Krause 2002a), study participants were asked whether they prayed for their own health problems or the health problems of significant others. Unpublished analyses of these qualitative data suggest that a number of people did not pray for their health. In fact, they indicated that it is wrong to do so because they believe that the purpose of prayer is to thank God, praise God, and request that God's will be done. So if these individuals were to derive health benefits from the ties they maintain with their fellow church members, these benefits would represent a latent function of church-based social ties.

The Potential Influence of Response Bias

Response bias refers to the tendency to give answers to survey questions in a way that is other than truthful. Although there are a number of different types of response bias, social desirability is one that has been a concern among researchers who study religion. Social desirability refers to the tendency to give answers to survey questions that place the respondent in a socially favorable light. So, for example, evidence of social desirability response bias would be found if a study participant indicates that he or she engages in a socially valued type of behavior (e.g., going to church every Sunday) even if the participant does not actually do so. Researchers have argued for decades that the problem of response bias may be especially evident in interviews with older people because they were raised during a time when appearances and propriety were valued more highly than they are today (Bradburn & Sudman 1981).

Batson, Schoenrade, and Ventis (1993) have been especially troubled by social desirability response bias in studies on religion: "We strongly believe the psychology of religion needs to re-examine its use of self-report questionnaires when measuring value-laden psychological and social correlates of religion. Methods are needed to distinguish among the way people present themselves, the way they honestly believe themselves to be, and the way they actually are" (383). Although it is not possible to know with any certainty, it is likely that social desirability response bias may affect the way some older people respond to questions about social relationships in the church. For example, questions about negative interaction with fellow church members, and especially questions about negative interaction with the clergy, are likely to be subject to socially desirable reporting bias because these unpleasant social encounters stand out in sharp contrast to officially sanctioned teachings about social relationships in the church.

A number of different strategies have been devised to confront the problem of social desirability response bias. Some investigators have developed scales that are thought to identify study participants who are especially prone to respond to sensitive questions in a socially desirable manner. Perhaps the most famous scale is the Marlowe-Crowne Social Desirability Scale (Crowne & Marlowe 1964). Cast within the context of the current volume, the use of this scale would entail the following strategy. Assume a researcher is interested in studying the relationship between negative interaction in the church and depression. He or she may be concerned that answers to questions on negative interaction and depression may be affected by social desirability. If this concern is valid, then the relationship between negative interaction in the church and depression will be biased. In an effort to confront this problem, the investigator may also administer a social desirability scale at the same time that information on negative interaction and depression is obtained. Then, when the data are analyzed, the researcher would statistically partial out the effects of social desirability from both negative interaction and depression. Doing so presumably eliminates the unwanted influence of this type of response bias. Although this strategy initially appears to make sense, it has not been all that successful in practice. Problems have arisen for a number of reasons. For example, there are a number of problems with the way that social desirability has been measured (see King & Bruner 2000, for a review of this issue).

Other researchers maintain that, whenever possible, researchers should instead rely on behavioral measures of religion rather than self-reports (e.g., Batson et al. 1993). Although it is hard to argue against obtaining behavioral measures of religiousness, doing so is not always feasible. For example, it is difficult to envision how an investigator might obtain a behavioral measure of negative interaction in the church. In contrast, it is possible to obtain behavioral measures of participation in formal church relationships, such as Bible study groups and prayer groups, by assessing how often people attend them. But merely knowing that an older person attended these groups provides little insight into the nature of the relationships that arise within them.

A third strategy to confront problems associated with social desirability response bias arises from efforts to think more carefully about the fundamental nature of this construct. Early investigators, such as Crowne and Marlowe (1964), viewed social desirability as a personality trait, but this view changed in subsequent years as investigators began to realize that social desirability might arise from the way a survey is designed and conducted. More specifically, this latter group of researchers argue that the way in which survey questions are phrased may affect the odds that socially desirable responses will be forthcoming (DeMaio 1984). Other investigators maintain that social desirability can be reduced if study participants are properly motivated and interviewers create an open and welcoming environment in which honest answers are explicitly encouraged and reinforced (Cannell, Miller, & Oksenberg 1981). Although there is relatively little hard evidence to support these views, the author's experience with the qualitative item-development phase of the RAH Survey suggests they may be of some merit (Krause 2002a). The responses of study participants were thoughtful, forthright, and open when time was taken to impress the importance of the study upon them and when they were told how their input would fit into, and be essential for, the successful realization of the wider aims of the study.

A fourth way of dealing with social desirability is sometimes referred to as audio computer-assisted self-interviewing (ACASI) (Groves, Fowler, Couper, Lepkowski, Singer, & Tourangeau 2004). Here, the study participant operates a laptop computer; the computer displays the question on the screen and plays a recording of the question to the respondent. The respondent then types his or her answer into the computer. The underlying assumption is that social desirability response bias is reduced if a study participant hears the question and provides an answer without actually having openly to report sensitive behaviors during a face-to-face dialog with an interviewer. It is less clear, however, whether these procedures work well with members of the current cohort of older adults who may be less familiar or less comfortable with using modern computer technology.

Although there is no foolproof way of dealing with social desirability response bias, perhaps the best strategy is to try to eliminate or reduce it before it arises, which is perhaps best accomplished by carefully wording questions in a neutral way and motivating study participants by helping them see the value of the study and the important role they play in it.

Effect Sizes in Research on Church-Based Social Ties and Health

The last methodological problem to be examined in this book involves the expectations that some researchers may have regarding the size of the relationships they expect to see in empirical studies of church-based social relationships and health. This issue is important for investigators who conduct empirical research, and it is important for the scholars who review their work. Time and time again, reviewers have raised issues about effect size as the author has gone through the process of publishing papers from the RAH Survey. Specifically, these reviewers have questioned whether the size of the relationships that are found are sufficiently large. Consequently, the purpose of the discussion that follows is to address this issue by exploring a question that gets right to the heart of the matter: can seemingly small effects be substantively and clinically meaningful? Because the wide majority of investigators who study church-based social ties and health rely on regression-based procedures to analyze their data, the discussion provided below deals with effect sizes as they are reflected in correlations and the proportion of variance explained (i.e., multiple R-squared).

During the past several decades, psychologists have devoted considerable effort to demonstrating that seemingly small effect sizes are important. Consider the titles from two key articles in this literature: "When Small Effects Are Impressive" (Prentice & Miller 1992) and "A Variance Explanation Paradox: When a Little Is a Lot" (Abelson 1985). Although the conclusions based on these titles may initially appear to be somewhat counterintuitive, there are sound reasons that seemingly small effects are important. Ahadi and Diener (1989) conducted a Monte Carlo simulation in order to identify important constraints on effect sizes. Their findings reveal, "It is a simple property of effect sizes that as the number of independent determinants of some behavior increases, the magnitude of the correlations between any one of the determinants and the behavior must decrease" (Ahadi & Diener 1989, 398). They focused on the correlations between personality traits and behaviors in their study. A specific finding from their work helps to bring their conclusions into sharper focus: "When a behavior had only three determinants, we found that there appeared to be an upper bound correlation of approximately .50 for the prediction of a specific behavior from a specific trait" (Ahadi & Diener 1989, 403).

Research by Strube (1991) reveals that the conclusions reached by Ahadi and Diener (1989) may not be as straightforward as these investigators suggest. In support of Ahadi and Diener (1989), Strube (1991) demonstrates that as the number of determinants of a construct increases, the correlation between any one determinant and the outcome decreases. However, Strube (1991) goes on to show that this correlation is also affected by the reliability of the constructs under consideration as well as the average correlation among the determinants. More specifically, Strube (1991) demonstrates that when the determinants are measured with error (i.e., when the reliability of the determinants declines), the correlation declines between the determinants and the outcome. In addition, his analyses reveal that as the average correlation among determinants increases, the correlation increases between any one determinant and the outcome. Put the other way around, increasing the number of independent determinants lowers the correlation between any one determinant and the outcome.

Despite these additional complicating factors, the analysis by Strube (1991) nevertheless reveals that there are clear limits to the size of the correlations obtained in the social and behavioral sciences. His findings indicate, for example, that the correlation between a determinant and an outcome is .53 when there are five determinants of an outcome, the average reliability among them is .80, and the correlation among the determinants is .30.

Using the figures provided by Strube (1991) as a benchmark, it is instructive to reflect on the number of factors that determine a person's health in late life. Doing so is likely to reveal that the number of determinants of health is overwhelming. When the genetic, environmental (e.g., air pollution), lifestyle (e.g., exercise and diet), social, and psychological determinants of health that have been identified in the literature are taken into consideration, it is not hard to see why the impact of any one factor is likely to be modest, especially when the effects of measurement error in these determinants are taken into account. Nevertheless, modest or even low correlations may be substantively meaningful. Evidence of this may be found in a revealing review of the literature by Rutledge and Loh (2004). They report that the bivariate correlation between smoking and mortality is .04 and the bivariate correlation between the daily use of aspirin and the subsequent development of a myocardial infarction is .03. Yet few clinicians would argue that avoiding tobacco and taking an aspirin daily are not clinically significant health behaviors.

Abelson (1985) provides yet another reason that study findings can be meaningful even though the proportion of explained variance is modest. He illustrates this critical point by using baseball batting averages as an example. He calculated the percentage of variance in a single at-bat that is explained by skill differentials among Major League Baseball players. Abelson's (1985) calculations reveal that knowing a player's level of skill explains less than 1 percent of the variance in any single batting performance (i.e., whether they get a hit at any one point in time). But he goes on to show that it is the *cumulative process* through which variables operate in the real world that is the critical factor; batting skills are an important determinant of performance across multiple times at bat. Abelson (1985) concludes, "Thus, one should not necessarily be scornful of minuscule values for percentage variance explanation, provided there is statistical assurance that these values are significant above zero, and that the degree of potential cumulation is substantial" (133). The effects of a number of the constructs that are discussed in the current volume are likely to accumulate slowly over fairly extensive periods of time. So, for example, the effects of stress that are discussed in chapter 2 are best viewed by assessing not one, but cumulative exposure to a range of life events over fairly lengthy periods of time (see Wheaton 1994, for an illuminating empirical demonstration of this possibility). Similarly, it is unlikely that either one or a small number of supportive acts in church are likely to have an appreciable impact on the health of an older person. Instead, the continued provision of assistance over the natural history of a stressor is likely to have the greatest effect. Unfortunately, the cumulative effect of church-based social support will be difficult to detect in studies that rely on cross-sectional designs.

Concerns about seemingly modest effect sizes are especially likely to arise when tests are performed for statistical interaction effects. A number of literature reviews of social and behavioral research reveal that interaction effects in surveys typically explain between 1 percent and

3 percent of the variance in an outcome (Auginis 2004; Chaplin 1991; Evans 1991), for at least two reasons. As discussed in chapter 6, the first may be found by reflecting on how tests for interaction effects are performed. Here, researchers create a cross-product term by multiplying the two independent variables that are thought to constitute the interaction effect (e.g., stress and church-based emotional support). Then some health-related outcome is regressed on this multiplicative term and other pertinent study measures. However, as research by Bohrnstedt and Marwell (1978) demonstrates conclusively, the reliability of the cross-product term is often quite a bit lower than the reliability of either of the component parts that are used to create it, and when the reliability of measures is low, study effect sizes will often be attenuated. The second reason why the amount of variance explained by interaction terms is likely to be low has been discussed at length by McClelland and Judd (1993). They show that the amount of variance that is explained by multiplicative terms is determined by joint distribution of the variables that are used to create it. Their work suggests that the amount of explained variance is maximized when the joint distributions of half the observations fall at the extreme values of the component constructs. However, this is rarely the case for variables that are measured in large nationwide probability samples. For this reason the amount of variance explained by interaction terms that are based on this type of data is quite modest.

The broader message that emerges from this discussion of effect size issues is twofold. First, investigators should not lose heart when the analyses they conduct suggest that constructs like church-based social relationships appear to explain fairly modest amounts of variance in health-related outcomes. Failing to move forward with the publication of results because the effect size appears to be modest will not help advance the field. Second, researchers who review papers on church-based social ties and health for scholarly journals must be aware of the basic principles and findings that are discussed in this section so that they do not reject studies that provide theoretically and clinically meaningful results.

Casting a Broader Net: Delving into the Dark Morass of Subjectivity

Although a wide range of conceptual and methodological challenges have been examined throughout the current volume, there is an even broader, more abstract issue that must be met head-on. This issue involves problems that arise from the highly subjective nature of research on religion. Two ways in which subjectivity has influenced the discussion of church-based social ties in this volume are examined below: the first has to do with the nature of the sources that have been used throughout this book to document and bolster key theoretical points and conceptual arguments, whereas the second involves potential problems that arise from the subjective nature of religion itself.

A deliberate attempt has been made throughout this volume to turn to a wide range of sources in order to derive greater insight into the nature and functioning of church-based social relationships. This odyssey has led to disciplines and sources that are either unfamiliar or that may seem unusual to some social and behavioral scientists. Included among these unconventional sources were works in literature, drama, poetry, ethics, history, and philosophy. Throughout, the intent has been to leave no stone unturned. This approach is consistent with the views of Heraclitus, a Greek philosopher who lived from 544 BCE to 484 BCE. Heraclitus observed, "Friends of wisdom (philosophers) must be enquirers into many things" (as quoted in Bakalis 2005, 35). What unites the diverse disciplines and academic traditions that are examined in this volume is a burning desire on the part of the authors to know themselves, their social world, and their place in it. These are not issues that emerged only with the advent of the social and behavioral sciences 150 years or so ago. Instead, these issues have occupied the thoughts of brilliant men and women since the beginning of civilization itself. As noted in chapter 1, if so many great minds in so many fields find these fundamental issues of human social existence to be so important, then we have no recourse other than to examine their work closely. By viewing the same issues from often dramatically different perspectives, the work of these interdisciplinary scholars provides a way of finding fresh new insights into social relationships in the church and helps bolster our confidence in the findings that emerge from research on them.

Still, some traditional social and behavioral scientists may feel that crossing over into sources like literature and poetry somehow diminishes the scientific nature of our enterprise and that these sources have no place in the work we do. Cooley (1927) tackled this issue head-on more than eighty years ago. He maintained, "We hear it questioned whether sociology is a science or a philosophy. It is both, and an art also" (Cooley 1927, 160). Some might object and argue that only insights that emerge from empirical research can be trusted because conclusions that are reached in the humanities and elsewhere are simply too subjective. Once again, Cooley (1927) had a compelling reply to these detractors:

All books dealing largely with human questions are speculative, those abounding in statistics and laboratory observations as much so as any. You may always see, if you look closely, vast chasms bridged by conjecture: we know so little that it cannot be otherwise. Not method, chiefly, but sagacity, insight, breadth of knowledge, humble honesty, and real love of the truth are our guarantee for the value of these speculations; and we must judge whether we can trust our author very much as we do in the case of the doctor, lawyer, or plumber. (157–158)

As the conceptual and methodological challenges that have been identified throughout this volume reveal, the vast chasms discussed long ago by Cooley (1927) are still with us today, and his solution to them is just as valid. Empirical methods are only as good as the ideas they are designed to evaluate. And there are no boundaries to the sources of good ideas. It is the hope of the author that using a wide range of somewhat unconventional sources encourages students as well as established scholars to do the same. They might be surprised and enlightened by what they find. Seemingly "new" social scientific insights may turn out to be not so new after all, and perspectives and hypotheses that have yet to be evaluated lie buried in the back lot and dark corners of what are considered by some to be obscure works. Whether following this strategy has produced anything of value in the current volume is, of course, best left to the reader. Hopefully, he or she will find something to be gained by taking this unbridled and uninhibited approach to thinking about social relationships in the church and health in late life.

As noted above, there is a second way in which presumed problems arise with subjectivity in the study of religion. Some investigators may feel that the foundations upon which religious beliefs rest (e.g., the existence of God or heaven) cannot be verified scientifically, and as a result, religious phenomena fall outside the proper purview of the social and behavioral sciences. At one level, the study of social relationships in the church avoids this conceptual morass because it doesn't matter if the things that people believe about religion are valid or true. Instead, as W. I. Thomas pointed out some time ago, "If men define situations as real, they are real in their consequences" (Thomas & Thomas 1928, 572); the potential health-related effects of church-based social ties are very real indeed. Viewed from this perspective, it doesn't matter if Jesus actually taught that unconditional forgiveness is a key prerequisite for attaining the kingdom of heaven. In fact, it doesn't even matter if there is a heaven at all. All that is necessary is that a person believes it is so, and if they do, then the concrete health-related implications of these highly subjective beliefs can be examined in a relatively objective manner.

But at a different level, sidestepping a thorough examination of the subjective aspects of religion may be ill-advised, for two reasons. First, at least some research on religion and health can be explained only by exploring highly subjective and mystical phenomena. Recall the compelling findings that have emerged from a number of studies on intercessory prayer (e.g., Harris et al., 1999). Investigators who study intercessory prayer evoke the direct intervention of God as a way of explaining the health-related changes they have observed. Second, in order to understand truly the concrete implications of leading a religious life, religious beliefs must be grasped firmly, and researchers must develop a deep appreciation for how these subjective beliefs arise and operate in daily life. Some useful insight into this issue may be found by returning to Albert Schweitzer's (1933/1990) concept of the Reverence for Life. This construct was evoked in chapter 2 to explain why people at church may be especially inclined to help each other. Schweitzer went to some lengths to explain how a Reverence for Life emerges: "If our will to live begins to meditate about itself and the universe, we will become sensitive to life around us and will then, insofar as it is possible, dedicate through our actions our own will to live to that of the infinite will to live" (237). Following this, Schweitzer (1933/1990) went on to ground his conceptual framework firmly in the most subjective phenomena possible when he argued that, "Rational thinking, if it goes deep, ends of necessity in the irrational realm of mysticism" (237). So if the logical end point of reflection on religion leads to the mystical and the numinous, researchers may have no choice but to follow it all the way down to that level.

But in addition to the insights provided by Schweitzer (1933/1990), something important happens when subjective beliefs about religion become the focal point of scholarly examination. More specifically, pursuing this line of inquiry takes the study of church-based relationships beyond the realm of the individual into a higher-order social phenomenon that emerges when subjective views of religion are shared with others. The outcome of this group process is perhaps best captured by turning to a well-known story in the New Testament. In the Gospel according to Luke, it is told that the Pharisees demanded to know when the kingdom of God will come. Jesus told them, "Behold, the kingdom of God is within you" (Luke 17:21, King James Version). But there is another way to translate Jesus' response. In addition to his well-known work on human development, Erik Erikson spent a good deal of time studying the life of Martin Luther. Erikson reports a very interesting account of how Martin Luther translated Jesus' response to the question that the Pharisees posed. Instead of saying it is within you, Luther translated Jesus' response to say, "Behold the kingdom of God is in the midst of you" (as reported in Hoare 2002, 109; see also Coe 1902, 166). This is a very interesting choice of words because it takes the discussion of the kingdom of God out of the realm of the individual psyche (i.e., it is within you) and locates it in a larger, higher-order social phenomenon that only emerges at the group level (i.e., it is in the midst of you). According to this alternative translation, the kingdom of God (i.e., heaven) is not something that each individual creates on his or her own. Instead, it is something that may be found in the relationships that are formed with those who share the faith. It emerges not from within the individual unconscious, as James (1902/1997) maintained, but is instead a subjective social product. But more than this, the collective view of paradise that is highlighted by Luther suggests that heaven is (or at least can be) present in the here and now, and that it is not some abstract realm of existence that is only accessible upon death. This, in turn, boldly underscores the potential that social relationships in the church have to improve the quality of this life for the faithful. By providing a detailed examination of the precise ways in which these benefits may arise, the intent of the author has been to take highly subjective discussions of things like heaven down to the level at which many older people live their lives on a daily basis. By doing so, it is possible to see how church-based social ties are very real in their consequences.

Appendix

Technical Details of the Religion, Aging, and Health (RAH) Survey

A number of unpublished analyses are presented throughout this volume. The data that were used in these analyses are from the Religion, Aging, and Health (RAH) Survey that was conducted by the author. The purpose of this appendix is to provide technical detail on the RAH Survey.

This study was executed in two phases. Funds for both phases of this project were provided by grants to the author from the National Institute on Aging (RO1 AG014749 and RO1 AG026259). The first phase was concerned with developing closed-ended survey measures of religion that reflect the way older people think about, describe, and practice their faith in daily life. This was accomplished by devising and executing a comprehensive item-development program that took three years to complete. This item-development program consisted of seven steps that were primarily qualitative in nature. More specifically, this item-development strategy involved conducting eight focus groups, conducting 131 individual in-depth interviews, drafting a preliminary set of closed-ended items, having the items reviewed by a distinguished panel of experts, testing the closed-ended items with 85 cognitive interviews, and conducting a pilot study of 98 older adults (see Krause 2002a, for a detailed discussion of this item-development program).

Once a good set of closed-ended survey measures of religion were in place, the second phase of the study was devoted to conducting a nationwide longitudinal survey of older people. The participants in this nationwide survey have now been interviewed a total of three times. All interviewing was conducted by Harris Interactive, New York (formerly Louis Harris and Associates).

The study population was defined as all household residents who are either African American or white, English-speaking, and sixty-six years of age or older at the time of the baseline survey. Geographically, the study population is restricted to eligible residents residing in the coterminous United States (i.e., residents of Alaska and Hawaii were excluded). Finally, the study was restricted to individuals who were either currently practicing Christians, people who were Christian in the past but no longer practice any religion, and individuals who were not affiliated with any faith at any point in their lifetime. The goal of the RAH Survey was to devise and test a comprehensive battery of items to assess religion in late life. Older people who were practicing a religion other than Christianity (e.g., Jews or Muslims) were excluded because it would have been too difficult to devise a comprehensive set of religion measures that would be suitable for persons of all faiths.

The sampling frame for the RAH Survey consisted of all eligible persons contained in the Health Care Finance Administration (HCFA) Medicare Beneficiary Eligibility List (HCFA is now called the Center for Medicare and Medicaid Services (CMS). This list contains the name, address, sex, and race of virtually every older person in the United States. It should be emphasized that people are included in this list even if they are not receiving Social Security benefits. Even so, some older individuals are not included in this database because they do not have a Social Security number. This may be due to factors such as undocumented immigration.

A five-step process was used to draw the sample. First, each year, researchers at HCFA draw a 5 percent sample of the names in their master file using a simple random sampling procedure. The sampled names include individuals who are at least sixty-five years of age. However, by the time the field period for the RAH Survey began, subjects in the 5 percent file were at least sixty-six years of age. It is for this reason that the study population was defined as including individuals who were sixty-six years of age or older. In the second step of the sampling procedure, the 5 percent file was split into two subfiles—one containing older whites and one containing older blacks. Each file was sorted separately by county, and then by ZIP codes within each county. In the third step, an nth interval was calculated for each subfile based on the total number of eligible records. Following a random start, seventy-five nth selections were made in each file. In the fourth step of the sampling strategy, primary sampling units (PSUs) were formed by selecting approximately twenty-five additional names above and twenty-five additional names below each case identified in step three. Finally, in the last stage, sampled persons within each PSU were recruited for an interview with the goal of obtaining approximately ten completed interviews per PSU.

Interviewing for the Wave 1 survey took place in 2001. A total of 1,500 interviews were completed successfully. Older African Americans were oversampled so that sufficient statistical power would be available for exploring race differences in religion. More specifically, the final sample contained 748 older whites and 752 older black people. The overall response rate for the baseline survey was 62 percent. Preliminary analyses reported by Krause (2002b) reveal that the average age of the study participants was 74.4 years (SD = 6.3 years), approximately 38 percent were older men, and the average number of years of schooling that were completed successfully by the study participants was 11.6 years (SD = 3.4 years).

Once the Wave 1 data became available, an extensive amount of time was spent using state-of-the-art quantitative data analytic procedures to assess the factor structure and psychometric properties of the newly devised measures of religion. This work revealed that the measures crafted during the phase-one, item-development program were empirically sound. The Wave 2 survey was conducted in 2004. A total of 1,024 of the original 1,500 study participants were reinterviewed successfully, 75 refused to participate, 112 could not be located, 70 were too ill to be interviewed, 11 had moved to a nursing home, and 208 were deceased. Not counting those who had died or were placed in a nursing home, the re-interview rate for the Wave 2 survey was 80 percent.

The Wave 3 interviews took place in 2006–2007. In the process of conducting these interviews, an effort was made to reinterview all older people who participated at Wave 1, with the obvious exception of those who were dead (1,500 – 208 = 1,292). A total of 969 older people participated in the Wave 3 interviews, 33 refused to be interviewed, 17 were too ill to take part in the survey, 118 could not be located, and an additional 155 former study participants had died. Not counting those who had died, the reinterview rate for the Wave 3 survey was 85 percent.

Funds are available for a fourth wave of interviews. These interviews will be conducted in 2008.

References

Abelson, R. P. (1985). Variance explanation paradox: When a little is a lot. *Psychological Bulletin, 97*, 128–133.

Adams, R. G., Blieszner, R., & De Vries, B. (2000). Definitions of friendship in the third age: Age, gender, and study location effects. *Journal of Aging Studies, 14*, 117–133.

Adler, A. (1933/1956). *The individual psychology of Alfred Adler: A systematic presentation in selections from his writings* (H. L. Ansbacher & R. R. Ansbacher, Eds.). New York: Basic Books.

Ahadi, S., & Diener, E. (1989). Multiple determinants of effect size. *Journal of Personality and Social Psychology, 56*, 398–406.

Ainsworth, M. D. S. (1985). Attachment across the lifespan. *Bulletin of the New York Academy of Medicine, 61*, 792–812.

Allport, G. W. (1950). *The individual and his religion.* New York: Macmillan.

Allport, G. W. (1966). The religious context of prejudice. *Journal for the Scientific Study of Religion, 5*, 447–457.

American Psychiatric Association (1994). *Diagnostic and statistical manual of mental disorders: Fourth Edition.* Washington, DC: American Psychiatric Association.

Andersson, L. (1998). Loneliness research and interventions: A review of the literature. Ageing & Society, 2, 264–274.

Aneshensel, C. S. (2002). *Theory-based data analysis for the social sciences.* Thousand Oaks, CA: Pine Forge Press.

Aneshensel, C. S., Rutter, C. M., & Lachenbruch, P. A. (1991). Social structure, stress, and mental health: Competing conceptual and analytic models. *American Sociological Review, 56*, 166-178.

Antonucci, T. C. (1985). Personal characteristics, social support, and social behavior. In R. H. Binstock & E. Shanas (Eds.), *Handbook of aging and the social sciences* (pp. 94–128). New York: Van Nostrand Reinhold.

Antonucci, T. C. (2001). Social relationships: An examination of social networks, social support, and sense of control. In J. E. Birren & K. W. Schaie (Eds.), *Handbook of the psychology of aging* (pp. 427–451). San Diego, CA: Academic Press.

Argue, A., Johnson, D. R., & White, L. K. (1999). Age and religiosity: Evidence from a three-wave panel analysis. *Journal for the Scientific Study of Religion, 38*, 423–435.

Aron, A. (2003). Self and close relationships. In M. R. Leary & J. P. Tangney (Eds.), *Handbook of self and identity* (pp. 442–461). New York: Guilford.

Auginis, H. (2004). *Regression analysis for categorical moderators.* New York: Guilford.

Bachelor, A., & Horvath, A. (1999). The therapeutic relationship. In M. A. Hubble, B. L. Duncan, & S. D. Miller (Eds.), *The heart and soul of change: What works in therapy* (pp. 133–178). Washington, DC: American Psychological Association.

Bahr, H. M. (1970). Aging and religious disaffiliation. *Social Forces, 49,* 59–71.

Bakalis, N. (2005). *Handbook of Greek philosophy.* Victoria, British Columbia: Trafford Publishing.

Baldwin, J. A., & Hopkins, R. (1990). African American and European American cultural differences as assessed by the Worldviews Paradigm: An empirical analysis. *Western Journal of Black Studies, 14,* 38–52.

Baldwin, J. M. (1902). *Fragments in philosophy and science of being: Collected essays and addresses.* New York: Charles Scribner's Sons.

Baltes, P. B. (1991). The many faces of aging: Toward a psychology of old age. *Psychological Medicine, 21,* 837–854.

Baltes, P. B., & Smith, J. (1999). Multilevel and systemic analysis of old age: Theoretical and empirical evidence for a fourth age. In V. L. Bengston & K. W. Schaie (Eds.), *Handbook of theories of aging* (pp. 153–173). New York: Springer.

Baltes, P. B., & Smith, J. (2003). New frontiers in the future of aging: From successful aging of the young old to the dilemmas of the Fourth Age. *Gerontology, 49,* 123–135.

Bandura, A. (1982). Self-efficacy mechanism in human agency. *American Psychologist, 37,* 122–147.

Barefoot, J. C., Maynard, K. E., Beckham, J. C., Brummett, B. H., Hooker, K., & Siegler, I. C. (1998). Trust, health, and longevity. *Journal of Behavioral Medicine, 21,* 517–526.

Barna, G. (2002). *The state of the church 2002.* Ventura, CA: Issachar Resources.

Barnes, L. L., & Sered, S. S. (2005). *Religion and healing in America.* New York: Oxford University Press.

Barney, J. B., & Hansen, M. H. (1994). Trustworthiness as a source of competitive advantage. *Strategic Management Journal, 15,* 175–216.

Barrera, M. (1986). Distinctions between social support concepts, measures, and models. *American Journal of Community Psychology, 14,* 413–425.

Bartel, M. (2004). What is spiritual? What is spiritual suffering? *The Journal of Pastoral Care & Counseling, 58,* 187–201.

Bartkowski, J. P. (2000). Breaking walls, raises fences: Masculinity, intimacy, and accountability among Promise Keepers. *Sociology of Religion, 61,* 33–53.

Bartkowski, J. P., & Matthews, T. L. (2005). Race/ethnicity. In H. R. Ebaugh (Ed.), *Handbook of religion and social institutions* (pp. 163–183). New York: Springer.

Barusch, A. S. (1999). Religion, adversity, and age: Religious experience among low-income elderly women. *Journal of Sociology and Social Welfare, 26,* 125–142.

Batson, C. D., Schoenrade, P., & Ventis, W. L. (1993). *Religion and the individual: A social-psychological perspective.* New York: Oxford University Press.

Battista, J., & Almond, R. (1973). The development of meaning in life. *Psychiatry, 36,* 409–427.

Baumeister, R. F. (1991). *Meanings of life.* New York: Guilford.

Baumeister, R. F., Tice, D. M., & Hutton, D. G. (1989). Self-presentation motivations and personality differences in self-esteem. *Journal of Personality, 57,* 547–579.

Beal, C. (2006). Loneliness in older women: A review of the literature. *Issues in Mental Health Nursing, 27,* 795–813.

Becker, E. (1973). *The denial of death.* New York: Free Press.

Becker, P. E. (1999). *Congregations in conflict: Cultural models of local religious life.* New York: Cambridge University Press.

Beit-Hallahmi, B., & Argyle, M. (1997). *The psychology of religious behavior, belief, and experience.* New York: Routledge.

Belle, D. (1982). Social ties and social support. In D. Belle (Ed.), *Lives in stress: Women and depression* (pp. 133–144). Beverly Hills, CA: Sage.

Benore, E. R., & Park, C. L. (2004). Death-specific religious beliefs and bereavement: Belief in an afterlife and continued attachment. *The International Journal for the Psychology of Religion, 14,* 1–22.

Bentler, P. M., & Bonett, D. G. (1980). Significance tests and goodness-of-fit in the analysis of covariance structures. *Psychological Bulletin, 88,* 588–600.

Berger, P. L. (1967). *The sacred canopy: Elements of a sociological theory.* New York: Doubleday.

Berger, P. L., & Luckman, T. (1966). *The social construction of reality: A treatise in the sociology of knowledge.* New York: Anchor Books.

Berger, P. L., & Pullberg, S. (1965). Reification and sociological critique of consciousness. *History and Theory, 4,* 196–211.

Berkman, L. F., Glass, T., Brissette, I., & Seeman, T. (2000). From social integration to health: Durkheim in the new millennium. *Social Science and Medicine, 51,* 843–857.

Berrenberg, J. L. (1987). The Belief in Personal Control Scale: A measure of God-mediated and exaggerated control. *Journal of Personality Assessment, 51,* 194–206.

Bettencourt, B. A., & Sheldon, K. (2001). Social roles as mechanisms for psychological need satisfaction within groups. *Journal of Personality and Social Psychology, 81,* 1131–1143.

Bidwell, D. R. (2001). Maturing religious experience and the postmodern self. *Pastoral Psychology, 49,* 277–290.

Bierhoff, H. W. (1992). Trust and trustworthiness. In L. Montada, S. H. Flipp, &

J. J. Lerner (Eds.), *Life crises and experiences of loss in adulthood* (pp. 411–433). Hillsdale, NJ: Lawrence Erlbaum.

Black, H. K., & Rubinstein, R. L. (2000). *Old souls: Aged women, poverty, and the experience of God.* New York: Aldine De Gruyter.

Blackbird, T., & Wright, P. H. (1985). I: Project overview and an exploration of the pedestal effect. *Journal of Psychology & Theology, 13,* 274–283.

Blalock, H. M. (1982). *Conceptualization and measurement in the social sciences.* Beverly Hills, CA: Sage.

Blank, M. B., Mahmood, M., Fox, J. C., & Guterbock, T. (2002). Alternative mental health services: The role of the black church in the South. *American Journal of Public Health, 92,* 1668–1672.

Blazer, D. G. (2002). *Depression in late life* (3rd ed.). New York: Springer.

Bohrnstedt, G. W. (1983). Measurement. In P. H. Rossi, J. D. Wright, & A. B. Anderson (Eds.), *Handbook of survey research* (pp. 70–121). New York: Academic Press.

Bohrnstedt, G. W., & Marwell, G. (1978). The reliability of products of two random variables. In K. Schuessler (Ed.), *Sociological methodology, 1978* (pp. 254–273). San Francisco: Jossey-Bass.

Bollen, K. A. (1989). *Structural equations with latent variables.* New York: Wiley.

Bolles, R. C. (1957). Occam's razor and the science of behavior. *Psychological Reports, 3,* 321–324.

Bowlby, J. (1969). *Attachment and loss: Vol. 1. Attachment.* New York: Basic Books.

Bowlby, J. (1973). *Attachment and loss: Vol. 2. Separation.* New York: Basic Books.

Bowlby, J. (1980). *Attachment and loss: Vol. 3. Loss.* New York: Basic Books.

Bradburn, N., & Sudman, S. (1981). *Improving interview method and questionnaire design.* San Francisco: Jossey-Bass.

Bradley, W. J., & Schaefer, K. C. (1998). *The uses and misuses of data and models: The mathematization of the human sciences.* Thousand Oaks, CA: Sage.

Brady, F. (1965). Introduction. In A. Pope, *An essay on man* (pp. vii–xvii). New York: Macmillan.

Brown, H. O. (1997). Godly sorrow, sorrow of the world: Some Christian thoughts on repentance. In A. Etzioni (Ed.), *Repentance: A comparative perspective* (pp. 31–42). Lanham, MD: Rowman & Littlefield.

Brown, L. B. (1994). *The human side of prayer.* Birmingham, AL: Religious Education Press.

Burton, R. (2003). Spiritual pain: A brief overview and an initial response within the Christian tradition. *The Journal of Pastoral Care & Counseling, 57,* 437–446.

Byrd, R. C. (1988). Positive therapeutic effects of intercessory prayer in a coronary care unit population. *Southern Medical Journal, 81,* 826–829.

Cacioppo, J. T., Hughes, M. E., Waite, L. J., Hawkley, L. C., & Thisted, R. A.

(2006). Loneliness as a specific risk factor for depressive symptoms: Cross-sectional and longitudinal analysis. *Psychology and Aging, 21,* 140–151.

Cannell, C. F., Miller, P. V., & Oksenberg, L. (1981). Research in interviewing techniques. In S. Leinhardt (Ed.), *Sociological methodology, 1981* (pp. 389–437). San Francisco: Jossey-Bass.

Caplan, G. (1981). Mastery of stress. *American Journal of Psychiatry, 138,* 413–420.

Carrier, H. (1965). *The sociology of religious belonging.* New York: Herder and Herder.

Carstensen, L. L. (1992). Social and emotional patterns in adulthood: Support for socioemotional selectivity theory. *Psychology and Aging, 7,* 331–338.

Cassel, J. (1964). Social science theory as a source of hypotheses in epidemiological research. *American Journal of Public Health, 25,* 256–282.

Chaiken, S., Wood, W., & Eagly, A. H. (1996). Principles of persuasion. In E. T. Higgins & A. W. Kruglanski (Eds.), *Social psychology: Handbook of basic principles* (pp. 702–742). New York: Guilford.

Chalfant, H., Roberts, P. A., Heller, P. L., Briones, D., Aguirre-Hochbaum, S., & Farr, W. (1990). The clergy as a resource for those encountering psychological distress. *Review of Religious Research, 31,* 305–315.

Chaplin, W. F. (1991). The next generation of moderator research in personality psychology. *Journal of Personality, 59,* 143–178.

Chochinov, H. M., & Cann, B. J. (2005). Interventions to enhance the spiritual aspects of dying. *Journal of Palliative Medicine, 8,* supplement, S103–S115.

Clark, D. B. (2000). Working with groups, families, and couples: Clergy as systems analysts. In G. Ahlskog & H. Sands (Eds.), *The guide to pastoral counseling and care* (pp. 243–273). Madison, CT: Psychosocial Press.

Clark, W. H. (1958). *The psychology of religion.* New York: Macmillan.

Cocking, D., & Kennett, J. (1998). Friendship and the self. *Ethics, 108,* 502–527.

Coe, G. A. (1902). *The religion of the mature mind.* London: Fleming H. Revell Company.

Coe, J. H. (2000). Musings on the dark night of the soul: Insights from St. John of the Cross and a developmental spirituality. *Journal of Psychology and Theology, 28,* 293–307.

Cohen, J., Cohen, P., West, S. G., & Aiken, L. S. (2003). *Applied multiple regression/correlation analysis for the behavioral sciences* (3rd ed.). Mahwah, NJ: Lawrence Erlbaum.

Cohen, S. (2004). Social relationships and health. *American Psychologist, 59,* 676–684.

Colbert, S. J., & Krause, N. (2007). Witnessing violence across the life course, depressive symptoms, and alcohol use among older persons. *Health Education & Behavior* (in press).

Collins, N. L., & Miller, L. C. (1994). The disclosure-liking link: From meta-analysis toward a dynamic conceptualization. *Psychological Bulletin, 116,* 457–475.

Cooley, C. H. (1902/2003). *Human nature and the social order.* New Brunswick, NJ: Transaction Publishers.

Cooley, C. H. (1909/2003). *Social organization.* New Brunswick, NJ: Transaction Publishers.

Cooley, C. H. (1927). *Life and the student.* New York: Alfred A. Knopf.

Cooper, T. D. (2003). *Sin, pride, and self-acceptance.* Downers Grove, IL: InterVarsity Press.

Coopersmith, S. (1967). *The antecedents of self-esteem.* San Francisco: W. H. Freeman and Company.

Corporation for National and Community Service. (2006). Volunteer growth in America: A review of trends since 1974. From the following website: http://www.nationalservice.gov.

Coward, H. (1986). Intolerance in the world's religions. *Studies in Religion, 15,* 419-431.

Coyne, J. C., & Racioppo, M. W. (2000). Never the twain shall meet: Closing the gap between coping research and clinical intervention. *American Psychologist, 55,* 655–664.

Coyne, J. C., Wortman, C. B., & Lehman, D. R. (1988). The other side of support: Emotional overinvolvement and miscarried helping. In B. H. Gottlieb (Ed.), *Marshaling social support: Formats, processes, and effects* (pp. 305–350). Newbury Park, CA: Sage.

Crowne, D., & Marlowe, D. (1964). *The approval motive.* New York: John Wiley and Sons.

Crystal, S. (1986). Measuring income and inequality among the elderly. *The Gerontologist, 26,* 56–59.

Cutrona, C. E., Suhr, J. A., & MacFarlane, R. (1990). Interpersonal transactions and the psychological sense of support. In S. Duck (Ed.), *Personal relationships and social support* (pp. 30–45). Newbury Park, CA: Sage.

Das, T. K., & Teng, B. S. (2004). The risk-based view of trust: A conceptual framework. *Journal of Business and Psychology, 19,* 85–116.

Davidson, J. D. (1972). Patterns of belief at the denominational and congregational levels. *Review of Religious Research, 13,* 197–205.

Davidson, J. D., & Pyle, R. E. (2005). Social class. In H. R. Ebaugh (Ed.), *Handbook of religion and social institutions* (pp. 185–205). New York: Springer.

Debats, D. (1999). Sources of meaning: An investigation of significant commitments in life. *Journal of Humanistic Psychology, 39,* 30–57.

DeMaio, T. J. (1984). Social desirability and survey measurement: A review. In C. F. Turner & E. Martin (Eds.), *Surveying subjective phenomena, vol. 2* (pp. 257–282). New York: Russell Sage Foundation.

Denney, N. W. (1988). A reanalysis of the influence of the Friendly Visitor Program. *American Journal of Community Psychology, 16,* 409–425.

Department of Labor. (2002). Volunteering in the United States. From the following website: http://www.bls.gov/cps.

DeShon, R. P. (1998). A cautionary note on measurement error correlations in structural equation models. *Psychological Methods, 3,* 412–423.

Dewey, J. (1922/1950). *Human nature and conduct: An introduction to social psychology.* New York: Random House.

Donini, L. M., Savina, C., & Cannella, C. (2003). Eating and appetite control in the elderly: Anorexia of aging. *International Psychogeriatrics, 15,* 73–87.

Du Bois, W. E. B. (2000). *Du Bois on religion* (P. Zuckerman, Ed.). New York: Alta Mira Press.

Durkheim, E. (1897/1951). *Suicide: A study in sociology* (J. Spaulding & G. Simpson, Trans.). New York: Free Press.

Durkheim, E. (1915/1965). *Elementary forms of religious life.* London: George, Allen Unwin, Ltd.

du Toit, M., & du Toit, S. (2001). *Interactive LISREL: User's guide.* Lincolnwood, IL: Scientific Software International.

Dyer, D. R. (2000). *Jung's thoughts on God: Religious depths of the psyche.* York Beach, ME: Nicolas-Hayes.

Eckenrode, J., & Wethington, E. (1990). The process and outcome of mobilizing social support. In S. Duck (Ed.), *Personal relationships and social support* (pp. 83–103). Newbury Park: Sage.

Edwards, A. C., Nazroo, J. Y., & Brown, G. W. (1998). Gender differences in marital support following a shared life event. *Social Science and Medicine, 46,* 1077–1085.

Edwards, J. (1746/2004). *The religious affections.* Carlisle, PA: The Banner of Truth Trust.

Ehmann, C. (1999). The age factor in religious attitudes and behavior. Available on the following website: http//www.gallup.com.

Ekwall, A. K., Sivberg, B., & Hallberg, I. R. (2005). Loneliness as a predictor of quality of life among older caregivers. *Journal of Advanced Nursing, 49,* 23–32.

Eliade, M. (1978). *A history of religious ideas: Vol. 1. From the Stone Age to the Eleusinian mysteries.* Chicago: University of Chicago Press.

Eliassen, A. H., Taylor, J., & Lloyd, D. A. (2005). Subjective religiosity and depression in transition to adulthood. *Journal for the Scientific Study of Religion, 44,* 187–199.

Ellison, C. G. (1995). Rational choice explanations of individual religious behavior: Notes on the problem of social embeddedness. *Journal for the Scientific Study of Religion, 34,* 89–97.

Ellison, C. G., Boardman, J. D., Williams, D. R., & Jackson, J. S. (2001). Religious involvement, stress, and mental health: Findings from the 1995 Detroit Area Study. *Social Forces, 80,* 215–249.

Ellison, C. G., Flannelly, K. J., & Weaver, A. J. (2006). The clergy as a source of mental health assistance: What Americans believe. *Review of Religious Research, 48,* 190–211.

Ellison, C. G., & George, L. K. (1994). Religious involvement, social ties, and social support in a southeastern community. *Journal for the Scientific Study of Religion, 33,* 46–61.

Ellison, C. G., Krause, N. M., Shepherd, B. C., & Chaves, M. A. (2007). Congregational characteristics, anticipated support, and negative interaction in the church. Under review.

Ellison, C. G., & Levin, J. S. (1998). The religion-health connection: Evidence, theory, and future directions. *Health Education & Behavior, 25,* 700–720.

Ellison, C. G., & Sherkat, D. E. (1995). The "semi-voluntary institution" revisited: Regional variations in church participation among Black Americans. *Social Forces, 73,* 1415–1437.

Ellison, C. G., Zhang, W., Krause, N., & Marcum, J. P. (2007). Does negative interaction in the church increase depression? Longitudinal findings from the Presbyterian Panel Survey. Under review.

Emerson, R. W. (1841/1983). *Ralph Waldo Emerson: Essays and lectures.* New York: Literary Classics of the United States.

Emmons, R. A., & Crumpler, C. A. (2000). Gratitude as a human strength: Appraising the evidence. *Journal of Social and Clinical Psychology, 19,* 56–69.

Emmons, R. A., & McCullough, M. E. (2003). Counting blessings versus burdens: An experimental investigation of gratitude and subjective well-being in daily life. *Journal of Personality and Social Psychology, 84,* 377–389.

Emmons, R. A., & McCullough, M. E. (2004). *The psychology of gratitude.* New York: Oxford University Press.

Enright, R. D. (1996). Counseling within the forgiveness triad: On forgiving, receiving forgiveness, and self-forgiveness. *Counseling & Values, 40,* 107–127.

Enright, R. D., Freedman, S., & Rique, J. (1998). The psychology of interpersonal forgiveness. In R. D. Enright & J. North (Eds.), *Exploring forgiveness* (pp. 46–62). Madison: University of Wisconsin Press.

Erikson, E. (1959). *Identity and the life cycle.* New York: International University Press.

Euripides. (1960). Hippolytus. In M. Hadas & J. McLean (Trans.), *Ten plays by Euripides* (pp. 65–98). New York: Bantam Books.

Evans, M. G. (1991). The problem of analyzing multiplicative composites: Interactions revisited. *American Psychologist, 46,* 6–15.

Everson-Rose, S. A., & Lewis, T. T. (2005). Psychosocial factors and cardiovascular disease. *Annual Review of Public Health, 26,* 469–500.

Exline, J. J., & Rose, E. (2005). Religious and spiritual struggles. In R. F. Paloutzian & C. L. Park (Eds.), *Handbook of the psychology of religion and spirituality* (pp. 315–330). New York: Guilford.

Exline, J. J., Yali, A. M., & Sanderson, W. C. (2000). Guilt, discord, and alienation: The role of religious strain in depression and suicidality. *Journal of Clinical Psychology, 56,* 1481–1496.

Federal Interagency Forum on Aging Related Statistics. (2004). *Older Americans 2004: Key indicators of well-being.* Washington DC: U.S. Government Printing Office.

Feldman, P. J., & Steptoe, S. (2004). How neighborhoods and physical functioning are related: The roles of neighborhood socioeconomic status, perceived neighborhood strain, and individual health risk factors. *Annals of Behavioral Medicine, 27,* 91–99.

Fetzer Institute/National Institute on Aging Working Group. (1999). *Multidimensional measurement of religiousness/spirituality for use in health research.* Kalamazoo, MI: John E. Fetzer Institute.

Fiala, W. E., Bjorck, J. P., & Gorsuch, R. (2002). The religious support scale: Construction, validation, and cross-validation. *American Journal of Community Psychology, 20,* 761–86.

Folkman, S., & Moskowitz, J. T. (2004). Coping: Pitfalls and promise. *Annual Review of Psychology, 55,* 745–774.

Fowler, J. W. (1981). *Stages of faith: The psychology of human development and the quest for meaning.* New York: Harper & Row.

Frank, J. D. (1961). *Persuasion and healing: A comparative study of psychotherapy.* Baltimore: The Johns Hopkins Press.

Frank, J. D., & Frank, J. B. (1991). *Persuasion and healing* (3rd ed.). Baltimore: Johns Hopkins University Press.

Frankel, E. (1998). Repentance, psychotherapy, and healing through a Jewish lens. *American Behavioral Scientist, 41,* 814–833.

Frankl, V. E. (1959/1985). *Man's search for meaning.* New York: Washington Square Press.

Fremantle, A. (1954). *The age of belief.* New York: Mentor Books.

Freud, S. (1913). *Totem and taboo: Some points of agreement between the mental lives of savages and neurotics.* London: Routledge.

Friedman, M., & Rosenman, R. H. (1974). *Type A behavior and your heart.* Greenwich, CT: Fawcett.

Fries, J. F. (1980). Aging, natural death, and the compression of morbidity. *New England Journal of Medicine, 303,* 130–135.

Fuller, R. C. (2001). *Spiritual but not religious: Understanding the unchurched in America.* New York: Oxford University Press.

Gallup, G., & Lindsay, D. M. (1999). *Surveying the religious landscape: Trends in U.S. beliefs.* Harrisburg, PA: Morehouse Publishing.

Genia, V. (1996). I, E, quest, and fundamentalism as predictors of psychological and spiritual well-being. *Journal for the Scientific Study of Religion, 35,* 56–64.

George H. Gallup International Institute. (1997). *Spiritual beliefs and the dying process.* Princeton, NJ.

George, L. K. (1981). Subjective well-being: Conceptual and methodological issues. *Annual Review of Gerontology and Geriatrics, 2,* 345–382.

George, L. K. (2004). Social and economic factors related to psychiatric disorders in late life. In D. G. Blazer, D. C. Steffens, & E. W. Busse (Eds.), *The American psychiatric textbook of geriatric psychiatry* (3rd ed.) (pp. 139–161). Washington DC: American Psychiatric Association.

George, L. K., Hays, J. C., Flint, E. P., & Meador, K. G. (2004). Religion and health in life course perspective. In K. W. Schaie, N. Krause, & A. Booth (Eds.), *Religious influences on health and well-being in the elderly* (pp. 246–282). New York: Springer.

George, L. K., Landerman, R., Blazer, D. G., & Anthony, J. C. (1991). Cognitive impairment. In L. N. Robins & D. A. Rogier (Eds.), *Psychiatric disorders in America: The Epidemiologic Catchment Area Study* (pp. 281–327). New York: Free Press.

George, L. K., Larson, D. B., Koenig, H. G., & McCullough, M. E. (2000). Spirituality and health: What we know and what we need to know. *Journal of Social and Clinical Psychology, 19,* 102–116.

Goffman, E. (1959). *The presentation of self in everyday life.* New York: Anchor Books.

Goldhaber, D. E. (2000). *Theories of human development: Integrative perspectives.* Mountain View, CA: Mayfield Publishing Company.

Gordon, T., & Mitchell, D. (2004). A competency model for the assessment and delivery of spiritual care. *Palliative Medicine, 18,* 646–651.

Gottlieb, B. H. (1997). Conceptual and measurement issues in the study of coping with chronic stress. In B. H. Gottlieb (Ed.), *Coping with chronic stress* (pp. 3–40). New York: Plenum.

Groves, R. M., Fowler, F. J., Couper, M. P., Lepkowski, J. M., Singer, E., & Tourangeau, R. (2004). *Survey methodology.* New York: Wiley Interscience.

Gurland, B. J. (2004). Epidemiology of psychiatric disorders. In J. Sadavoy, L. F. Jarvik, G. T. Grossberg, & R. S. Meyers (Eds.), *Comprehensive textbook of geriatric psychiatry* (3rd ed.) (pp. 3–37). New York: W. W. Norton.

Gutmann, D. (1987). *Reclaimed powers: Toward a new psychology of men and women in later life.* New York: Basic Books.

Haight, B. K., & Webster, J. D. (1995). *The art and science of reminiscing: Theory, research, methods, and applications.* Washington, DC: Taylor & Francis.

Hall, G. S. (1922). *Senescence: The last half of life.* New York: D. Appleton and Company.

Hall. G. S. (1923). *Jesus the Christ in the light of psychology.* New York: D. Appleton and Company.

Hall, J. H., & Fincham, F. D. (2005). Self-forgiveness: The stepchild of forgiveness research. *Journal of Social and Clinical Psychology, 24,* 621–637.

Hansson, R. O., & Carpenter, B. N. (1990). Relational competence and adjustments in older adults: Implications for the demands of aging. In M. A. P.

Stephens, J. H. Crowther, S. E. Hobfoll, & D. L. Tennenbaum (Eds.), *Stress and coping in later life families* (pp. 131–151). Washington DC: Hemisphere Publishing.

Harris, W. S., Gowda, M., Kolb, J. W., Strychacz, C. P., Bacek, J. L., Jones, P. G., Forker, A., O'Keefe, J. H., & McCallister B. D. (1999). A random, controlled trial of the effects of remote, intercessory prayer on outcomes in patients admitted to the coronary care unit. *Archives of Internal Medicine, 159,* 2273–2278.

Hartman, W. J. (1976). *Membership trends: A study of decline and growth in the United Methodist Church, 1949–1975.* Nashville: Discipleship Resources.

Havighurst, R. J., Neugarten, B. L., & Tobin, S. S. (1968). Disengagement and patterns of aging. In B. L. Neugarten (Ed.), *Middle age and aging* (pp. 161–172). Chicago: University of Chicago Press.

Hawkley, L. C., Masi, C. M., Berry, J. D., & Cacioppo, J. T. (2006). Loneliness as a unique predictor of age-related differences in systolic blood pressure. *Psychology and Aging, 21,* 152–164.

Hayes, J. C., Landerman, L. R., Blazer, D. G., Koenig, H. G., Carroll, J. W., & Musick, M. A. (1998). Age, health, and the "electronic church." *Journal of Aging and Health, 10,* 458–482.

Hecht, J. M. (2003). *Doubt: A history.* San Francisco: Harper San Francisco.

Heiler, F. (1932). *Prayer: A study in the history and psychology of prayer.* New York: Oxford University Press.

Henretta, J. S. (2001). Work and retirement. In R. H. Binstock & L. K. George (Eds.), *Handbook of aging and the social sciences* (5th ed.) (pp. 255–271). San Diego, CA: Academic Press.

Herd, D. (1996). The influence of religious affiliation on sociocultural predictors of drinking among black and white Americans. *Substance Use and Misuse, 31,* 35–63.

Heyer-Grey, Z. A. (2000). Gender and religious work. *Sociology of Religion, 61,* 467–471.

Hill, D. (2002). The grieving Christian mother: What are her needs? *Journal of Pastoral Counseling, 37,* 50–73.

Hill, P. C., & Hood, R. W. (1999). *Measures of religiosity.* Birmingham, AL: Religious Education Press.

Hill, T. D., Angel, J. L., Ellison, C. G., & Angel, R. J. (2005). Religious attendance and mortality: An 8-year follow-up of older Mexican Americans. *Journal of Gerontology: Social Sciences, 60B,* S102–S109.

Hill, T. D., Burdette, A. M., Ellison, C. G., & Musick, M. A. (2006). Religious attendance and health behaviors of Texas adults. *Preventive Medicine, 42,* 309–312.

Hoare, C. H. (2002). *Erikson on development in adulthood: New insights from the unpublished papers.* New York: Oxford University Press.

Hobfoll, S. E. (1998). *Stress, culture, and community: The psychology and philosophy of stress.* New York: Plenum.

Hobfoll, S. E., & Stokes, J. P. (1988). The process and mechanics of social support. In S. Duck, D. F. Hayes, S. E. Hobfoll, W. Ickes, & B. M. Montgomery (Eds.), *Handbook of personal relationships: Theory, research, and intervention* (pp. 497–511). London: Wiley.

Hodges, E. V., Finnegan, R. A., & Perry, D. G. (1999). Skewed autonomy-relatedness in preadolescents' conceptions of their relationships with mother, father, and best friend. *Developmental Psychology, 35,* 737–748.

Hoge, D. R. (1972). A validated intrinsic religious motivation scale. *Journal for the Scientific Study of Religion, 11,* 369–376.

Hogg, J. R., & Heller, K. (1990). A measure of relational competence for community-dwelling elderly. *Psychology and Aging, 5,* 580–588.

Hohmann, A. A., & Larson, D. B. (1993). Psychiatric factors predicting use of clergy. In E. L. Worthington Jr. (Ed.), *Psychotherapy and religious values* (pp. 71–84). Grand Rapids: Baker Book House.

Holmes, T. H., & Rahe, R. H. (1967). The Social Readjustment Rating Scale. *Journal of Psychosomatic Research, 11,* 213–218.

House, J. S., & Kahn, R. L. (1985). Measures and concepts of social support. In S. Cohen & S. L. Syme (Eds.), *Social support and health* (pp. 83–108). New York: Academic Press.

House, J. S., Landis, K. R., & Umberson, D. (1988). Social relationships and health. *Science, 241,* 540–545.

Hoyle, R. H., Kernis, M. H., Leary, M. R., & Baldwin, M. W. (1999). *Selfhood: Identity, esteem, and regulation.* Boulder, CO: Westview Press.

Hubble, M. A., Duncan, B. L., & Miller, S. D. (1999). *The heart and soul of change: What works in therapy.* Washington DC: American Psychological Association.

Hughes, C. C., Tremblay, M. A., Rapoport, R. N., & Leighton, A. (1960). *People of Cove and Woodlot.* New York: Basic Books.

Hummer, R. A., Benjamins, M. R., & Rogers, R. G. (2004). Racial and ethnic disparities in health and mortality among the U.S. elderly population. In N. B. Anderson, R. A. Bulatao, & B. Cohen (Eds.), *Critical perspectives on racial and ethnic differences in health in late life* (pp. 53–94). Washington DC: The National Academic Press.

Hummer, R., Rogers, R., Nam, C., & Ellison, C. G. (1999). Religious involvement and U.S. adult mortality. *Demography, 36,* 273–285.

Hunsberger, B. S., McKenzie, B., Pratt, M., & Pancer, S. M. (1993). Religious doubt: A social psychological analysis. *Research in the Social Scientific Study of Religion, 5,* 27–51.

Hunsberger, B. S., Pratt, M., & Pancer, S. M. (2002). A longitudinal study of religious doubt in high school and beyond: Relationships, stability, and searching for answers. *Journal for the Scientific Study of Religion, 41,* 255–266.

Iannaccone, L. R. (1995). Voodoo economics? Reviewing the rational choice approach to religion. *Journal for the Scientific Study of Religion, 34,* 76–89.

Idler, E. L., & Kasl, S. V. (1997). Religion among disabled and nondisabled persons I: Cross-sectional patterns in health practices, social activities, and well-being. *Journal of Gerontology: Social Sciences, 52B,* S294–S305.

Ingersoll-Dayton, B., Krause, N., & Morgan, D. L. (2002). Religious trajectories and transitions over the life course. *International Journal of Aging and Human Development, 55,* 51–70.

Ingram, R. E. (1990). Self-focused attention in clinical disorders: Review and conceptual model. *Psychological Bulletin, 107,* 156–176.

Jacobi, Y., & Hull, R. F. C. (1953). *C. G. Jung psychological reflections: A new anthology of his writings 1905–1961.* Princeton, NJ: Princeton University Press.

James, W. (1892/1961). *Psychology: The briefer course.* New York: Harper & Row.

James, W. (1902/1997). *Selected writing—William James.* New York: Book-of-the-Month Club.

Jammer, M. (1999). *Einstein and religion.* Princeton, NJ: Princeton University Press.

Jeon, Y. H., Brodaty, H. & Chesterson, J. (2005). Respite care for caregivers of people with severe mental illness. *Journal of Advanced Nursing, 49,* 297–306.

Jourard, S. M. (1959). Health personality and self-disclosure. *Journal of Mental Hygiene, 43,* 499-507.

Kahn, J. R., & Fazio, E. M. (2005). Economic status over the life course and racial disparities in health. *Journal of Gerontology: Social Sciences (special issue), 60B,* 76–84.

Kanner, A. D., Coyne, J. C., Schaefer, C., & Lazarus, R. S. (1981). Comparison of two modes of stress measurement: Daily hassles and uplifts versus major life events. *Journal of Behavioral Medicine, 4,* 1–39.

Kaplan, A. (1964). *The conduct of inquiry.* San Francisco: Chandler Publishing Company.

Kaplan, H. B. (1975). *Self-attitudes and deviant behavior.* Pacific Palisades, CA: Goodyear Publishing Company.

Kelcourse, F. B. (2002). Pastoral counseling in the life of the church. *Encounter, 63,* 137–146.

Kelloway, E. K. (1998). *Using LISREL for structural equation modeling.* Thousand Oaks, CA: Sage.

Kessler, R. C. (1979). A strategy for studying differential vulnerability to the psychological consequences of stress. *Journal of Health and Social Behavior, 20,* 100–108.

Kessler, R. C., & Greenberg, D. (1981). *Linear panel analysis: Models of quantitative change.* New York: Academic Press.

Kessler, R. C., McLeod, J. D., & Wethington, E. (1985). The costs of caring: A perspective on the relationship between sex and psychological distress. In I. G. Sarason & B. R. Sarason (Eds.), *Social support: Theory, research, and applications* (pp. 491–506). The Hague, the Netherlands: Martinus Nijhoff.

King, M. F., & Bruner, G. C. (2000). Social desirability bias: A neglected aspect of validity testing. *Psychology & Marketing, 17*, 79–103.

Kirkpatrick, L. A. (2005). *Attachment, evolution, and the psychology of religion.* New York: Guilford.

Kirschenbaum, H., & Henderson, V. L. (1989). *The Carl Rogers reader.* Boston: Houghton Mifflin Company.

Kline, R. B. (2005). *Principles and practice of structural equation modeling.* New York: Guilford.

Knapp, J. L. (2001). The impact of congregation-related variables on programs for senior adult members. *Journal of Applied Gerontology, 20*, 24–38.

Koenig, H. G. (1994). *Aging and God.* New York: Haworth Pastoral Press.

Koenig, H. G. (1999). *The healing power of faith: Science explores medicine's last great frontier.* New York: Simon & Schuster.

Koenig, H. G., & Cohen, H. J. (2002a). Psychosocial factors, immunity, and wound healing. In H. G. Koenig & H. J. Cohen (Eds.), *Psychoneuroimmunology and the faith factor* (pp. 124–138). New York: Oxford University Press.

Koenig, H. G., & Cohen, H. J. (2002b). *The link between religion and health: Psychoneuroimmunology and the faith factor.* New York: Oxford University Press.

Koenig, H. G., McCullough, M. E., & Larson, D. B. (2001). *Handbook of religion and health.* New York: Oxford University Press.

Kohlberg, L. (1973). Stages and aging in moral development - some speculations. *The Gerontologist, 13*, 497–502.

Koltko-Rivera, M. E. (2006). Rediscovering the later version of Maslow's Hierarchy of Needs: Self-transcendence and opportunities for theory, research, and unification. *Review of General Psychology, 10*, 302–317.

Krause, N. (1987). Understanding the stress process: Linking social support with locus of control beliefs. *Journal of Gerontology, 42*, 589–593.

Krause, N. (1993). Neighborhood deterioration and social isolation in late life. *International Journal of Aging and Human Development, 36*, 9–38.

Krause, N. (1994). Stressors in salient social roles and well-being in late life. *Journal of Gerontology: Psychological Sciences, 49*, P137–P148.

Krause, N. (2001). Social support. In R. H. Binstock & L. K. George (Eds.), *Handbook of aging and the social sciences* (5th ed.) (pp. 272–294). San Diego, CA: Academic Press.

Krause, N. (2002a). A comprehensive strategy for developing closed-ended survey items for use in studies of older adults. *Journal of Gerontology: Social Sciences, 57B*, S263–S274.

Krause, N. (2002b). Exploring race differences in a comprehensive battery of church-based social support measures. *Review of Religious Research, 44*, 126–149.

Krause, N. (2002c). Church-based social support and health in old age: Exploring variations by race. *Journal of Gerontology: Social Sciences, 57B,* S332–S347.

Krause, N. (2003a). The social foundations of personal control in late life. In S. H. Zarit, L. I. Pearlin, & K. W. Schaie (Eds.), *Personal control in social and life course contexts* (pp. 45–70). New York: Springer.

Krause, N. (2003b). Religious meaning and subjective well-being in late life. *Journal of Gerontology: Social Sciences, 58B,* S160–S170.

Krause, N. (2003c). Praying for others, financial strain, and physical health status in late life. *Journal for the Scientific Study of Religion, 42,* 377–391.

Krause, N. (2003d). A preliminary assessment of race differences in the relationship between religious doubt and depressive symptoms. *Review of Religious Research, 45,* 93–115.

Krause, N. (2003e). Exploring race differences in the relationship between social interaction with the clergy and feelings of self-worth in late life. *Sociology of Religion, 64,* 183–205.

Krause, N. (2004a). Stressors in highly valued roles, meaning in life, and the physical health status of older adults. *Journal of Gerontology: Social Sciences, 59B,* S287–S297.

Krause, N. (2004b). Assessing the relationship among prayer expectancies, race, and self-esteem in late life. *Journal for the Scientific Study of Religion, 65,* 35–56.

Krause, N. (2005a). God-mediated control and psychological well-being in late life. *Research on Aging, 27,* 136–164.

Krause, N. (2005b). Negative interaction and heart disease in late life: Exploring variations by socioeconomic status. *Journal of Aging and Health, 17,* 28–55.

Krause, N. (2006a). Social Relationships. In R. H. Binstock & L. K. George (Eds.), *Handbook of aging and the social sciences* (pp. 181–200). San Diego: Academic Press.

Krause, N. (2006b). Exploring the stress-buffering effects of church-based social support and secular social support on health in late life. *Journal of Gerontology: Social Sciences, 61B,* S35–S43.

Krause, N. (2006c). Gratitude toward God, stress, and health in late life. *Research on Aging, 28,* 163–183.

Krause, N. (2006d). Church-based social support and mortality. *Journal of Gerontology: Social Sciences, 61B,* S140–S146.

Krause, N. (2006e). Religious doubt and psychological well-being: A longitudinal investigation. *Review of Religious Research, 47,* 287–302.

Krause, N. (2006f). Religion and health in late life. In J. E. Birren & K. W. Schaie (Eds.), *Handbook of the psychology of aging* (6th ed.) (pp. 499–518). San Diego: Academic Press.

Krause, N. (2006g). Exploring race and sex differences in church involvement during late life. *International Journal for the Psychology of Religion, 16,* 127–144.

Krause, N. (2007a). Evaluating the stress-buffering function of meaning in life among older people. *Journal of Aging and Health* 19, 792–812.

Krause, N. (2007b). Social involvement in religious institutions and God-mediated control beliefs: A longitudinal investigation. *Journal for the Scientific Study of Religion* 46, 519-537.

Krause, N. (2007c). The social foundation of religious meaning in life. *Research on Aging*, in Press.

Krause, N. (2007d). Self-expression and depressive symptoms in late life. *Research on Aging, 29,* 187–206.

Krause, N. (2008). Lifetime trauma, prayer, and psychological distress in late life. Under review at the *International Journal for the Psychology of Religion*.

Krause, N., & Bastida, E. (2007). Core religious beliefs and providing support to others in late life. Under review at *Mental Health, Religion, and Culture*.

Krause, N., & Borawski-Clark, E. (1994). Clarifying the functions of social support in late life. *Research on Aging, 16,* 251–279.

Krause, N., & Borawski-Clark, E. (1995). Social class differences in social support among older adults. *The Gerontologist, 35,* 498–508.

Krause, N., Chatters, L. M., Meltzer, T., & Morgan, D. L. (2000a). Using focus groups to explore the nature of prayer in late life. *Journal of Aging Studies, 14,* 191–212.

Krause, N., Chatters, L. M., Meltzer, T., & Morgan, D. L. (2000b). Negative interaction in the church: Insights from focus groups with older adults. *Review of Religious Research, 41,* 510–533.

Krause, N., & Ellison, C. G. (2003). Forgiveness by God, forgiveness of others, and psychological well-being in late life. *Journal for the Scientific Study of Religion, 42,* 77–93.

Krause, N., & Ellison, C. G. (2007). The doubting process: A longitudinal study of the precipitants and consequences of religious doubt. Under review at the *Journal for the Scientific Study of Religion*.

Krause, N., Ellison, C. G., & Marcum, J. P. (2002). The effects of church-based emotional support on health: Do they vary by gender? *Sociology of Religion, 63,* 21–47.

Krause, N., Ellison, C. G., Shaw, B. A., Marcum, J. P., & Boardman, J. (2001). Church-based social support and religious coping. *Journal for the Scientific Study of Religion, 40,* 637–656.

Krause, N., Ellison, C. G., & Wulff, K. M. (1998). Church-based social support, negative interaction, and psychological well-being: Findings from a national sample of Presbyterians. *Journal for the Scientific Study of Religion, 37,* 725–741.

Krause, N., Herzog, A. R., & Baker, E. (1992). Providing support to others and well-being in later life. *Journal of Gerontology: Psychological Sciences, 47,* P300–P311.

Krause, N., Ingersoll-Dayton, B., Ellison, C. G., & Wulff, K. M. (1999). Aging, religious doubt, and psychological well-being. *The Gerontologist, 39,* 525–533.

Krause, N., Liang, J., & Yatomi, N. (1989). Satisfaction with social support and depressive symptoms: A longitudinal analysis. *Psychology and Aging, 4,* 88–97.

Krause, N., Newsom, J. T., & Rook, K. S. (2008). Financial strain, negative interaction, and health: Evidence from two nationwide longitudinal surveys. Under review.

Krause, N., & Rook, K. S. (2003). Negative interaction in late life: Issues in stability and generalizability of conflict across relationships. *Journal of Gerontology: Psychological Sciences, 58B,* P88–P99.

Krause, N., & Shaw, B. A. (2000). Giving social support to others, socioeconomic status, and changes in self-esteem in late life. *Journal of Gerontology: Social Sciences, 55B,* S323–S333.

Krause, N., Shaw, B. A., & Cairney, J. (2004). A descriptive epidemiology of lifetime trauma and the physical health status of older adults. *Psychology and Aging, 19,* 637–648.

Krause, N., & Wulff, K. M. (2004). Religious doubt and health: Exploring the potential dark side of religion. *Sociology of Religion, 65,* 35–56.

Krause, N., & Wulff, K. M. (2005). Church-based social ties, a sense of belonging in a congregation, and physical health status. *The International Journal for the Psychology of Religion, 15,* 73–93.

La Gaipa, J. J. (1990). The negative effects of informal support systems. In S. Duck (Ed.), *Personal relationships and social support* (pp. 122–139). Newbury Park, CA: Sage.

LaMothe, R. (2005). An analysis of pride systems and the dynamics of faith. *Pastoral Psychology, 53,* 239–253.

Langner, T. S., & Michael, S. T. (1963). *Life stress and mental health.* New York: Free Press.

Lao-tzu. (400 BCE/1988). *Tao Te Ching* (S. Mitchell, Trans.). New York: Harper Perennial.

Larson, D. G., & Chastain, R. L. (1990). Self-concealment: Conceptualization, measurement, and health implications. *Journal of Social and Clinical Psychology, 8,* 439–455.

Lazarus, R. S., & Folkman, S. (1984). *Stress, appraisal, and coping.* New York: Springer.

Lee, B. Y., & Newberg, A. B. (2005). Religion and health: A review and critical analysis. *Zygon, 40,* 443–468.

Lee, G. (1985). Kinship and social support of the elderly: The case of the United States. *Ageing and Society, 5,* 19–38.

Lenski, G. (1961). *The religious factor: A sociological study of religion's impact on politics, economics, and family life.* New York: Doubleday.

Lepore, S. J. (1995). Measurement of chronic stressors. In S. Cohen, R. C. Kessler, & L. U. Gordon (Eds.), *Measuring stress: A guide for health and social scientists* (pp. 102–120). New York: Oxford University Press.

Levenson, M. R., Jennings, P. A., Aldwin, C. M., & Shiraishi, R. W. (2005). Self-transcendence: Conceptualization and measurement. *International Journal of Aging and Human Development, 60,* 127–143.

Levin, J. S. (1996a). How prayer heals: A theoretical model. *Alternative Therapies, 2,* 66–73.

Levin, J. S. (1996b). How religion influences morbidity and health: Reflections on natural history, salutogenesis, and host resistance. *Social Science and Medicine, 43,* 849–864.

Levin, J. S. (2001). *God, faith, and health: Exploring the spirituality-healing connection.* New York: Wiley.

Levin, J. S. (2004). Prayer, love, and transcendence: An epidemiologic perspective. In K. W. Schaie, N. Krause, & A. Booth (Eds.), *Religious influences on health and well-being in the elderly* (pp. 69–95). New York: Springer.

Levin, J. S., Taylor, R. J., & Chatters, L. M. (1994). Race and gender differences in religiosity among older adults: Findings from four national surveys. *Journal of Gerontology: Social Sciences, 49,* S137–S145.

Lewis, C. S. (1942/2001). *Mere Christianity.* San Francisco: Harper.

Lewis, M. A., & Rook, K. S. (1999). Social control in personal relationships: Impact on health behaviors and psychological distress. *Health Psychology, 18,* 63–71.

Liebow, E. (1967). *Talley's Corner: A study of negro streetcorner men.* Boston: Little Brown.

Loveland, M. T. (2003). Religious switching: Preference development, maintenance, and change. *Journal for the Scientific Study of Religion, 42,* 147–157.

Luoh, M. C., & Herzog, A. R. (2002). Individual consequences of volunteer and paid work in old age: Health and mortality. *Journal of Health and Social Behavior, 43,* 490–509.

Maimonides, M. (1190/2004). *The guide for the perplexed.* New York: Barnes and Noble.

Maltby, J., Macaskill, A., & Day, L. (2001). Failure to forgive self and others: A replication and extension of the relationships between forgiveness, personality, social desirability, and general health. *Personality and Individual Differences, 30,* 881–885.

Marmot, M., & Wilkinson, R. G. (2006). *Social determinants of health.* New York: Oxford University Press.

Marques, A. H., & Sternberg, E. M. (2007). The biology of positive emotions and health. In S. G. Post (Ed.), *Altruism and health: Perspectives from empirical research* (p. 149–188). New York: Oxford University Press.

Maslow, A. H. (1954). *Motivation and personality.* New York: Harper.

Maslow, A. H. (1971). *The farther reaches of human nature.* New York: Viking Press.

Maton, K. I. (1989). The stress-buffering role of spiritual support: Cross-sectional and prospective investigations. *Journal for the Scientific Study of Religion, 28,* 310–323.

Mattis, J. S., & Jagers, R. J. (2001). A relational framework for the study of religiosity and spirituality in the lives of African Americans. *Journal of Community Psychology, 29,* 519–539.

Mattlin, J. A., Wethington, E., & Kessler, R. C. (1990). Situational determinants of coping and coping effectiveness. *Journal of Health and Social Behavior, 31,* 103–122.

Maves, P. B. (1960). Aging, religion, and the church. In C. Tibbitts (Ed.), *Handbook of social gerontology* (pp. 698–749). Chicago: University of Chicago Press.

Maynard-Reid, P. U. (2000). *Diverse worship: African-American, Caribbean & Hispanic perspectives.* Downers Grove, IL: InterVarsity Press.

McAdams, D. P., Aubin, E., & Logan, R. L. (1993). Generativity among young, midlife, and older adults. *Psychology and Aging, 8,* 221–230.

McCarty, R., & Childre, D. (2004). The grateful heart: The psychophysiology of appreciation. In R. A. Emmons & M. E. McCullough (Eds.), *The psychology of gratitude* (pp. 230–255). New York: Oxford University Press.

McClelland, G. H., & Judd, C. M. (1993). Statistical difficulties of detecting interactions and moderator effects. *Psychological Bulletin, 114,* 376–390.

McCullough, M. E., Enders, C. K., Brion, S. L., & Jain, A. R. (2005). The varieties of religious development in adulthood: A longitudinal investigation of religion and rational choice. *Journal of Personality and Social Psychology, 89,* 78–89.

McCullough, M. E., & Larson, D. B. (1999). Prayer. In W. R. Miller (Ed.), *Integrating spirituality into treatment: Resources for practitioners* (pp. 85–110). Washington, DC: American Psychological Association.

McCullough, M. E., Pargament, K. I., & Thoresen, C. E. (2000). *Forgiveness: Theory, research, and practice.* New York: Guilford.

McDowell, I., & Newell, C. (1996). *Measuring health: A guide to rating scales and questionnaires.* New York: Oxford University Press.

McFadden, S. H. (1999). Religion, personality and aging: A life span perspective. *Journal of Personality, 67,* 1081–1104.

McFadden, S. H. (2005). Points of connection: Gerontology and the psychology of religion. In R. F. Paloutzian & C. L. Park (Eds.), *Handbook of the psychology of religion and spirituality* (pp. 162–176). New York: Guilford.

McFadden, S. H., Knepple, A. M., & Armstrong, J. A. (2003). Length and locus of friendship influence, church members' sense of social support, and comfort with sharing emotions. *Journal of Religious Gerontology, 15,* 39–55.

McGrath, P. (2002). Creating a language for "spiritual pain" through research: A beginning. *Supportive Care in Cancer, 10,* 637–646.

McKay, B., & Musil, L. A. (2005). The "Spiritual Healing Project": A study of the meaning of spiritual healing in the United Church of Christ. In L. L. Barnes & S. S. Sered (Eds.), *Religion and healing in America* (pp. 49–57). New York: Oxford University Press.

McMillen, J. C. (1999). Better for it: How people benefit from adversity. *Social Work, 44,* 455–468.

McPherson, M., Smith-Lovin, L., & Cook, J. M. (2001). Birds of a feather: Homophily in social networks. *Annual Review of Sociology, 27,* 415–444.

Mead, G. H. (1934/1962). *Mind, self, and society from the standpoint of a social behaviorist.* Chicago: University of Chicago Press.

Meller, I., Fichter, M. M., & Schroppel, H. (2004). Mortality risk in the octo and nonagenarians according to psychic symptoms, cause and place of death: Longitudinal results of an epidemiological follow-up community study. *European Journal of Psychiatry, 18,* 44–59.

Mendes de Leon, C. F. (2005). Why do friendships matter for survival? *Journal of Epidemiology and Community Health, 59,* 538–539.

Meredith, G. E., & Schewe, C. D. (2002). *Defining markets defining moments: America's 7 generational cohorts, their shared experiences, and why business should care.* New York: Hungry Minds, Inc.

Merton, R. K. (1949). *Social theory and social structure: Toward the codification of theory and research.* Glencoe, IL: Free Press.

Midlarsky, E. (1991). Helping as coping. In M. C. Clark (Ed.), *Prosocial behavior: Review of personality and social psychology. Vol. 12* (pp. 238–264). Newbury Park, CA: Sage.

Mills, C. W. (1959). *The sociological imagination.* New York: Oxford University Press.

Mirowsky, J. (1995). Age and sense of control. *Social Psychology Quarterly, 58,* 31–43.

Mirowsky, J., & Ross, C. E. (2003). *Education, social status, and health.* New York: Aldine De Gruyter.

Moadel, A., Morgan, C., Fatone, A., Grennan, J., Carter, J., & Laruffa, G. (1999). Seeking meaning and hope: Self-reported spiritual and existential needs among an ethnically-diverse cancer patient population. *Psycho-Oncology, 8,* 378–385.

Montaigne, Michel de. (2003). *Michel de Montaigne: The complete works* (D. M. Frame, Trans.). New York: Alfred Knopf.

Musick, M. A., Herzog, A. R., & House, J. S. (1999). Volunteering and mortality among older adults: Findings from a national sample. *Journal of Gerontology: Social Sciences, 54B,* S173–S180.

Musick, M. A., & Wilson, J. (2003). Volunteering and depression: The role of psychological and social resources in different age groups. *Social Science and Medicine, 56,* 259–269.

Naydler, J. (2000). *Goethe on science: An anthology of Goethe's writings.* Edinburgh: Floris Books.

Neighbors, H. W., Musick, M. A., & Williams, D. R. (1998). The African American minister as a source of help for series personal crises: Bridge or barrier to mental health care? *Health Education and Behavior, 25,* 759–777.

Nelsen, H. M., & Nelsen, A. K. (1975). *Black church in the sixties.* Lexington: University of Kentucky Press.

Nelson, E. A., & Dannefer, D. (1992). Aged heterogeneity: Fact or fiction? The fate and diversity in gerontological research. *The Gerontologist, 32,* 17–23.

Neugarten, B. L. (1965/1996). Personality changes in the aged. In D. A. Neugarten (Ed.), *The meanings of age: Selected papers of Bernice L. Neugarten* (pp. 256–269). Chicago: University of Chicago Press.

New American Webster Dictionary (1982). Chicago: New American Library.

Newby-Clark, I. R. (2004). Getting ready for the bad times: Self-esteem and anticipatory coping. *European Journal of Social Psychology, 34,* 309–316.

Newport, F. (2004). A look at Americans and religion today. Available on the following website: http://poll.gallup.com.

Newsom, J. T., Mahan, T. L., Rook, K. S., & Krause, N. (2008). Stable negative social exchanges and health. *Health Psychology 27,* 78–86.

Newsom, J. T., Rook, K. S., Nishishiba, M., Sorkin, D. H., & Mahan, T. L. (2005). Understanding the relative importance of positive and negative exchanges: Examining specific domains and appraisals. *Journal of Gerontology: Psychological Sciences, 60B,* P304–P312.

Niebuhr, R. (1964). *The nature and destiny of man, Vol. 1.* New York: Charles Scribner's Sons.

Nielsen, M. E. (1998). An assessment of religious conflicts and their resolutions. *Journal for the Scientific Study of Religion, 37,* 379–391.

Nietzsche, F. (1895/1999). *The anti-Christ.* Tucson, AZ: See Sharp Press.

Nunn, K. P. (1996). Personal hopefulness: A conceptual review of the relevance of the perceived future to psychiatry. *British Journal of Medical Psychology, 69,* 227–245.

Nunnally, J. C., & Bernstein, I. H. (1994). *Psychometric theory* (3rd ed.). New York: McGraw-Hill.

Oates, W. E. (1997). The theological context of pastoral counseling. *Review and Expositor, 94,* 521–530.

Oden, T. (1969). *The structure of awareness.* Nashville: Abingdon.

Okun, M. A., & Keith, V. M. (1998). Effects of positive and negative social exchanges from various sources on depressive symptoms in younger and older adults. *Journal of Gerontology: Psychological Sciences, 53B,* P4–P20.

Okun, M. A., & Michel, J. (2006). Sense of community and being a volunteer among the young-old. *Journal of Applied Gerontology, 25,* 173–188.

Olson, D. V. A. (1989). Church friendships: Boon or barrier to church growth? *Journal for the Scientific Study of Religion, 28,* 432–447.

Olson, J. M., Roese, N. J., Zanna, M. P. (1996). Expectancies. In E. T. Higgins & A. W. Kruglanski (Eds.), *Social psychology: Handbook of basic principles* (pp. 211–238). New York: Guilford.

Oman, D., & Thoresen, C. E. (2005). Do religion and spirituality influence health? In R. F. Paloutzian & C. L. Park (Eds.), *Handbook of the psychology of religion and spirituality* (pp. 435–459). New York: Guilford.

Oman, D., Thoresen, C. E., & McMahon, K. (1999). Volunteerism and mortality among the community-dwelling elderly. *Journal of Health Psychology, 4,* 301–316.

Oppenheimer, J. E., Flannelly, K. J., & Weaver, A. J. (2004). A comparative analysis of the psychological literature on collaboration between clergy and mental-health professionals—Perspectives from secular and religious journals: 1970–1999. *Pastoral Psychology, 53,* 153–162.

Orsi, R. A. (2005). *Between heaven and earth: The religious worlds people make and the scholars who study them.* Princeton, NJ: Princeton University Press.

Pargament, K. I. (1997). *The psychology of religious coping: Theory, research, and practice.* New York: Guilford.

Pargament, K. I., Koenig, H. G., & Perez, L. M. (2000). The many methods of religious coping: Development and initial validation of the RCOPE. *Journal of Clinical Psychology, 56,* 519–543.

Pargament, K. I., Magyar, G. M., Benore, E., & Mahoney, A. (2005). Sacrilege: A study of sacred loss and desecration and their implications for health and well-being in a community sample. *Journal for the Scientific Study of Religion, 44,* 59–78.

Pargament, K. I., Silverman, W., Johnson, S., Echemendia, R., & Snyder, S. (1983). The psychosocial climate of religious congregations. *American Journal of Community Psychology, 11,* 351–381.

Pargament, K. I., Zinnbauer, B. J., Scott, A. B., Butter, E. M., Zerowin, J., & Stanik, P. (1998). Red flags and religious coping: Identifying some religious warning signs among people in crisis. *Journal of Clinical Psychology, 54,* 77–89.

Park, C. L. (2005). Religion and meaning. In R. F. Paloutzian & C. L. Park (Eds.), *Handbook of the psychology of religion and spirituality* (pp. 295–314). New York: Guilford.

Patterson, B. R., Bettini, L., & Nussbaum, J. F. (1993). The meaning of friendship across the life span: Two studies. *Communication Quarterly, 41,* 145–160.

Paulson, D. S. (2004). The near death process and pastoral counseling. *Pastoral Psychology, 52,* 339–352.

Payne, B. P. (1994). Faith development among older men. In E. H. Thompson (Ed.), *Older men's lives* (pp. 85–103). Thousand Oaks, CA: Sage.

Payne-Stencil, B. (1997). Religion and faith development of older women. In J.

M. Coyle (Ed.), *Handbook of women and aging* (pp. 223–241). Westport, CT: Greenwood Press.

Pearlin, L. I., Menaghan, E., Lieberman, M., & Mullan, J. (1981). The stress process. *Journal of Health and Social Behavior, 22,* 337–356.

Pennebaker, J. W. (1995). *Emotion, disclosure, and health.* Washington DC: American Psychological Association.

Perry, R. B. (1954). *The thought and character of William James, briefer version.* New York: George Braziller.

Peterson, C., & Seligman, M. E. (2004). *Character strengths and virtues: A handbook and classification.* New York: Oxford University Press.

Peterson, C., Seligman, M. E., & Vaillant, G. E. (1988). Pessimistic explanatory style is a risk factor for physical illness: A thirty-five-year longitudinal study. *Journal of Personality and Social Psychology, 55,* 23–27.

Peterson, L. R., & Roy, A. (1985). Religiosity, anxiety, and meaning and purpose: Religion's consequences for well-being. *Review of Religious Research, 27,* 49–62.

Pineles, S. L., Street, A. E., & Koenen, K. C. (2006). The differential relationship between shame-proneness and guilt-proneness to psychological and somatization symptoms. *Journal of Social and Clinical Psychology, 25,* 688–704.

Plato & Eliot, C. W. (1909). *The Apology, Phaedo, and Crito of Plato; Golden Sayings of Epictetus; Mediations of Marcus Aurelius: Part 2, Harvard Classics.* New York: P. F. Collier and Son.

Poloma, M. M., & Gallup, G. H. (1991). *Varieties of prayer: A survey report.* Philadelphia: Trinity Press International.

Poloma, M. M., & Hoelter, L. F. (1998). The "Toronto Blessing": A holistic model of healing. *Journal for the Scientific Study of Religion, 37,* 257–272.

Pope, A. (1731/1965). *An essay on man.* New York: Macmillan.

Prentice, D. A., & Miller, D. T. (1992). When small effects are impressive. *Psychological Bulletin, 112,* 160–164.

Princeton Religion Research Center. (1994). *Religion in America (1994 Supplement).* Princeton, NJ: Gallup Poll.

Pyszczynski, T., Greenberg, J., Hamilton, J., & Nix, G. (1991). On the relationship between self-focused attention and psychological disorder: A critical reappraisal. *Psychological Bulletin, 110,* 538–543.

Radloff, L. S. (1977). The CES-D Scale: A self-report depression scale for research in the general population. *Applied Psychological Measurement, 1,* 385–401.

Raudenbush, S. W., & Bryk, A. S. (2002). *Hierarchical linear models: Applications and data analysis methods* (2nd ed.). Thousand Oaks, CA: Sage.

Raykov, T. (1998). A method for obtaining standard errors and confidence intervals of composite reliability for congeneric measures. *Applied Psychological Measurement, 22,* 369–374.

Reed, I. C. (2005). Creativity: Self-perceptions over time. *International Journal of Aging and Human Development, 60,* 1–18.

Reich, K. H. (1992). Religious development across the life span: Conventional and cognitive development approaches. In D. L. Featherman, R. H. Lerner, & M. Perlmutter (Eds.), *Life-span development and behavior* (pp. 145–188). Hillsdale, NJ: Lawrence Erlbaum.

Reis, H. T., & Collins, N. (2000). Measuring relationship properties and interactions relevant to social support. In S. Cohen, L. G. Underwood, & B. H. Gottlieb (Eds.), *Social support measurement and intervention* (pp. 136–192). New York: Oxford University Press.

Reissman, F. (1965). The "helper" therapy principle. *Social Work, 10,* 27–32.

Reker, G. T. (1997). Personal meaning, optimism, and choice: Existential predictors of depression in community and institutional elderly. *The Gerontologist, 37,* 709–716.

Richards, M. (2003). Caring for the caregiver. In M. A. Kimble & S. H. McFadden (Eds.), *Aging, spirituality, and religion, Vol. 2* (pp. 180–192). Minneapolis: Fortress Press.

Robb, C., Haley, W. E., Becker, M. A., Polivka, L. A., & Chwa, H. J. (2003). Attitudes toward mental health care in younger and older adults: Similarities and differences. *Aging & Mental Health, 7,* 142–152.

Roberts, J. D. (2003). *Black religion, black theology* (E. M. Goatley, Ed.). Harrisburg, PA: Trinity Press International.

Robins, R. W., Trzesniewski, K. H., Tracy, J. L., Gosling, S. D., & Potter, J. (2002). Global self-esteem across the lifespan. *Psychology and Aging, 17,* 423–434.

Rogers, C. (1986). A client-centered/person-centered approach to therapy. In H. Krischenbaum & V. L. Henderson (Eds.), *The Carl Rogers reader* (pp. 135–152). Boston: Houghton Mifflin Company.

Rook, K. S. (1984). The negative side of social interaction: Impact on psychological well-being. *Journal of Personality and Social Psychology, 46,* 1097–1108.

Rook, K. S. (1987). Social support versus companionship: Effects on life stress, loneliness, and evaluations by others. *Journal of Personality and Social Psychology, 52,* 1132–1147.

Rook, K. S. (1990). Stressful aspects of older adults' social relationships: Current theory and research. In M. A. P. Stephens, J. H. Crowther, S. E. Hobfoll, & D. L. Tennenbaum (Eds.), *Stress and coping in later life* (pp. 172–192). Washington, DC: Hemisphere.

Rook, K. S. (1991). Facilitating friendship formation in late life: Puzzles and challenges. *American Journal of Community Psychology, 19,* 103–110.

Rook, K. S., & Pietromonaco, P. (1987). Close relationships: Ties that heal or ties that bind? In W. H. Jones & D. Perlman (Eds.), *Advances in personal relationships* (pp. 1–35). Greenwich, CT: JAI Press.

Rorty, O. A. (1990). Pride produces the ideal of self: Hume on moral agency. *Australian Journal of Philosophy, 68,* 255–269.

Rosow, I. (1976). Status and role change through the life span. In R. H. Binstock

& E. Shanas (Eds.), *Handbook of aging and the social sciences* (pp. 457–482). New York: Van Nostrand Reinhold.

Ross, C. E., & Sastry, J. (1999). The sense of personal control: Social-structural causes and emotional consequences. In C. S. Aneshensel & J. C. Phalen (Eds.), *Handbook of the sociology of mental health* (pp. 369–394).

Ross, E. A. (1896). Social control V. *American Sociological Review, 2,* 433–445.

Ross, E. A. (1907). *Sin and society.* Boston: Houghton Mifflin Company.

Rost, R. A. (2003). Issues of grace and sin in pastoral care with older adults. In M. A. Kimble & S. H. McFadden (Eds.), *Aging, spirituality, and religion: A handbook, Vol. 2* (pp. 239–254). Minneapolis: Fortress Press.

Rowe, J. W., & Kahn, R. L. (1998). *Successful aging.* New York: Pantheon.

Royce, J. (1912/2001). *The sources of religious insight.* Washington, DC: Catholic University of America Press.

Rubin, L. B. (1976). *Worlds of pain: Life in the working-class family.* New York: Basic Books.

Russell, B. (1957/2000). A free man's worship. In E. D. Klemke (Ed.), *The meaning of life* (pp. 71–77). New York: Oxford University Press.

Rutledge, T., & Loh, C. (2004). Effect sizes and statistical testing in the determination of clinical significance in behavioral medicine research. *Annals of Behavioral Medicine, 27,* 138–145.

Rye, M. S., Pargament, K. I., Ali, M. A., Beck, G. L., Dorff, E. N., Hallisey, C., Narayanan, V., & Williams, J. G. (2000). Religious perspectives on forgiveness. In M. E. McCullough, K. I. Pargament, & C. E. Thoresen (Eds.), *Forgiveness: Theory, research, and practice* (pp. 17–40). New York: Guilford.

Ryff, C. D., & Singer, B. (1998). The contours of positive human health. *Psychological Inquiry, 9,* 1–28.

Sabate, J. (2004). Invited commentary: Religion, diet, and research. *British Journal of Nutrition, 92,* 199–201.

Saltzman-Chafetz, J. (2001). Theoretical understandings of gender: A third of a century of feminist thought in sociology. In J. H. Turner (Ed.), *Handbook of sociological theory* (pp. 613–631). New York: Plenum.

Schieman, S., Pudrovska, T., & Milkie, M. A. (2005). The sense of divine control and the self-concept. *Review of Religious Research, 27,* 165–196.

Schimmel, S. (2002). *Wounds not healed by time: The power of repentance and forgiveness.* New York: Oxford University Press.

Schlenker, B. R. (2003). Self-presentations. In M. R. Leary & J. P. Tangney (Eds.), *Handbook of self and identity* (pp. 492–518). New York: Guilford.

Schopenhauer, A. (1851/2004). *Essays and aphorisms.* New York: Penguin Books.

Schulz, J. H. (2001). *The economics of aging.* Westport, CT: Auburn House.

Schulz, R., & Heckhausen, J. (1996). A life span-model of successful aging. *American Psychologist, 51,* 702–714.

Schulz, R., & Martire, L. (2004). Family caregiving of persons with dementia:

Prevalence, health effects, and support strategies. *American Journal of Geriatric Psychiatry, 12,* 240–249.

Schulz, R., Newsom, J., & Mittelmark, M. (1997). Health effects of caregiving: The Cardiovascular Health Effects Study: An ancillary study of the Cardiovascular Health Study. *Annals of Behavioral Medicine, 19,* 110–116.

Schweitzer, A. (1933/1990). *Out of my life and thought.* Baltimore: The Johns Hopkins University Press.

Schweitzer, A. (1949). *The philosophy of civilization.* New York: Macmillan.

Seeman, T. E., Lusignolo, T. M., Albert, M., & Berkman, L. (2001). Social relationships, social support, and patterns of cognitive aging in healthy, high-functioning older adults: MacArthur Studies in Successful Aging. *Health Psychology, 20,* 243–255.

Seneca, L. A. (2004). *Letters from a Stoic.* New York: Penguin Books.

Seplaki, C. L., Goldman, N., Weinstein, M., & Lin, Y. H. (2004). How are biomarkers related to physical and mental well-being? *Journal of Gerontology: Biomedical Sciences and Medical Sciences, 59A,* M201–M217.

Shand, J. D. (2000). The effects of life experiences over a 50-year period on the certainty of belief and disbelief in God. *The International Journal for the Psychology of Religion, 10,* 85–100.

Sherman, E. (1991). *Reminiscence and the self in old age.* New York: Springer.

Sherman, N. (1993). Aristotle and the shared life. In N. K. Badhwar (Ed.), *Friendship: A philosophical reader* (pp. 91–107). Ithaca, NY: Cornell University Press.

Simmel, G. (1898/1997). A contribution to the sociology of religion. In H. J. Helle (Ed.), *Essays on religion—Georg Simmel* (pp. 101–120). New Haven, CT: Yale University Press.

Sinclair, U. (1918/2000). *The profits of religion.* Amherst, NY: Prometheus Books.

Sinnott, J. D., & Shifren, K. (2001). Gender and aging: Gender differences and gender roles. In J. E. Birren & K. W. Schaie (Eds.), *Handbook of the psychology of aging* (5th ed.) (pp. 454–476). San Diego: Academic Press.

Skinner, E. A. (1997). A guide to the construct of control. *Journal of Personality and Social Psychology, 71,* 549-570.

Sloan, R. P., & Bagiella, E. (2002). Claims about religious involvement and health outcomes. *Annals of Behavioral Medicine, 24,* 14–21.

Smith, A. (1759/2002). *The theory of moral sentiments.* Cambridge: Cambridge University Press.

Smith, A. (1776). *An inquiry into the nature and causes of the wealth of nations.* London: Strahan & Cadell.

Smith, C., & Faris, R. (2005). Socioeconomic inequality in the American religious system: An update and assessment. *Journal for the Scientific Study of Religion, 44,* 94–104.

Smith, H. (1991). *The world's religions.* New York: Harper Collins.

Snyder, C. R., Michael, S. T., & Cheavens, J. S. (1999). Hope as a psychotherapeutic foundation of common factors, placebos, and expectancies. In M. A. Hubble, B. L. Duncan, & S. D. Miller (Eds.), *The heart and soul of change: What works in therapy* (pp. 179–200). Washington, DC: American Psychological Association.

Sokolovsky, J., & Cohen, C. I. (1981). Measuring social interaction of the urban elderly: A methodological synthesis. *International Journal of Aging and Human Development, 13,* 233–244.

Sorkin, D., Rook, K. S., & Lu, J. (2002). Loneliness, lack of emotional support, lack of companionship, and the likelihood of having a heart condition in an elderly sample. *Annals of Behavioral Medicine, 24,* 290–298.

Sosis, R. (2000). Religion and intragroup cooperation: Preliminary results of a comparative analysis of utopian communities. *Cross-Cultural Research, 34,* 7–87.

Spilka, B., Hood, R. W., Hunsberger, B., & Gorsuch, R. (2003). *The psychology of religion* (3rd ed.). New York: Guilford.

Spinoza, B. D. (1677/2005). *Ethics and on the improvement of understanding.* New York: Barnes and Noble Books.

Stack, C. (1974). *All our kin: Strategies for survival in a black community.* New York: Harper & Row.

Starbuck, D. E. (1897). Contributions to the psychology of religion. *The American Journal of Psychology, 9,* 70–124.

Starbuck, D. E. (1899). *The psychology of religion.* New York: Charles Scribner's Sons.

Stark, R., & Bainbridge, W. S. (1987). *A theory of religion.* New Brunswick, NJ: Rutgers University Press.

Stark, R., & Finke, R. (2000). *Acts of faith: Explaining the human side of religion.* Berkeley: University of California Press.

Stark, R., & Glock, C. Y. (1968). *American piety: The nature of religious commitment.* Berkeley: University of California Press.

Stephens, J. (1976). *Loners, losers, and lovers: Elderly tenants in a slum hotel.* Seattle: University of Washington Press.

Sternberg, R. J., & Lubart, T. I. (2001). Wisdom and creativity. In J. E. Birrin & K. W. Schaie (Eds.), *Handbook of the psychology of aging* (pp. 500–522). San Diego: Academic Press.

Strube, M. J. (1991). Multiple determinants of effect size: A more general method of discourse. *Journal of Personality and Social Psychology, 61,* 1024–1027.

Strunk, O., Jr. (1965). *Mature religion: A psychological study.* New York: Abingdon Press.

Stryker, S. (2001). Traditional symbolic interactionism, role theory, and structural symbolic interactionism: The road to identity theory. In J. H. Turner (Ed.), *Handbook of sociological theory* (pp. 211–231). New York: Plenum.

Tallman, K., & Bohart, A. C. (1999). The client as a common factor: Clients as self-healers. In M. A. Hubble, B. L. Duncan, & S. D. Miller (Eds.), *The heart and soul of change: What works in therapy* (pp. 91–131). Washington, DC: American Psychological Association.

Tardy, C. H. (2000). Self-disclosure and health: Revisiting Sidney Jourard's hypothesis. In S. Petronio (Ed.), *Balancing the secrets of private disclosure.* Mahwah NJ: Lawrence Erlbaum.

Taylor, R. J., Chatters, L. M., & Levin, J. (2004). *Religion in the lives of African Americans: Social, psychological, and health perspectives.* Thousand Oaks, CA: Sage.

Taylor, R. J., Ellison, C. G., Chatters, L. M., Levin, J. S., & Lincoln, K. D. (2000). Mental health services in faith communities: The role of clergy in black churches. *Social Work, 45,* 73–87.

Taylor, S. (1991). Asymmetrical effects of positive and negative events. The mobilization-minimization hypothesis. *Psychological Bulletin, 110,* 67–85.

Tedeschi, R. G., & Calhoun, L. G. (2004). Posttraumatic growth: Conceptual foundations and empirical evidence. *Psychological Inquiry, 15,* 1–18.

Thoits, P. A. (1991). Merging identity theory with stress research. *Social Psychology Quarterly, 54,* 101–112.

Thoits, P. A., & Hewitt, L. N. (2001). Volunteer work and well-being. *Journal of Health and Social Behavior, 42,* 115–131.

Thomas, L. (1987). Friendship. *Synthese, 72,* 217–236.

Thomas, W. I., & Thomas, D. S. (1928). *The child in America: Behavioral problems and programs.* New York: Knopf.

Thornton, J. F., & Varenne, S. B. (2006). *John Calvin: Steward of God's covenant— Selected writings.* New York: Random House.

Tillich, P. (1987). *The essential Tillich: An anthology of the writing of Paul Tillich.* Chicago: University of Chicago Press.

Tocqueville, A. (1835/1960). *Democracy in America, Vol. 2.* New York: Vintage Books.

Tornstam, L. (2005). *Gerotranscendence: A developmental theory of positive aging.* New York: Springer.

Trinitapoli, J. (2005). Congregation-based services for elders: An examination of patterns and correlates. *Research on Aging, 27,* 241–264.

Trzesniewski, K. H., Donnellan, M. B., & Robins, R. W. (2003). Stability of self-esteem across the lifespan. *Journal of Personality and Social Psychology, 84,* 205–220.

Tucker, J. S., & Mueller, J. S. (2000). Spouse's social control of health behaviors: Use and effectiveness of specific strategies. *Personality and Social Psychology Bulletin, 26,* 1120–1130.

Turner, R. J., & Wheaton, B. (1995). Checklist measurement of stressful life events. In S. Cohen, R. C. Kessler, & L. U. Gordon (Eds.), *Measuring stress: A guide for health and social scientists* (pp. 29–53). New York: Oxford University Press.

Ueno, K., & Adams, R. G. (2006). Adult friendship: A decade review. In P. Noller & J. A. Feeney (Eds.), *Close relationships* (pp. 151–169). New York: Psychology Press.

Umberson, D. M., Chen, D., House, J. S., Hopkins, K., & Slaten, E. (1996). Gender differences in relationships and psychological well-being. *American Sociological Review, 61,* 837–857.

Underwood, L. G., & Teresi, J. A. (2002). The Daily Spiritual Experience Scale: Development, theoretical description, reliability, exploratory factor analysis, and preliminary construct validity using health-related data. *Annals of Behavioral Medicine, 24,* 22–33.

U.S. Bureau of the Census. (1975). *1970 Census of population and housing, evaluation, and research program: Accuracy of data for selected population characteristics as measured in the 1970 CPS-Census match.* Washington, DC: U.S. Government Printing Office.

U.S. Department of Health and Human Services. (1992). *Healthy people 2000: National health promotion and disease prevention objectives.* Boston: Jones and Bartlett.

U.S. Department of Health and Human Services. (2004). *Health, United States, 2004: Special Excerpt: Trend tables on 65 and older population.* Hyattsville, MD: Centers for Disease Control and Prevention.

Vacha-Haagse, T., Kogan, L. R., Tani, C. R., & Woodall, A. (2001). Reliability generalization: Exploring variation of reliability coefficients of the MMPI Clinical Scales scores. *Educational and Psychological Measurement, 61,* 45–59.

Vaillant, G. (2002). *Aging well: Surprising guideposts to a happier life.* Boston: Little, Brown, and Company.

Van Willigen, M. (2000). Differential benefits of volunteering across the life course. *Journal of Gerontology: Social Sciences, 55B,* S308–S318.

Vargas, C. M., Burt, V. L., Gillum, R. F., & Pamuk, E. R. (1997). Validity of self-reported hypertension in the National Health and Nutrition Examination Survey III: 1988–1991. *Preventive Medicine, 26,* 678–685.

Veroff, J., Douvan, E., & Kulka, R. (1981). *The inner American: A self portrait from 1957 to 1976.* New York: Basic Books.

Waern, M., Rubenowitz, E., & Wilhelmson, K. (2003). Predictors of suicide in the older elderly. *Gerontology, 49,* 328–334.

Wang, P. S., Berglund, P. A., Kessler, R. C. (2003). Patterns and correlates of contacting clergy for mental disorders in the United States. *Health Services Research, 38,* 647–673.

Ward, L. F. (1883). *Dynamic sociology or applied social science as based upon statistical sociology and the less complex sciences, Vol. 2.* New York: D. Appleton and Company.

Weber, M. (1922/1963). *The sociology of religion.* Berlin: J. C. B. Mohr.

Welch, M. R., Sikkink, D., Sartain, E., & Bond, C. (2004). Trust in God, trust in man: The ambivalent role of religion in shaping dimensions of social trust. *Journal for the Scientific Study of Religion, 43,* 317–343.

Wells, J. A., & Strictland, D. E. (1982). Physiogenic bias as invalidity in psychiatric symptom scales. *Journal of Health and Social Behavior, 23,* 235–252.

Westermeyer, J. F. (2004). Predictors and characteristics of Erikson's life cycle model among men: A 32-year longitudinal study. *International Journal of Aging and Human Development, 58,* 29–48.

Wethington, E., & Kessler, R. C. (1986). Perceived support, received support, and adjustment to stressful life events. *Journal of Health and Social Behavior, 27,* 78–89.

Wheaton, B. (1985). Personal resources and mental health: Can there be too much of a good thing? *Research in Community and Mental Health, 5,* 139–184.

Wheaton, B. (1994). Sampling the stress universe. In W. R. Avison & I. H. Gotlib (Eds.), *Stress and mental health: Contemporary issues and prospects for the future* (pp. 77–114). New York: Plenum.

Whitehead, A. N. (1917). *The organization of thought, educational and scientific.* London: Williams and Norgate.

Whitehead, A. N. (1926/1996). *Religion in the making.* New York: Fordham University Press.

Whitehouse, H., & McCauley, R. N. (2005). *Mind and religion: Psychological and cognitive foundations of religiosity.* Walnut Creek, CA: AltaMira Press.

Whitman, W. (1892/2001). *Leaves of grass.* New York: The Modern Library.

Williams, K. D., Forgas, J. P., & von Hippel, W. (2005). *The social outcast: Social exclusion, rejection, and bullying.* New York: Psychology Press.

Williams, R. B. (2002). Hostility, neuroendocrine changes, and health outcomes. In H. G. Koenig & H. J. Cohen (Eds.), *The link between religion and health: Psychoneuroimmunology and the faith factor* (pp. 160–173).

Wilson, J. (2000). Volunteering. *Annual Review of Sociology, 26,* 215–240.

Wink, P., & Dillon, M. (2001). Religious involvement and health outcomes in late adulthood: Findings from a longitudinal study of women and men. In T. G. Plante & A. C. Sherman (Eds.), *Faith and health: Psychological perspectives* (pp. 75–106). New York: Guilford.

Winseman, A. L. (2005). Friendship feeds the flock: People with best friends at church more spiritually committed. Paper posted at the following website: http://poll.gallup.com.

Woldoff, R. A. (2002). *The effects of local stressors on neighborhood attachment.* Social Forces, 81, 87–116.

Woodruff-Borden, J., Brothers, A. J., & Lister, S. C. (2001). Self-focused attention commonalities across psychopathologies and predictors. *Behavioural and Cognitive Psychotherapy, 29,* 169–178.

Worthington, E. L., Mazzeo, S. E., & Canter, D. E. (2005). Forgiveness-promoting approach: Helping clients REACH forgiveness through using a longer model that teaches reconciliation. In L. Sperry & E. P. Shafranske (Eds.), *Spiritually oriented psychotherapy* (pp. 235–257). Washington, DC: American Psychological Association.

Wortman, C. B., Silver, R. C., & Kessler, R. C. (1993). The meaning of loss and adjustment to bereavement. In M. S. Stroebe, W. Stroebe, & R. O. Hansson (Eds.), *Handbook of bereavement: Theory, research, and intervention* (pp. 349–366). New York: Cambridge University Press.

Wundt, W. (1915). *Volkerpsychologie: Band 6, Mythos and Religion.* Leipzig: Kroner.

Wuthnow, R. (1991). *Acts of compassion.* Princeton, NJ: Princeton University Press.

Wuthnow, R. (1994). *Sharing the journey: Support groups and America's new quest for community.* New York: Free Press.

Wuthnow, R. (1999). *Growing up religious: Christians and Jews and their journeys of faith.* Boston: Beacon Press.

Wuthnow, R. (2000). How religious groups promote forgiveness: A national study. *Journal for the Scientific Study of Religion, 39,* 125–139.

Wuthnow, R. (2003). Studying religion, making it sociological. In M. Dillon (Ed.), *Handbook of the sociology of religion* (pp. 16–30). New York: Cambridge University Press.

Wuthnow, R., Christiano, K., & Kuzlowski, J. (1980). Religion and bereavement: A conceptual framework. *Journal for the Scientific Study of Religion, 19,* 408–422.

Young, F. W. (2004). Social determinants, social support, and health: A critique. *Social Theory & Health, 2,* 142–152.

Zarit, S. H., Pearlin, L. I., & Schaie, K. W. (2003). *Personal control in social and life course contexts.* New York: Springer.

Zinnbauer, B. J., & Pargament, K. I. (2005). Religiousness and spirituality. In R. F. Paloutzian & C. L. Park (Eds.), *Handbook of the psychology of religion and spirituality* (pp. 21–42). New York: Guilford.

Index

Abelson, R. P., 260
ACASI (audio computer-assisted self-interviewing), 257–58
activity theory and volunteering, 140
Adams, R. G., 85
Adler, A., 24
adversity, growth through, 63–65
African American religious life, 192–202
African Americans. *See* race
afterlife, 5, 122–23
age as a factor of social structure, 187
Ahadi, S., 258–59
Ainsworth, M. D. S., 124
Albert, M., 252
Aldwin, C. M., 15
Allport, G. W., 142
Almond, R., 43
American Psychiatric Association, 73
Aneschensel, C. S., 231
anger and health, 164–65
anticipated support, 36, 65–66
anticipatory coping, 40
Argue, A., 18
Argyle, M., 207–8
Armstrong, J. A., 84–85, 242
Aron, A., 97
assumption of essentialism, 15–16
attachment theory in pastoral counseling, 123–25
Aubin, E., 141
audio computer-assisted self-interviewing (ACASI), 257–58
authority and the clergy, 172

Bahr, H. M., 15
Bainbridge, W. S., 113–14, 170
Baker, E., 143
Baldwin, J. A., 194
Baldwin, J. M., 23
Baldwin, M. W., 40
Baltes, P. B., 69

Bandura, A., 50
Barefoot, J. C., 100
Barna, G., 16, 20
Bastida, E., 236–39
Batson, C. D., 256
Battista, J., 43
Baumeister, R. F., 40, 92
Becker, E., 170
Becker, M. A., 117
Becker, P. E., 157
Beckham, J. C., 100
Beit-Hallahmi, B., 207–8
belief as a dimension of religion, 5, 235–36
Belle, D., 221, 224
belonging, 92–94
Benjamins, M. R., 187
Benore, E., 164
Benore, E. R., 123
Bentler-Bonett Normed Fit Index (NFI), 88
bereavement as a stressor, 73
Berger, P. L., 52, 58, 175
Berglund, P. A., 115–16
Berkeley Growth Studies, 18
Berkman, L., 252
Bernard of Chartres, 25–26
Bettencourt, B. A., 99
Bible study groups, 127–34
biomarkers of health status, 250–51
Bjorck, J. P., 93
Black, H. K., 221, 223
Blackbird, R., 111
Blalock, H. M., 8–9
Blazer, D. G., 252
Boardman, J. D., 34, 56
Bohart, A. C., 125
Bohrnstedt, G. W., 261
Bond, C., 100–101
Borawski-Clark, E., 223
Bowlby, J., 123
Bradley, W. J., 7

Brion, S. L., 18–19
Brothers, A. J., 101
Brown, G. W., 169
Brummett, B. H., 100
Burdette, A. M., 95
Butter, E. M., 158–59, 161

Cairney, J., 72
Calhoun, L. G., 62
Calvin, J., 66
Cann, B. J., 122
Caplan, G., 41–42, 49, 55
caregivers, 146–47
Carrier, H., 92–93
Carstensen, L. L., 102, 106, 172
Carter, J., 121
Cassel, J., 148–49
causality in research, 245–47
Center for Epidemiologic Studies
    Depression Scale, 199, 252
ceremony, religious, importance of,
    109
Chaiken, S., 182
Chatters, L. M.: on gender and church
    participation, 207; on negative
    interaction in the church, 167; on
    negative interaction with clergy,
    169–70; on prayers answered, 129–
    30; on private vs. group prayer, 133;
    on religion and health, 27; on use of
    pastoral counseling, 116
Chaves, M. A., 176–77
Cheavens, J. S., 120–21
Childre, D., 64
Chockinov, H. M., 122
Christians in research, 11
church attendance: belonging and,
    93; health and, 26; health behaviors
    and, 94–95; homebound assistance
    programs, 150; as a measure of
    religion, 4, 20; volunteering and, 142
church participation and gender,
    207–10
church-based companion friendship:
    conceptual and methodological
    challenges, 106–11; degree of
    closeness in, 110; development of,
    108–10; effects on health and well-
    being, 91–102; gender and health
    in late life, 211–12, 214; health
    and, 103–6; history and negative
    interaction in, 184–85; measuring,

85–91; overview, 79–85; race and
    health in late life, 196, 200–201;
    Rook's view, 29; socioeconomic
    status and health in late life, 225–26
church-based formal relationships:
    Bible study and prayer groups, 127–
    34; gender and health in late life,
    212, 214; homebound assistance
    programs, 145–51; measuring,
    151; motives for, 152–53; need
    for explication, 244–45; negative
    interaction with clergy, 169–71;
    pastoral counseling, 113–27; race
    and health in late life, 196–97, 201;
    socioeconomic status and health in
    late life, 226; volunteering, 134–44
church-based social relationships:
    definition, 28; effect size in research,
    258–61; limited benefits of, 248–50;
    manifest and latent functions of,
    254–55; need for a taxonomy, 244–
    45
church-based social support:
    anticipated support, 65–66; benefits
    of, 46–53; companion friendship
    and, 106–8; conceptual and
    methodological challenges, 75–78;
    denominational variation, 241–43;
    dimensions of, 36–38; forgiveness,
    59–61; gender and health in late
    life, 210–11, 213–14; gratitude to
    God, 61–65; limited benefits of,
    198–99; longitudinal research, 247;
    measuring, 35–39; overview, 33–
    35; pastoral counseling and, 126–
    27; prayer and, 57–59; providing
    support, 66–70; race and health in
    late life, 195, 199–200; religious
    beliefs and, 235–39; religious
    coping responses, 54–57; seeking
    and not seeking support, 44–46;
    social structural factors and, 189;
    socioeconomic status and, 223–25;
    theoretical underpinnings of, 53–
    65; types of stressors, 70–75. *See also
    under support*
Chwa, H. J., 117
Clark, W. H., 43
class. *See* socioeconomic status
clergy: companion friendship with,
    111; health effects of negative
    interaction on, 160; negative

interaction and race, 201–2; negative interaction in late life, 197–98; negative interaction with, 169–72
close companion friends, 29. *See also* church-based companion friendship
Cocking, D., 81–82
cognitive impairment, 188, 251–52
Cohen, C. I., 222
Cohen, H. J., 251
cohort effects, 17–18, 137
Colbert, S. J., 253
Collins, N., 114
companion friends, 29, 79
companion friendship: changes over time, 109–10; gender differences, 209; in secular and religious contexts, 80–85. *See also* church-based companion friendship
companionship contrasted with friendship, 79
compassion and providing support, 70
compensation and volunteering, 134–35, 142
competition and pride, 174
compression of morbidity, 249
conceptual and methodological challenges: assessing core religious values, 239–61; Bible study and prayer groups, 132–34; causality in research, 245–47; church-based companion friendship, 106–11; church-based social relationships, 244–45, 248–50, 254–55; church-based social support, 75–78; effect size, 258–61; exploring different beliefs, 240–43; homebound assistance programs, 149–51; interpreting longitudinal studies, 247–48; measuring health outcomes, 250–54; negative interaction in the church, 173–85; pastoral counseling, 125–27; social desirability response bias, 255–58; volunteering, 142–44
conceptual models of religion and health, 6–8
confidentiality and privacy, 126, 155, 173–75
conflict, institutional, 176–77
congregational climate, 175–77
connectedness. *See* spiritual connectedness
construct validity, 105–6

content validity, 10
control, feeling of: as a dimension of religion, 5; effects of stress, 41–42; need for, 232; primary and secondary, 50; providing support and, 69; restored by church-based social support, 49–52
control, God-mediated, 247–48
control, types of, 50–52
Cook, J. M., 83
Cooley, C. H.: on connectedness and interdependence, 237; on empathy, 109; on faith in social relationships, 23; on hostility, 183; on the looking-glass self, 47; on religion in society, 11–12; on self-disclosure, 97; on self-expresison, 98; on socioeconomic status, 216; on stress and religion, 33; on subjectivity in research, 262–63
Coopersmith, S., 39
coping, anticipatory, 40
coping responses, 54, 57–59
coping scale, religious, 51, 54–55, 58, 60
Corporation for National and Community Service, 136
counseling. *See* pastoral counseling
Coward, H., 45
creativity contrasted with self-expression, 98–99
cross-sectional research, 16–17, 161
Crowne, D., 257
Crumpler, C. A., 61
Crystal, S., 217
culture, 193–94
Current Population Surveys of 2005, 136

Dannefer, D., 20
Das, T. K., 100
Davidson, J. D., 236
Day, L., 60
death, beliefs about, 5
death anxiety, 170–72
Debats, D., 52
dementia, 188, 251–52
denominational variation, 241–43
depression, detection of, 252–53. *See also* mental health
determinant correlation, 259
Dewey, J., 32

Diener, E., 258–59
differential impact: compared with differential involvement, 190–91, 229–30; gender and health in late life, 213–15; race and health in late life, 199–202; socioeconomic status and health in late life, 227–28
differential involvement: compared with differential impact, 190–91, 229–30; gender and health in late life, 210–13; race and health in late life, 195–99; socioeconomic status and health in late life, 225–27
Dillon, M., 18
dimensions of religion, 5, 20, 235–36
divine, qualities of, 6
divine control, 51
divine healing through prayer groups, 132
doubt as a dimension of religion, 5. *See also* religious doubt
Douvan, E., 115
Du Bois, W. E. B., 193
Duncan, B. L., 125
Durkheim, E., 11, 22–23, 95
dyads, 108, 144, 179–80
Dyer, D. R., 13

Eagly, A. H., 182
Echemendia, R., 175–76
Eckenrode, J., 44, 117
education, 74, 219, 223
Edwards, A. C., 169
Edwards, J., 185
effect size in social relationship research, 258–61
ego. *See* self-esteem
ego and anticipated support, 65
Einstein, A., 230
Eliade, M., 232
Ellison, C. G.: on African American religious life, 198; on church attendance and health, 95; on forgiveness, 60, 131, 243; on forgiveness and race, 201–2; on gender and health, 204; on institutional conflict, 176–77; on negative interaction and health, 160–62, 244; on negative interaction in the church, 158; on rational choice theory, 84; on religion and health, 26; on religious coping

responses, 56; on religious doubt, 165–66; on stress and support, 34; on use of pastoral counseling, 116
Emerson, R. W., 81–82, 92
Emmons, R. A., 61, 64
emotional support: companion friendship and, 107; definition, 36; from inside and outside the church, 75; restorative quality of, 49; restoring, 53; spiritual connectedness and, 238
empathy in companion friendship, 109
Enders, C. K., 18–19
end-of-life care, 121–23
Enright, R. D., 60, 119
Epictetus, 62, 165
Epidemiologic Catchment Area surveys, 251
Erikson, E., 42, 141, 171
essentialism, assumption of, 15–16
ethical progress, 67
ethnic groups, absence of research data, 192
Euripides, 110
Everson-Rose, S. A., 164
exchange theory and volunteering, 140–41
Exline J. J., 74
extrinsic religious orientation, 142

faith: development with age, 14; exploring differences, 240–43; pastoral counseling and, 125–26; in social relationships, 22–23. *See also entries at religion*
Family Life Cycle, 15
Fatone, A., 121
Fazio, E. M., 218
Feldman, P. J., 221
Fetzer Institute: dimensions of religion, 5, 7; measuring church-based social support, 35–36; negative interaction in the church, 158–61; spirituality index, 10
Fiala, W. E., 93
Fincham, F. D., 119
Finke, R., 52
Finnegan, R. A., 110
Flannelly, K. J., 114, 116
Flint, E. P., 20
Folkman, S., 54
forgiveness: as a coping response, 59–

61; definition, 60; denominational variation, 243; as a dimension of religion, 5; group attendance and, 130–31; negative interaction and, 182–83; pastoral counseling and, 118–21; race and, 202; reflected in church-based social support, 48
Fowler, J. W., 14
Frank, J. B., 120
Frank, J. D., 120
Frankel, E., 243
Frankl, V. E., 42
Freedman, S., 60
Freud, S., 12
Friendly Visitor Program, 150
friendship: contrasted with companionship, 79; history and negative interaction, 184–85; volunteering and, 153. *See also* church-based companion friendship; companion friendship
Fries, J. F., 249
Fuller, R. C., 10
fundamental–liberal scale and spiritual support, 242–43

Gallup, G., 20–21, 57
Gallup International Institute, 121
gender: differences in church-based social support, 203–6; differential impact, 213–15; differential involvement, 210–13; as a factor of social structure, 187; health and, 187–88; mental health and, 253–54
gender roles, 204–5, 207–10
General Social Survey of 1996, 116
General Social Survey of 1999, 16
generativity and volunteering, 141
George, L. K., 9, 20, 188
gerontology, social, and volunteering, 140
gerontranscendence in late life, 102
Glock, C. Y., 235–36, 239
God, personal relationship with, 5
God, qualities of the divine, 6
God-mediated control, 51–52, 247–48
Goethe, J. W. von, 47
Goldhaber, D. E., 15–16
Gordon, T., 117
Gorsuch, R., 16, 93
Gottlieb, B. J., 72
gratitude, 61–65

Greenberg, D., 246–47
Grennan, J., 121
growth through adversity, 63–65
guilt and pastoral counseling, 118–21
Gurland, B. J., 188
Gutmann, D., 208–9

Haley, W. E., 117
Hall, G. S., 12, 16, 23–24
Hall, J. H., 119
Hartman, W. J., 168
hassles, daily, as stressors, 71
Hays, J. C., 20
health: belonging and, 94; Bible study and prayer groups and, 128–32; church-based companion friendships and, 103–6; cognitive impairment, 188, 251–52; commitment to faith and, 125–26; measuring, 250–54; negative interaction in the church and, 162–69; self-absorption and, 101–2; self-disclosure and, 97–98; self-expression and, 99–100; trust and, 100–101
health benefits: of Bible study and prayer group attendance, 133–34; of companion friendships, 94–97; of homebound assistance programs, 146–49; limits of, 248–50; of pastoral counseling, 117–25
Health Care Finance Administration, 268
Hecht, J. M., 73
Heckhausen, J., 49–50
helping, 155, 236
Herd, D., 96
Herzog, A. R., 139, 143
Hewitt, L. N., 138–39
Heyer-Grey, Z. A., 204–5
Hill, D., 122–23
Hill, P. C., 5, 35
Hill, T. D., 95
history, 110, 193–94
Hobfoll, S. E., 221
Hodges, E. V., 110
Hohmann, A. A., 114–15
Holmes, T. H., 59, 73, 156
homebound assistance programs, 145–51
homogeneity in church-based companion friendship, 83
homophily principle, 83

Hood, R. W., 5, 16, 35
Hooker, K., 100
hope through pastoral counseling, 120
Hopkins, R., 194
House, J. S., 27, 139, 152
Hoyle, R. H., 40
Hubble, M. A., 125
Hughes, C. C., 220
Hummer, R. A., 187
Hunsberger, B., 16
Hunsberger, B. S., 73
Hutton, D. G., 40

identity theory and negative
    interaction, 160
Idler, E. L., 94
IFI (Incremental Fit Index), 88–89
income as a socioeconomic factor,
    217–18
Incremental Fit Index (IFI), 88–89
independence and seeking support, 46
Index of Inconsistency, 217
indigence among older women, 116
individual and society, dialectic
    between, 31
Ingersoll-Dayton, B., 20
Ingram, R. E., 101
inspiration in companion friendship,
    82
instrument reliability, 90
intercessory prayer, 264
interdependency, 66–70
interpersonal conflict as a stressor, 156.
    See also negative interaction in the
    church
intimacy in companion friendship,
    87–90
intrinsic religious orientation, 142
isolation, 139, 146–47, 221, 224

Jackson, J. S., 34
Jain, A. R., 18–19
James, W.: on multiple selves, 47; on
    prayer, 57; on qualities of the divine,
    6; on religion, 12; on religion in late
    life, 13
Jennings, P. A., 15
Johnson, D. R., 18
Johnson, S., 175–76
Jourard, S. M., 97
Judd, C. M., 261
Jung, C., 12–13

Kahn, J. R., 218
Kahn, R. L., 27–28, 69
Kaplan, A., 28
Kaplan, H. B., 39–40
Kasl, S. V., 94
Kelcourse, F. B., 117
Kennett, J., 81–82
Kernis, M. H., 40
Kessler, R. C.: on anticipated support,
    65–66; on bereavement, 73; on
    interpreting data, 247; on religious
    coping responses, 72; on research
    practices, 246; on use of pastoral
    counseling, 115–16
kingdom of God, 264–65
Kirkpatrick, L. A., 124
Knepple, A. M., 84–85, 242
Koenig, H. G.: on growth through
    adversity, 63; RCOPE scale, 51, 54–
    55; on reactions to stress, 44; on
    religion and health, 251; on religion
    and spirituality, 9
Kogan, L. R., 90
Kohlberg, L., 14–15
Koltko-Rivera, M. E., 67
Krapp, J. L., 145
Krause, N.: on belonging, 93–94; on
    church-based social support, 36–38,
    49; on confidentiality in pastoral
    counseling, 126; on congregational
    cohesiveness, 176; on dimensions
    of religion, 5; on education, 223; on
    exposure to violence and gender,
    253; on forgiveness, 60, 131, 243;
    on forgiveness and race, 201–2;
    on gender and health, 204; on God-
    mediated control, 51–52, 247–
    48; on gratitude to God, 62, 64;
    on institutional conflict, 176–
    77; on interpersonal conflict, 186;
    on meaning in life, 42–44, 52–
    53, 122; on measuring companion
    friendship, 86–90; on negative
    spiritual support, 75; on negative
    interaction and health, 160–62, 178–
    79, 244; on negative interaction in
    the church, 156, 158–59, 167; on
    negative interaction over time, 163,
    165; on negative interaction with
    clergy, 169–70; on optimism, 120;
    on prayer and stress, 58; on prayers
    answered, 129–30; on praying for

others, 132; on private vs. group prayer, 133; on providing support, 70, 72; on racial differences in church-based social support, 195–202; on religious coping responses, 56; on religious development with age, 20; on religious doubt, 74, 165–66; on religious meaning, 43; on self-expresison, 99; social relationships, definition, 28; on social relationships in lower socioeconomic status, 220–22; on social skills in companion friendship, 108–9; on spiritual connectedness, 236–39; on stress in late life, 33; on support from inside and outside the church, 75, 77; on trauma, 72; on volunteering and mental health, 143
Kuhn, R. L., 152
Kulka, R., 115

LaMothe, R., 173–75
Landis, K. R., 27
Langner, T. S., 222
Lao-tzu, 68
Larson, D. B., 9, 114–15
Laruffa, G., 121
late life: companion friendships in, 102; negative interaction in the church, 171–73; personality changes in, 102; providing support, 69; self-esteem in, 41; social skills in, 109
latent functions of social relationships, 254–55
Lazarus, R. S., 54
Leary, M. R., 40
leaving congregations, 166–69, 178–79
Leighton, A., 220
Levenson, M. R., 15
Levin, J. S.: on church attendance and health, 26; on gender and church participation, 207; on religion and health, 27, 148; on use of pastoral counseling, 116
Lewis, C. S., 26, 121, 174
Lewis, T. T., 164
liberal–fundamental scale and spiritual support, 242–43
Lieberman, M., 40
life events as stressors, 71
Lincoln, K. D., 116
Lindsay, D. M., 20–21, 57

Lister, S. C., 101
Logan, R. L., 141
Loh, C., 260
loneliness, 139, 146–47, 221, 224
longitudinal research: causality in, 245; on gender and church-based social support, 204; interpreting findings, 247–48; on negative interaction and health, 178–79; on negative interaction in the church, 161; on religion and aging, 17–19
looking-glass self, 47
love, unconditional, 48
love as a dimension of religion, 236
Loveland, M. T., 167
Lu, J., 86, 93
Luckman, T., 175
Luoh, M. C., 139
Lusignolo, T. M., 252
Luther, M., 57, 265

Macaskill, A., 60
Magyar, G. M., 164
Mahan, T. L., 156
Mahoney, A., 164
Maimonides, M., 63
Maltby, J., 60
manifest functions of social relationships, 254–55
Marcum, J. P.: on gender and health, 204; on negative interaction and health, 158, 161–62; on religious coping responses, 56
Marlowe, D., 257
Marlowe-Crowne Social Desirability Scale, 256
Marmot, M., 188
Martire, L., 150–51
Marwell, G., 261
Maslow, A. H., 42, 67, 92
Maton, K. I., 34
Mattis, J. S., 193
Mattlin, J., 72
Maves, P. B., 16
Maynard, K. E., 100
Maynard-Reid, P. U., 194
McAdams, D. P., 141
McCarty, R., 64
McCauley, R. N., 148
McClelland, G. H., 261
McCullough, M. E.: on gratitude to God, 61, 64; on religion

and spirituality, 9; on religious development with age, 18–19
McFadden, S. H.: on companion friendship in and out of church, 84–85; on faith development, 14; on research inadequacies, 6; on spiritual support, 242
McGrath, P., 121
McKay, B., 132, 255
McKenzie, B., 73
McMahon, K., 139–40
McMillen, J. C., 62
McPherson, M., 83
Mead, G. H., 23, 181
Meador, K. G., 20
meaning, religious, 43
meaning as a dimension of religion, 5
meaning in life: effects of stress on, 42–44; need for, 232; restoring, 52–53; through end-of-life counseling, 121–23
measurement and theory, interplay between, 8–9, 233
measures: of companion friendships, 85–91; of formal relationships, 151; of healthy outcomes, 250–54; of negative interaction in the church, 157–60; reliability of, 261; of religion, 4–6, 20, 35, 257; of social support, 35–39; of socioeconomic status, 216–20; of spiritual support, 75; of spirituality, 9–10
media use, as a measure of religion, 20
medical expenses in late life, 13
Medicare Beneficiary Eligibility List, 268
Meltzer, T.: on negative interaction in the church, 167; on negative interaction with clergy, 169–70; on prayers answered, 129–30; on private vs. group prayer, 133
Menaghan, E., 40
mental health: cognitive impairment, 188, 251–52; research issues, 251–53; self-forgiveness and, 119–20; social structural factors and, 188. See also health
mental illness and pastoral counseling, 115–17
Meredith, G. E., 17
Merton, R. K., 233, 254

Mexican Americans, absence of research data, 192
Michael, S. T., 120–21, 222
Midtown Manhattan Study, 222
Milkie, M. A., 51, 230
Miller, S. D., 125
Mills, C. W., 192
Mirowsky, J., 74, 218–19
Mitchell, D., 117
Moadel, A., 121
Montaigne, M. de, 81
moral development with age, 14–15
morality from social relationships, 22
Morgan, C., 121
Morgan, D. L.: on negative interaction in the church, 167; on negative interaction with clergy, 169–70; on prayers answered, 129–30; on private vs. group prayer, 133; on religious development with age, 20
mortality and volunteering, 139–40
Mueller, J. S., 96–97
Mullan, J., 40
multiple selves, 48
Musick, M. A., 95, 138–39
Musil, L. A., 132, 255
Mystery, the, 122

National Congregations Survey, 145
National Institute on Aging: dimensions of religion, 5, 7; measuring church-based social support, 35–36; negative interaction in the church, 158–61; RAH Survey, 229–30, 267; spirituality index, 10
Nazroo, J. Y., 169
negative interaction in the church: benefits of, 182–84; characterizing, 177–78; with the clergy, 169–71; conceptual and methodological challenges, 173–85; conceptual linkages, 162–69; definition, 155; depression and, 245–46; gender and health in late life, 212–15; genesis of, 173–77; measuring, 157–60; perpetrators, 180–81; prior research, 160–62; race and health in late life, 197–99, 201–2; socioeconomic status and health in late life, 226; unjustified, 180
Nelsen, A. K., 193
Nelsen, H. M., 193

Nelson, E. A., 20
Neugarten, B. L., 102
"new life," Christianity as, 23–24
Newby-Clark, I. R., 40
Newsom, J. T., 156
NFI (Bentler-Bonett Normed Fit Index), 88
Niebuhr, R., 174
Nietzsche, F., 32
nomos (meaning in life), 52–53

Oates, W. E., 118
occupation as a socioeconomic factor, 218
Oden, T., 82–83
Olson, D. V. A., 168
Oman, D., 139–40
oneness. *See* spiritual connectedness
openness in companion friendship, 87–90
Oppenheimer, J. E., 114
optimism, 66, 120
orientation, religious, 142
originality, 25
Orsi, R. A., 241

Pancer, S. M., 73
parameters, research, 7, 9–11
Pargament, K. I.: on conceptual models, 6; on congregational climate, 175–76; on meaning in life, 43; on negative interaction in the church, 158–59, 161; RCOPE scale, 51, 54–55; on reactions to stress, 44; on sanctification theory, 164
Park, C. L., 123, 165–66
pastoral counseling: attachment theory, 123–25; conceptual and methodological challenges, 125–27; end-of-life care, 121–23; guilt and forgiveness, 118–21; health benefits, 117–25; overview, 113–15; race and, 196–97; use of services, 115–17
Paulson, D. S., 122
Pearlin, L. I., 40
pedestal effect, 111
Perez, L. M., 44, 51, 54–55
period effects in research, 17–18
Perry, D. G., 110
personal control. *See* control, feeling of
personal growth in companion friendship, 82

personal relationship with God, 5
persuasion and negative interaction, 182
Peterson, C., 66
Peterson, L. R., 43
philosophy and religion, 24–25
Pietromonaco, P., 162–63
Polivka, L. A., 117
Pope, A., 68
power and pride, 174
Pratt, M., 73
prayer: beliefs about answers, 129–30; as a coping response, 57–59, 73; group contrasted with private, 133; intercessory, 264; measure of, 8; as a measure of religion, 20; for others, 131–32, 238
prayer groups, 127–34, 255
pride and negative interaction, 173–75
primary and secondary control, 50
privacy and confidentiality, 126, 155, 173–75
providing support, benefits of, 66–70
proxy control, 50
psychiatry and religion, 12–13
psychology, 9–10, 23–24
Pudrovska, T., 51, 230
Pullberg, S., 58

qualities of the divine, 6

race: in church-based companion friendship, 83; differential impact, 199–202; differential involvement, 195–99; as a factor of social structure, 187; health and, 187, 192; historic and cultural influences, 193–94; mental health and, 253–54; negative interaction in the church, 212–13
RAH Survey: on Bible study and prayer groups, 133; on denominational variation, 241–43; on dimensions of church-based social support, 36–38; effects of stress, 107; on family income, 217; on forgiveness, 61, 119, 131; on gender differences in church-based social support, 210–14; on group attendance, 128; on health and church-based companion friendships, 103–6; on homebound assistance programs, 145, 147–48;

RAH Survey *(cont'd.)*
measuring companion friendship,
86–90; on negative interaction in
the church, 159–60; on negative
interaction with clergy, 171;
overview, 31, 267–69; on prayer, 59,
73; on prayers answered, 130; on
racial differences in church-based
social support, 195–202; on religious
doubt, 165–66; on socioeconomic
differences in church-based social
support, 225–28; on spiritual
connectedness, 239
Rahe, R. H., 59, 73, 156
Rapoport, R. N., 220
rational choice theory, 84
RCOPE scale, 51, 54–55, 58, 60
Reich, K. H., 14
Reis, H. T., 114
Reissman, F., 68–69
Reker, G. T., 42–43
religion: beliefs and church-based
social relationships, 235–39;
ceremony, importance of, 109;
contrasted with spirituality, 9–10,
15; definition, 23; dimensions of, 5,
235–36; exploring differences, 240–
43; measures of, 4–6, 35; reasons
to study, 11–13; satisfying human
needs, 232; as social or solitary,
23–24; socioeconomic status and,
189; subjectivity in research, 261–
65; various views, 32; vertical and
horizontal dimensions of, 236
Religion, Aging, and Health Survey. *See*
RAH Survey
religion and aging: research, 16–22;
theories, 14–16
religion and health: conceptual
models, 6–8; current knowledge, 4–
9, 22–28; homebound assistance
programs, 148–49; inadequate
research tools, 5–6; pastoral
counseling, 125–26
religious contrasted with secular
support, 76–77
religious coping scale, 51, 54–55, 58, 60
religious development, 14, 16–20
religious doubt, 5, 73–75, 165–66
religious life, African American,
192–202
religious meaning, 43

religious orientation, 142
religious self, 48, 84
reminiscence therapy, 122
research, conducting, 7, 9–11, 28
research issues: assessing core religious
values, 239–61; Bible study and
prayer groups, 132–34; causality
in research, 245–47; church-based
companion friendship, 106–11;
church-based social relationships,
244–45, 248–50, 254–55; church-
based social support, 75–78; effect
size, 258–61; exploring different
beliefs, 240–43; gender, social ties,
and health, 203–6; homebound
assistance programs, 149–51;
interpreting longitudinal studies,
247–48; linkages between social
relationships and health, 233–34;
measuring health outcomes, 250–54;
negative interaction in the church,
173–85; pastoral counseling, 125–27;
social desirability response bias, 255–
58; volunteering, 142–44
respite care, 147
response bias, 255–58
retrospective research on religion and
aging, 19–20
Reverence for Life, 67, 264
Richards, M., 147
Rique, J., 60
ritual for the homebound, 148
RMSEA (root mean square error of
approximation), 89
Robb, C., 117
Roberts, J. D., 193
Rogers, C., 70
Rogers, R. G., 187
role losses, 140, 172–73
Rook, K. S.: on belonging, 93; on close
companion friends, 29, 79–80; on
friendship and volunteering, 153;
on interpersonal conflict, 186; on
measuring companion friendship,
85–86; on negative interaction,
156, 162–63, 165; on sharing in
friendship, 81–82; on social control,
95
root mean square error of
approximation (RMSEA), 89
Rose, E., 74
Rosow, I., 69

Ross, C. E., 74, 218–19
Ross, E. A.: on church-based companion friendship, 83; on church-based social support, 48–49; on negative interaction in the church, 179; religion, definition, 23; on religious basis of support, 45; on spiritual connectedness, 236–37
Rost, R. A., 119
Rowe, J. W., 27–28, 69
Roy, A., 43
Royce, J., 24, 63, 237
Rubin, L. B., 220
Rubinstein, R. L., 221, 223
Russell, B., 238
Rutledge, T., 260
Ryff, C. D., 64

sanctification theory, anger in, 164
Sartain, E., 100–101
Schaefer, K. C., 7
Schewe, C. D., 17
Schieman, S., 51, 230
Schlenker, B. R., 109
Schoenrade, P., 256
Schopenhauer, A., 62, 156, 238
Schulz, J. H., 116
Schulz, R., 49–50, 150–51
Schweitzer, A., 67, 264
Scott, A. B., 158–59, 161
secondary control, 50
secular contrasted with religious support, 76–77
Seeman, T. E., 252
self, religious, 84
self, selves, 47–48
self-absorption and church-based companion friendship, 101–2
self-development in companion friendship, 82, 87–90
self-disclosure in companion friendship, 81, 97–98
self-esteem: anticipated support and, 65; definition, 39; effects of stress, 39–41; providing support and, 68–69; restored by church-based social support, 47–49; seeking support and, 44–46
self-expression in church-based companion friendship, 98–100
self-forgiveness through pastoral counseling, 118–19

self-transcendence, 15, 67
Seligman, M. E., 66
Seneca, 153
SES. See socioeconomic status
shame and health, 181
Shand, J. D., 17–18
sharing in companion friendship, 81–82
Shaw, B. A., 72, 221–22
Sheldon, K., 99
Shepherd, B. C., 176–77
Sherkat, D. E., 198
Sherman, N., 82–83
Shifren, K., 208
Shiraishi, R. W., 15
Siegler, I. C., 100
Sikkink, D., 100–101
Silver, R. C., 73
Silverman, W., 175–76
Simmel, G., 22, 64
Sinclair, U., 32
Singer, B., 64
Sinnott, J. D., 208
Skinner, E. A., 50
Smith, A.: on expectations of relationship, 163; on the looking-glass self, 47; on negative interaction in the church, 179; on positive and negative interactions, 156; on solitude, 101; on unjustified negative interaction, 180
Smith, J., 69
Smith-Lovin, L., 83
Snyder, C. R., 120–21
Snyder, S., 175–76
social control, 95–97
social desirability response bias, 255–58
social feelings, 24
social gerontology and volunteering, 140
Social Readjustment Rating Scale, 59
social relationships: among lower socioeconomic status, 220–22; health and, 27–28, 233; latent and manifest functions of, 254–55; reasons to study, 22–28; religious beliefs and, 236; role of, 31
social skills in companion friendship, 108–9
social structural factors: gender in late life, 203–16; overview, 187–91; race

social structural factors *(cont'd.)*
in late life, 192–202; socioeconomic
status in late life, 216–29
social structure, 187
social support compared with
organized volunteering, 143–44
sociality, 58, 232
society and individual, dialectic
between, 31
socioeconomic status (SES): among
older women, 116; in church-
based companion friendship, 83;
differences in church-based social
support, 220–25; as a factor of social
structure, 187; health and, 188;
measuring in late life, 216–20
socioemotional selectivity in late life,
102
sociology and religion, 11–12, 22–23
Sokolovsky, J., 222
solitude and self-absorption, 101
Sorkin, D., 86, 93
Spilka, B., 16
Spinoza, B. D., 180–81
spiritual connectedness, 236–39
spiritual support: definition, 36;
measuring, 75; restorative quality of,
49; restoring, 53
spirituality, 9–10, 15
Stanik, P., 158–59, 161
Starbuck, D. E., 13, 19
Stark, R.: on belief and religion, 239;
on clergy as intermediary with God,
170; on dimensions of religion, 235–
36; on God-mediated control, 52; on
pastoral counseling, 113–14
Stephens, J., 220
Steptoe, S., 221
Stirling County Study, 220
strains, chronic, as stressors, 71
stress: benefits of, 61–62; companion
friendship and, 106; definition, 73;
effects of, 39–44; overview, 33–35;
prayer and, 57–58
stressors, types of, 70–75
Strictland, D. E., 252–53
Strube, M. H., 259
subjectivity in research on religion,
261–65
support: anticipated, 36, 65–66;
providing, 66–70; religious or
secular, 76–77; satisfaction with, 36–

39; seeking and not seeking, 44–46;
tangible, 36, 238
support, emotional: companion
friendship and, 107; definition,
36; from inside and outside the
church, 75; restorative quality of, 49;
restoring, 53; spiritual connectedness
and, 238
support, spiritual: definition, 36;
measuring, 75; restorative quality of,
49; restoring, 53
support bank in companion
friendship, 110
symbolic interactionism, 11–12

Tallman, K., 125
tangible support, 36, 238
Tani, C. R., 90
Tardy, C. H., 98
Taylor, R. J., 27, 116, 207
Taylor, S., 156
Tedeschi, R. G., 62
Teng, B. S., 100
Terman Study, 18
terror management theory, 170
theory and measurement, interplay
between, 8–9, 233
third parties, role in negative
interaction, 181–82
Thoits, P. A., 138–39
Thomas, W. I., 263
Thoresen, C. E., 139–40
Tice, D. M., 40
Tillich, P., 26, 58, 166
Tocqueville, A. de, 12, 101
Tornstam, L., 102, 106, 172
trauma as a stressor, 71–72
Tremblay, M. A., 220
Trinitapoli, J., 145
trust: broken, 169, 182–83; in church-
based companion friendship, 100–
101; in companion friendship, 81;
confidentiality and privacy, 126,
155, 173–75
truthfulness in companion friendship,
81
Tucker, J. S., 96–97
type A personality, health effects of,
164

Ueno, K., 85
Umberson, D., 27

unconditional love in church-based
social support, 48
universal attitudes and social
structures, 23
U.S. Bureau of the Census, 136, 217
U.S. Congregational Life Survey, 161
U.S. Department of Labor, 135–37

Vacha-Haagse, T., 90
Vaillant, G. E., 66, 141
Van Willigen, M., 138
variables, research, 7
Ventis, W. L., 256
Veroff, J., 115
volunteering: conceptual and
methodological challenges, 142–
44; definitions, 134–35; exchange
theory and, 140–41; health and,
138–42; individual contrasted with
organized, 141–42; in late life, 135–
37; secular contrasted with church-
based, 142–43

Wang, P. S., 115–16
Ward, L. F., 12
wealth as a socioeconomic factor,
218–19
Weaver, A. J., 114, 116
Weber, M., 11
Welch, M. R., 100–101
Wells, J. A., 252–53
Wethington, E.: on anticipated support,
65–66; on religious coping responses,
72; on seeking support, 44; on use of
pastoral counseling, 117

White, L. K., 18
Whitehead, A. N., 24–25
Whitehouse, H., 148
Whitman, W., 184
Wilkinson, R. G., 188
Williams, D. R., 34
Williams, R. B., 164
Wilson, J., 134, 138–40
Wink, P., 18
Winseman, A. L., 94
Woldoff, R. A., 221
Wood, W., 182
Woodall, A., 90
Woodruff-Bordon, J., 101
Wortman, C. B., 73
Wright, P. H., 111
Wulff, K. M.: on belonging and health,
93–94; on God-mediated control,
247–48; on negative interaction and
health, 160–61, 244
Wundt, W., 12
Wuthnow, R.: on Bible study and
prayer groups, 128–32; on church-
based social support, 153; on
compassion, 70; on religion and
socioeconomic status, 189; on
religious ceremony, 109

Young, F. W., 222

Zerowin, J., 158–59, 161
Zhang, W., 158, 161–62
Zinnbauer, B. J., 158–59, 161